Mechanical Circulatory
Support Therapy In

# ADVANCED
# HEART FAILURE

# Mechanical Circulatory Support Therapy In
# ADVANCED HEART FAILURE

## MARIO C. DENG
## YOSHIFUMI NAKA

*Columbia University, USA*

Imperial College Press

ICP

*Published by*

Imperial College Press
57 Shelton Street
Covent Garden
London WC2H 9HE

*Distributed by*

World Scientific Publishing Co. Pte. Ltd.

5 Toh Tuck Link, Singapore 596224

*USA office:* 27 Warren Street, Suite 401-402, Hackensack, NJ 07601

*UK office:* 57 Shelton Street, Covent Garden, London WC2H 9HE

**Library of Congress Cataloging-in-Publication Data**
Deng, Mario C.
    Mechanical circulatory support therapy in advanced heart failure / Mario C. Deng,
Yoshifumi Naka.
        p. cm.
    Includes bibliographical references
    ISBN-13 978-1-86094-728-5 -- ISBN-10 1-86094-728-X
    ISBN-13 978-1-86094-773-5 (pbk) -- ISBN-10 1-86094-773-5 (pbk)
        1. Blood, Circulation, Artificial--Instruments. 2. Heart, Mechanical. 3. Heart failure--
Treatment. I. Title. II. Naka, Yoshifumi.

    RD598.35.A77 M4356 2007
    617.4'12--dc22

                                                                                2006049707


**British Library Cataloguing-in-Publication Data**
A catalogue record for this book is available from the British Library.

Typeset by Stallion Press
Email: enquiries@stallionpress.com




Printed by Fulsland Offset Printing (S) Pte Ltd, Singapore

# PREFACE

This book provides a state-of-the-art overview of mechanical circulatory support devices and their role in the care of patients with advanced heart failure. It is aimed at healthcare teams around the world who are involved in the patient care, research, and teaching of advanced heart failure; those in training; and the interested lay public. Situations in which a patient with advanced heart failure is evaluated as well as cared for before and after the implantation of mechanical circulatory support have to be described in a complementary way by the professional teams and their patients. Therefore, these perspectives are presented alongside to provide a comprehensive overview of the care process in its entire scope. In particular, the evidence-based medicine perspectives of not only expert cardiologists, cardiac surgeons, nurses, coordinators, social workers, psychologists, and physical therapists, but also (and equally important) patients and their relatives, are portrayed.

# ACKNOWLEDGMENTS

This work was supported by the National Heart, Lung, and Blood Institute (NHLBI)–Specialized Center for Clinically Oriented Research (SCCOR) grant HL 077096-01, named "The Biology of Human Long-Term Mechanical Circulatory Support".

# CONTENTS

# CHAPTER 1

# ADVANCED HEART FAILURE

## EPIDEMIOLOGY

### Epidemiological Scope

*Epidemiological Transition.* In less industrialized countries, the epidemiological transition is associated with a reduced risk of mortality from communicable diseases and an increased risk of death from cardiovascular diseases, including heart failure (Redfield, 2002; Cappuccio, 2004). Improved management of acute coronary syndromes and improved longevity of the population have resulted in a growing number of patients with heart failure. In industrialized countries, the prevalence and incidence of heart failure are estimated to be around 1.5% and 0.15% of the population, respectively (Hunt *et al.*, 2005; Deng, 2002). An estimated 10% of persons with heart failure are in advanced stages. In the United States and Europe alone, with >700 million inhabitants and >7 million patients with heart failure, the prevalence of advanced heart failure — constituting between 1%–10% of the heart failure population — is estimated to total between 70 000 and 700 000 patients (Deng, 2005).

*Evolution of Treatment Options.* Correspondingly, the evolution of treatment options for advanced heart failure patients over the last few decades has been impressive. It includes medical treatment (angiotensin-converting enzyme inhibitors, beta-blockade), defibrillator therapy, heart transplantation, and most recently mechanical circulatory support devices (MCSDs). The comparison of outcomes between different therapies for advanced heart failure is challenging. For example, heart transplantation has never been tested in a randomized clinical trial because of the obvious survival advantage in the 1970s in comparison to medical therapy, which has been questioned during the last decade. Therefore, the clinical decision-making

1

algorithm is subject to continuing debate and consensus processes, as exemplified by the recent guideline development initiative of the International Society for Heart and Lung Transplantation (Mehra *et al.*, 2006).

## Classification and Staged Therapy of Advanced Heart Failure

***Definition.***    The terminology of chronic heart failure in its advanced stages is not very precise. The terms "advanced", "severe", "congestive", "refractory", and "end-stage" heart failure are used in largely exchangable ways. End-stage heart failure reflects the impaired prognosis associated with it, and has been incorporated into the recent staging system for heart failure (Hunt *et al.*, 2001; Hunt *et al.*, 2005). However, the term advanced heart failure will be used in this book to express the more recent insight into the partial reversibility of the heart failure remodeling process.

***Classification.***    The New York Heart Association (NYHA) classification of heart failure has been complemented by a staging system of heart failure (Hunt *et al.*, 2001; Hunt *et al.*, 2005). This staging system has the advantages of including asymptomatic stages (risk factors, structural heart disease) and reflecting the progressive nature of the heart failure syndrome. It bears a resemblance with the classification of tumors, a similarly malignant group of conditions (Fig. 1).

## Prognosis of Advanced Heart Failure

***Epidemiological Data.***    The contemporary incidence and prognosis of heart failure are not well known. To describe the survival of a population-based cohort of patients with incident, i.e. new-onset heart failure and the clinical features associated with mortality, an observational study was conducted in a population of 151 000 served by 82 general practitioners in west London. New cases of heart failure were identified by daily surveillance of acute hospital admissions to the local district general hospital, and by general practitioner referral of all suspected new cases of heart failure to a rapid access clinic. All patients with suspected heart failure underwent clinical assessment; and chest radiography, ECG, and echocardiogram were

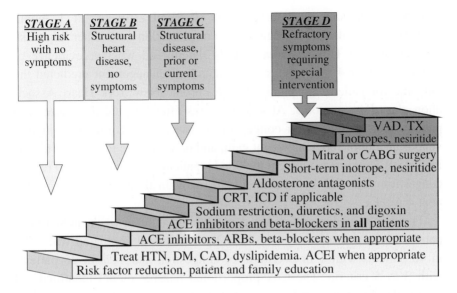

| STAGE A | STAGE B | STAGE C | STAGE D |
|---|---|---|---|
| High risk with no symptoms | Structural heart disease, no symptoms | Structural disease, prior or current symptoms | Refractory symptoms requiring special intervention |

VAD, TX
Inotropes, nesiritide
Mitral or CABG surgery
Short-term inotrope, nesiritide
Aldosterone antagonists
CRT, ICD if applicable
Sodium restriction, diuretics, and digoxin
ACE inhibitors and beta-blockers in **all** patients
ACE inhibitors, ARBs, beta-blockers when appropriate
Treat HTN, DM, CAD, dyslipidemia. ACEI when appropriate
Risk factor reduction, patient and family education

**Fig. 1.** Staging of heart failure and associated interventions (adapted from Hunt *et al.*, 2005).

performed. A panel of three cardiologists reviewed all the data and determined whether the definition of heart failure had been met. Patients were subsequently managed by the general practitioner in consultation with the local cardiologist or admitting physician. Death, overall and from cardiovascular causes, served as the main outcome measure.

There were 90 deaths (83 cardiovascular deaths) in the cohort of 220 patients with incident heart failure over a median follow-up of 16 months. Survival was 81% at 1 month, 75% at 3 months, 70% at 6 months, 62% at 12 months, and 57% at 18 months. Lower systolic blood pressure, higher serum creatinine concentration, and greater extent of crackles on auscultation of the lungs were independently predictive of cardiovascular mortality (all $p < 0.001$). The authors concluded that mortality is high in the first few weeks after diagnosis for patients with new heart failure, and that simple clinical features can identify patients at especially high risk of death (Cowie *et al.*, 2000).

***Response to Therapy and Prognosis.*** Class IV symptoms predict high mortality rates, but the outcome is not known for patients who improve to establish freedom from congestion. Revised estimates at 1 month could facilitate decisions regarding transplantation and other high-risk interventions. A UCLA/Harvard study determined whether evidence of congestion after 4 to 6 weeks of heart failure management predicted the outcome for patients hospitalized with chronic New York Heart Association class IV symptoms. At 4 to 6 weeks after hospital discharge, 146 patients were evaluated for congestion by five criteria (orthopnea, jugular venous distention, edema, weight gain, and new increase in baseline diuretics). Heart failure management included inpatient therapy tailored to relieve congestion, followed by adjustments to maintain fluid balance during the next 4 weeks.

Freedom from congestion was demonstrated at 4 to 6 weeks in 80 (54%) patients, who subsequently had 87% 2-year survival compared with 67% in 40 patients with 1 or 2 criteria of congestion and 41% in 26 patients with 3 to 5 criteria. The Cox proportional hazards model identified left ventricular dimension, pulmonary wedge pressure on therapy, and freedom from congestion as independent predictors of survival. The persistence of orthopnea predicted 38% 2-year survival (without urgent transplantation) versus 77% in 113 patients without orthopnea. Serum sodium was lower and blood urea nitrogen and heart rate were higher when orthopnea persisted. The authors concluded that the ability to maintain freedom from congestion identifies a population with good survival despite previous class IV symptoms. At 4 to 6 weeks of heart failure management, patients with persistent congestion may be considered for high-risk intervention (Lucas *et al.*, 2000).

## MANAGEMENT OVERVIEW

| | |
|---|---|
| **Ted L (born 1943)**<br><br>**Living with heart failure: preoperative perspective** | **My Early Years**<br>I was born with a congenital heart disease that kept me from keeping up with my little playmates. But as I reached my high school years, I began to outgrow the problem and went on to enjoy college intramural sports and upon graduation skiing, squash, sky diving, and golf.<br>    After graduating from Rollins College, I went to Wall Street to make my fame and fortune. I spent 20 hectic years in a bond-trading room, jumping up and down, |

yelling "buy!" "sell!" "you're done!" Then, I spent 16 years working as a financial planner with individuals and their corporations to develop a plan to cover all of life's contingencies.

During this time, in 1973, I met Trina Richner and within 5 weeks we were engaged. Since I had not seen a heart specialist in 20 years, I thought it best to get an updated diagnosis for my future bride and myself. Dr Steve Scheidt at New York Presbyterian Hospital–Cornell Medical Center was recommended to me, and I spent several days undergoing diagnostic tests. His conclusion: I had a form of cardiomyopathy called idiopathic hypertrophic subaortic stenosis — an enlarged heart muscle. But since I was asymptomatic, there was little I needed to do. I had annual checkups with him for the next 20 odd years.

## My Medical Journey

In the early 1990s, I experienced my first heart problem: dizzy spells and skipped heart beats. Over the next decade, my cardiologist mixed and matched various medications as the problems grew progressively worse. By early 2003, I knew I was really in trouble as I was having difficulty walking a New York City block, having to stop four or five times to catch my breath. I developed the typical symptoms of a person with chronic heart failure. I had shortness of breath and edema that was particularly obvious when one looked at my ankles. Dr Steve Scheidt came to the conclusion that I should have a consultation with a leading heart specialist in cardiomyopathy, Dr Barry Maron at the Minneapolis Heart Institute. In May 2003, I spent a day undergoing tests with his team of six, and late in the afternoon we convened in his office to hear the results.

Let me read a few sentences from a recent correspondence of his.

> Dear Ted ... I often think about the day of our consultation and how awkward I felt about hitting you with such bad news that I know you didn't expect ... and using such severe medical terms as "end-stage hypertrophic cardiomyopathy" to emphasize the

point that you needed to move fast ... which you did ... fortunately. Best Regards, Barry Maron.

I only had one question for Dr Maron: "The words 'end-stage' don't sound good to me. Just what are you telling me?" "Ted, you have 6 months to a year to live with that heart of yours."

Within a week upon return, I was interviewed by members of the Columbia Presbyterian Hospital's heart transplant team. I was told that I would make a good transplant candidate, but at that moment I was too healthy to be put on the heart transplant list. They would be most happy to follow my case. In 5 days, I went from "go home, move fast, you are dying and need a heart transplant" to "you're too healthy to be put on the list." Go figure!

At first I got mad, then I got angry and went into denial. But reality finally came upon me, and I began to ask God "why me?" Hadn't I spent the last 20 years as an active member of my church being as good a Christian as I could? I was even helping my community by serving on my cooperative building's Board of Trustees.

I also began to question my own body. Why had my body suddenly deserted me? For my entire life, my heart, mind, and body had all gone along together. If something bad happened to me, my body took care of it. Now, it was going off in a different direction and I had no control over it.

I began an emotional journey that has continued to this day. Once I began to learn about organ transplantation, I found that one out of three persons die while waiting for a new heart. Would I live long enough to get a new heart? I felt sorry for myself. Would the new heart take if I got one? How would it work? How long would it last? I thought a lot about my wife. If I died, was I leaving her in good financial shape? Who would she turn to for help? We had to make plans together.

One day, I came to the sudden realization that for me to live someone else had to die. I had been praying for God to get me a new heart from the beginning, but I couldn't imagine asking God to have someone else die so that I could live. I came around to the realization that if God wanted me to live, then he had a plan for me. What was it? If I was to get a new heart, what did he want me to do with it? That began a dialog between us that has continued right up to the present.

Dr Maron was right. My heart deteriorated rapidly to the point where I was having trouble walking from my bedroom to my kitchen by March 2004. Due to chronic heart failure, my body filled with 30 pounds of fluid surrounding my heart, lungs, and other bodily functions. It was most pronounced to the casual observer in my very swollen ankles.

## Clinical Presentation and Pathophysiology of Heart Failure

The introduction of newer modes of therapy into medical practice, and into the management of heart failure in particular, requires continuous evaluation of evidence according to established criteria. The distinction between evidence based on randomized clinical trials, all-or-none studies, outcomes research, cohort studies, case-control studies, case series, and investigational procedures allows differentiating between different levels of enthusiasm for clinical recommendations (http://www.cebm.net/levels_of_evidence.asp).

***Definition.*** Chronic heart failure is defined as a clinical syndrome in which, secondary to impaired function of the heart, a performance commensurate with the metabolic needs of the body cannot be maintained or can only be maintained at the expense of elevated filling pressures of the left and right ventricles (Braunwald, 1992).

***Compensatory Mechanisms.*** In increasing stages of heart failure, the adrenergic system, renin-angiotensin system, antidiuretic hormone system, and atrial natriuretic peptide system are chronically activated. These chronic neurohormonal changes lead to compensatory elevation of afterload, preload, heart rate, contractility, and cardiac hypertrophy. The New York Heart Association functional class IV is characterized by a flattening and rightward shift of the cardiac function curve to the point where reduced cardiac output does not fulfill the metabolic requirements of the body, capillary wedge pressure reaches a level at which pulmonary edema ensues, or both happen (Braunwald, 2002).

*Maladaptive Nature of Chronic Neurohormonal Activation.*   The discovery that neurohormonal mechanisms can exert a detrimental effect in individuals with advanced heart failure brings up the question of their evolutionary role. These mechanisms evolved for situations that coincide with acute volume losses in otherwise healthy persons. Of highest priority in these situations would be the maintenance of an adequate cardiac output, peripheral vascular resistance, and arterial perfusion pressure as well as consecutive regulation of blood volume. A temporary activation of the described neurohormonal mechanisms with intact cardiac function presumably does not initiate the vicious cycle encountered in heart failure. While an evolutionary optimization of acute cardiovascular regulation must be assumed, there is no need for optimization of regulatory mechanisms in chronic heart failure because it usually manifests beyond the reproductive age (Braunwald, 1992).

## Specific Underlying Disease Conditions in Heart Failure

*Cardiomyopathy WHO Classification.*   The 1995 World Health Organization classification of cardiomyopathies distinguishes between the following:

- dilated cardiomyopathies (ischemic and nonischemic);
- hypertrophic cardiomyopathies;
- restrictive cardiomyopathies;
- arrhythmogenic right ventricular cardiomyopathies;
- specific cardiomyopathies; and
- unclassified cardiomyopathies (Richardson *et al.*, 1996).

***Giant Cell Myocarditis.*** Among the unclassified cardiomyopathies is myocarditis. Among the group of myocarditis, the entity of giant cell myocarditis is the rarest but most devastating disease that usually affects young, otherwise healthy individuals. Associations with thymoma, inflammatory bowel disease, and a variety of autoimmune disorders have been reported. The rate of death or heart transplantation is approximately 70% at 1 year. Data from a Lewis rat model and from observational human studies suggest that giant cell myocarditis is mediated by T lymphocytes, and may respond to treatment aimed at attenuating T-cell function.

Recent findings from the Giant Cell Myocarditis Registry, a clinical and pathological database from 63 cases of giant cell myocarditis gathered from 36 medical centers, include the following: the sensitivity of endomyocardial biopsy for giant cell myocarditis for patients who undergo transplantation or autopsy is 82% to 85%. Registry subjects who received cyclosporine in combination with steroid, azathioprine, or muromonab-CD3 have prolonged transplant-free survival (12.6 months vs. 3.0 months for no immunosuppression). Posttransplantation survival is approximately 71% at 5 years, despite a 25% rate of giant cell infiltration in the donor heart. To confirm and extend these findings, randomized trials of immunosuppression included muromonab-CD3, cyclosporine, and steroids (Cooper *et al.*, 1997; Cooper, 2000).

***Other Forms of Myocarditis/Heart Muscle Disease.*** There has been controversy over the extent to which patients with unclassified dilated cardiomyopathies should undergo diagnostic endomyocardial biopsy testing. In a series of 100 consecutive patients, the pathological diagnostic information obtained was judged to be useful to the clinician in 54 patients and not useful in 46 patients. In 74 patients with congestive heart failure of unknown etiology and a dilated heart, useful pathological diagnoses included myocarditis, vasculitis, doxorubicin cardiomyopathy, and congestive cardiomyopathy. In most of the patients with biopsy findings of myocarditis, there were no other clinical or laboratory findings indicating the presence of this disease, and the diagnosis of myocarditis would have been overlooked without a biopsy. In 26 patients in whom there was clinical evidence of constrictive or restrictive cardiovascular physiological characteristics, useful biopsy diagnoses included radiation-induced cardiomyopathy, endomyocardial fibrosis, amyloidosis, or no myocardial disease; in the patients without myocardial disease, thoracotomies were performed for constrictive pericarditis. Transvenous endomyocardial biopsy can provide clinically useful information in the evaluation of diseases of the myocardium. The Dallas classification of myocarditis is based on EMB findings (Aretz *et al.*, 1987).

## Risk Stratification in Advanced Heart Failure

Risk stratification of patients with end-stage congestive heart failure is a critical component of the selection process for the best treatment; for example, if the choice between optimal medical therapy, heart transplantation, or chronic mechanical circulatory support has to be made. Accurate identification of individuals most likely to survive without a transplant would facilitate more efficient use of scarce donor organs.

*Heart Failure Survival Score (HFSS).* In a landmark collaboration between the University of Pennsylvania and Columbia University from 1987 to 1995, multivariable proportional hazards survival models were developed with the use of data on 80 clinical characteristics from 268 ambulatory patients with advanced heart failure (derivation sample). Invasive and noninvasive models (with and without catheterization-derived data) were constructed. A prognostic score was determined for each patient from each model. Stratum-specific likelihood ratios were used to develop three prognostic-score risk groups. The models were prospectively validated on 199 similar patients (validation sample) by calculation of the area under the receiver operating characteristic curve for 1-year event-free survival, the censored c-index for event-free survival, and comparison of event-free survival curves for prognostic-score risk strata. Outcome events were defined as urgent transplant or death without transplant.

The noninvasive model performed well in both samples, and increased performance was not attained by the addition of catheterization-derived variables. Prognostic-score risk groups derived from the noninvasive model in the derivation sample effectively stratified the risk of an outcome event in both samples (1-year event-free survival for derivation and validation samples, respectively: low risk, 93% and 88%; medium risk, 72% and 60%;

high risk, 43% and 35%). The authors concluded that the selection of candidates for cardiac transplantation may be improved by use of this noninvasive risk stratification model (Aaronson *et al.*, 1997). The beauty of this score resides not only in its powerful predictive value, but also in its easy bedside implementation by the equation $HFSS = [(0.69 \times CAD: YES = 1; NO = 0) + (0.022 \times HR) + (-0.046 \times LVEF) + (-0.026 \times mBP) + (0.61 \times IVCD: YES = 1; NO = 0) + (-0.055 \times VO_2) + (-0.047 \times Na)]$.

Heart failure has an annual mortality rate ranging from 5% to 75%. The purpose of the Seattle Heart Failure Model study was to develop and validate a multivariate risk model to predict 1-, 2-, and 3-year survival in heart failure patients with the use of easily obtainable characteristics relating to clinical status, therapy (pharmacological as well as device), and laboratory parameters. The Seattle Heart Failure Model was derived in a cohort of 1125 heart failure patients with the use of a multivariate Cox model. For medications and devices not available in the derivation database, hazard ratios were estimated from published literature. The model was prospectively validated in five additional cohorts totaling 9942 heart failure patients and 17307 person-years of follow-up.

The accuracy of the model was excellent, with respective predicted versus actual 1-year survival rates of 73.4% vs. 74.3% in the derivation cohort and 90.5% vs. 88.5%, 86.5% vs. 86.5%, 83.8% vs. 83.3%, 90.9% vs. 91.0%, and 89.6% vs. 86.7% in the five validation cohorts. For the lowest score, the 2-year survival was 92.8% compared with 88.7%, 77.8%, 58.1%, 29.5%, and 10.8% for scores of 0, 1, 2, 3, and 4, respectively. The overall receiver operating characteristic area under the curve was 0.729 (95% CI, 0.714 to 0.744). The model also allowed estimation of the benefit of adding medications or devices to an individual patient's therapeutic regimen. The authors concluded that the Seattle Heart Failure Model provides an accurate estimate of 1-, 2-, and 3-year survival with the use of easily obtained clinical, pharmacological, device, and laboratory characteristics (Levy *et al.*, 2002).

## Behavioral Interventions in Advanced Heart Failure

***Randomized Clinical Trials.*** The management of patients with heart failure, independent of the specific types of interventions anticipated, improves with multidisciplinary, patient-oriented, flexible care (Fonarow *et al.*, 1997; Shah *et al.*, 1998; Philbin, 1999). Since behavioral factors, such as poor compliance with treatment, frequently contribute to exacerbations of heart failure, a prospective randomized trial of the effect of a nurse-directed multidisciplinary intervention on rates of readmission within 90 days of hospital discharge, quality of life, and costs of care for high-risk patients 70 years of age or older who were hospitalized with congestive heart failure was conducted by Rich *et al.* (1995). The intervention consisted of comprehensive education of the patient and family, a prescribed diet, social service consultation and planning for an early discharge, a review of medications, and intensive follow-up.

Survival for 90 days without readmission, the primary outcome measure, was achieved in 91 of the 142 patients in the treatment group, as compared with 75 of the 140 patients in the control group who received conventional care ($P = 0.09$). There were 94 readmissions in the control group and 53 in the treatment group (risk ratio, 0.56; $P = 0.02$). The number of readmissions for heart failure was reduced by 56.2% in the treatment group (54 vs. 24, $P = 0.04$), whereas the number of readmissions for other causes was reduced by 28.5% (40 vs. 29, $P$ not significant). In the control group, 23 (16.4%) patients had more than one readmission, as compared with 9 (6.3%) patients in the treatment group (risk ratio, 0.39; $P = 0.01$). In a subgroup of 126 patients, quality-of-life scores at 90 days improved more from baseline for patients in the treatment group ($P = 0.001$). Because of the reduction in hospital admissions, the overall cost of care was $460 less per patient in the treatment group. It was concluded that a nurse-directed, multidisciplinary intervention can improve quality of life and reduce hospital admission and medical costs for elderly patients with congestive heart failure (Rich *et al.*, 1995).

## Pharmacological Treatment

***Randomized Clinical Trials of Renin-Angiotensin System Blockade.*** The first randomized prospective medical trial demonstrating a survival benefit from medical treatment in advanced heart failure was the CONSENSUS I trial (Swedberg, 1987). A total of 256 patients in NYHA class

IV heart failure were randomized to either enalapril or placebo. While the 1-year placebo mortality rate was 64%, it was reduced to 46% in the enalapril group. At 10-year follow-up, five patients, all in the enalapril group, were long-term survivors ($P = 0.004$). This study is unique in that it was the first heart failure trial not only in unselected NYHA class IV patients, but also in examining extended survival (Swedberg *et al.*, 1999).

In the RALES trial, 1663 patients who had severe heart failure and a left ventricular ejection fraction of <35%, and who were being treated with an angiotensin-converting enzyme inhibitor, a loop diuretic, and in most cases digoxin, were randomly assigned to receive 25 mg of spirono-lactone daily or placebo. After a mean follow-up period of 24 months, there was a 46% mortality rate in the placebo group and a 35% mortality rate in the spironolactone group (Pitt *et al.*, 1999). The angiotensin II type 1 receptor blocker valsartan significantly reduced the combined endpoint of mortality and morbidity, and improved clinical signs and symptoms in patients with heart failure. However, the *post hoc* observation of an adverse effect on mortality and morbidity in the subgroup receiving valsartan, an ACE inhibitor, and a beta-blocker raised concern about the potential safety of this specific combination (Cohn and Tognoni, 2001).

To determine whether the angiotensin receptor blocker (ARB) candesar-tan decreases cardiovascular mortality, morbidity, and all-cause mortality in patients with CHF and depressed LVEF, a prespecified analysis of the com-bined Candesartan in Heart Failure Assessment of Reduction in Mortal-ity and Morbidity (CHARM) low-LVEF trials was performed. CHARM is a randomized, double-blind, placebo-controlled, multicenter, international trial program. The New York Heart Association (NYHA) class II through IV CHF patients with an LVEF of ≤40% were randomized to candesartan or placebo in two complementary parallel trials (CHARM-Alternative, for patients who could not tolerate ACE inhibitors; and CHARM-Added, for patients who were receiving ACE inhibitors).

Mortality and morbidity were determined in 4576 low-LVEF patients (2289 on candesartan and 2287 on placebo), titrated as tolerated to a tar-get dose of 32 mg once daily, and observed for 2 to 4 years (median, 40 months). The primary outcome (time to first event by intention to treat) was cardiovascular death or CHF hospitalization for each trial, with all-cause mortality a secondary endpoint in the pooled analysis of the low-LVEF trials. Of the 2289 patients in the candesartan group, 817 (35.7%) experienced cardiovascular death or CHF hospitalization as compared with 944 (41.3%) in the placebo group (HR, 0.82; 95% CI, 0.74 to 0.90; $P < 0.001$), with reduced risk for both cardiovascular deaths [521 (22.8%) vs. 599 (26.2%); HR, 0.84 (95% CI, 0.75 to 0.95); $P = 0.005$] and CHF hospitalizations [516 (22.5%) vs. 642 (28.1%); HR, 0.76 (95% CI, 0.68 to 0.85); $P < 0.001$]. It is important to note that all-cause mortality was also significantly reduced by candesartan [642 (28.0%) vs. 708 (31.0%); HR, 0.88 (95% CI, 0.79 to 0.98); $P = 0.018$]. No significant heterogeneity for the beneficial effects of candesartan was found across prespecified and subsequently identified subgroups, including treatment with ACE inhibitors, beta-blockers, an aldosterone antagonist, or their combinations. The study drug was discontinued because of adverse effects exhibited by 23.1% of patients in the candesartan group and 18.8% in the placebo group, such as increased creatinine (7.1% vs. 3.5%, respectively), hypotension (4.2% vs. 2.1%), and hyperkalemia (2.8% vs. 0.5%) (all $P < 0.001$).

The authors concluded that candesartan significantly reduces all-cause mortality, cardiovascular death, and heart failure hospitalizations in patients with CHF and LVEF of ≤40% when added to standard therapies including ACE inhibitors, beta-blockers, and an aldosterone antagonist. Routine monitoring of blood pressure, serum creatinine, and serum potassium is warranted (Young *et al.*, 2004). The accompanying editorial concluded that angiotensin II receptor blockers are now a reasonable alternative to angiotensin-converting enzyme (ACE) inhibitors as first-line agents for HF. Angiotensin II receptor blockers or ACE inhibitors are useful to prevent HF in selected stage A and B patients (Fig. 1), and candesartan can improve outcomes in patients with impaired cardiac function who are intolerant of ACE inhibitors (Young *et al.*, 2004).

***Randomized Clinical Trials of Adrenergic System Blockade.*** The MERIT Study Group (1999) investigated whether metoprolol controlled release/extended release (CR/XL) once daily, in addition to standard therapy, would lower mortality in patients with decreased ejection fraction and symptoms of heart failure. The MERIT Study Group enrolled 3991 patients with chronic heart failure in New York Heart Association (NYHA) functional class II–IV and with ejection fraction of 0.40 or less, stabilized with optimum standard therapy, in a double-blind randomized controlled study. Randomization was preceded by a 2-week single-blind placebo run-in period. Of the 3991 patients, 1990 were randomly assigned metoprolol CR/XL 12.5 mg (NYHA III–IV) or 25.0 mg once daily (NYHA II), and 2001 were assigned placebo. The target dose was 200 mg once daily, and doses were uptitrated over 8 weeks. The primary endpoint was all-cause mortality, analyzed by intention to treat. The study was stopped early on the recommendation of the independent safety committee. The mean follow-up time was 1 year.

All-cause mortality was lower in the metoprolol CR/XL group than in the placebo group [145 (7.2% per patient-year of follow-up) vs. 217 deaths (11.0%), relative risk 0.66 (95% CI 0.53–0.81); $p = 0.00009$ or adjusted for interim analyses $p = 0.0062$]. There were fewer sudden deaths in the metoprolol CR/XL group than in the placebo group [79 vs. 132, relative risk 0.59 (95% CI 0.45–0.78); $p = 0.0002$], and fewer deaths from worsening heart failure [30 vs. 58, relative risk 0.51 (95% CI 0.33–0.79); $p = 0.0023$]. The authors concluded that metoprolol CR/XL once daily, in addition to optimum standard therapy, improves survival. The drug was well tolerated (MERIT, 1999).

The CIBIS-II Study Group (1999) investigated the efficacy of bisoprolol, a beta1-selective adrenoceptor blocker, in decreasing all-cause mortality in chronic heart failure. In a multicenter double-blind randomized placebo-controlled trial in Europe, they enrolled 2647 symptomatic patients in New York Heart Association class III or IV with a left ventricular ejection fraction of 35% or less that were receiving standard therapy with diuretics and angiotensin-converting enzyme inhibitors. They randomly assigned patients bisoprolol 1.25 mg ($n = 1327$) or placebo ($n = 1320$) daily, the drug being progressively increased to a maximum of 10 mg per day. Patients were followed up for a mean of 1.3 years. Analysis was by intention to treat. CIBIS-II was stopped early, after the second interim analysis, because bisoprolol showed a significant mortality benefit.

All-cause mortality was significantly lower with bisoprolol than with placebo [156 (11.8%) vs. 228 (17.3%) deaths, with a hazard ratio of 0.66

(95% CI 0.54–0.81, $p < 0.0001$)]. There were significantly fewer sudden deaths among patients on bisoprolol than in those on placebo [48 (3.6%) vs. 83 (6.3%) deaths, with a hazard ratio of 0.56 (95% CI 0.39–0.80, $p = 0.0011$)]. Treatment effects were independent of the severity or cause of heart failure. The authors concluded that beta-blocker therapy has benefits for survival in stable heart failure patients (CIBIS-II, 1999).

The COPERNICUS trial demonstrated beneficial effects on mortality in NYHA class IV patients with chronic heart failure. In this trial, the placebo 1-year mortality rate of 19.6% was reduced to 11% by carvedilol. All subgroups, including those with the most advanced heart failure, showed the same beneficial direction of effect (Packer *et al.*, 2001). The Carvedilol or Metoprolol European Trial (COMET) reported a significant survival benefit for carvedilol — a beta1-, beta2-, and alpha1-blocker — vs. metoprolol tartrate — a beta1-selective blocker — in patients with mild-to-severe chronic heart failure (Poole-Wilson *et al.*, 2003).

***Randomized Clinical Trials of Positive Inotropes/Vasodilators.*** Trials using positive inotropes such as vesnarinone (Feldman *et al.*, 1993; Cohn *et al.*, 1998), xamoterol (Ryden, 1990), ibopamine (Hampton *et al.*, 1997) and milrinone (Packer *et al.*, 1991) or vasodilators such as epoprostenol did not demonstrate a survival benefit; in fact, they showed an adverse mortality effect (Califf *et al.*, 1997). Over the past few years, a large clinical development program with the phosphodiesterase III inhibitor enoximone has yielded promising preliminary results during periods of concomitant cardioprotection with beta-blockers and ICDs. The phase II results of the Oral Enoximone in Intravenous Inotrope-Dependent Subjects (EMOTE) study showed promise (Lowes *et al.*, 2005).

However, the phase III Studies of Oral Enoximone Therapy in Advanced Heart Failure (ESSENTIAL) trials demonstrated a lack of statistically significant differences in all predefined endpoints (Cleland *et al.*, 2005). Time to all-cause mortality and time to first cardiovascular hospitalization were similar in the enoximone and placebo study groups (hazard ratios 0.97 and 0.98, respectively). Interestingly, both all-cause mortality and mortality or cardiovascular hospitalization rates were lower with enoximone in the last one-half of follow-up (beyond 16.4 months)

(5.4% with enoximone vs. 8.8% with placebo, $p = 0.045$; and 12.5% with enoximone vs. 17.4% with placebo, $p = 0.09$). Furthermore, patients with LVEF <20% had greater improvement in 6-min walk test distance in the enoximone group. High hopes are also being placed on the results of two phase III trials of another inodilator drug, levosimendan: "Survival in Patients with Acute Heart Failure in Need of Intravenous Inotropic Support" (SURVIVE) and "Second Randomized Multicenter Evaluation of Intravenous Levosimendan Efficacy vs. Survival in the Short Term Treatment of Decompensated Heart Failure" (REVIVE-II) (Cleland *et al.*, 2006).

***Randomized Clinical Trials of Antiarrhythmics in Ventricular Tachyarrythmias.*** Sudden death accounts for one third to one half of the deaths in patients with heart failure. With respect to antiarrhythmic treatment, class I antiarrhytmic drugs have been disappointing. Amiodarone and beta-blockers are the only interventions that have not been shown to increase mortality risks in patients with congestive heart failure. The GESICA trial evaluated the effect of low-dose amiodarone on 2-year mortality in patients with severe heart failure. This prospective multicenter trial included 516 patients on optimal standard treatment for heart failure. Patients were randomized to 300 mg/day amiodarone (260 patients) or to standard treatment (256 patients). Intention-to-treat analysis showed 87 deaths in the amiodarone group (33.5%) compared with 106 in the control group (41.4%) ($p = 0.024$) (Doval *et al.*, 1994).

The CHF-STAT investigators used a double-blind, placebo-controlled protocol, in which 674 patients with symptoms of congestive heart failure, cardiac enlargement, 10 or more premature ventricular contractions per hour, and a left ventricular ejection fraction of 40% or less were randomly assigned to receive amiodarone (336 patients) or placebo (338 patients). There was no significant difference in overall mortality between the two treatment groups ($P = 0.6$). The 2-year actuarial survival rate was 69.4% for the patients in the amiodarone group and 70.8% for those in the placebo group. There was a trend toward a reduction in overall mortality among the patients with nonischemic cardiomyopathy who received amiodarone (Singh *et al.*, 1995). Recent studies using beta-adrenergic blockers in patients with reduced systolic function and heart failure symptoms have shown significant reductions in overall mortality rates, with a combined relative risk reduction for sudden death of 38% (Teerlink and Massie, 2000).

## Resynchronization

*Randomized Clinical Trials.*   A growing body of evidence suggests that the use of implantable devices to resynchronize ventricular contraction may be a beneficial adjunct in the treatment of chronic heart failure. One third of patients with chronic heart failure have electrocardiographic evidence of a major intraventricular conduction delay, which may worsen left ventricular systolic dysfunction through asynchronous ventricular contraction. Uncontrolled studies suggest that multisite biventricular pacing improves hemodynamics and well-being by reducing ventricular asynchrony.

The MUSTIC trial assessed the clinical efficacy and safety of this new therapy. Sixty-seven patients with severe heart failure (New York Heart Association class III) due to chronic left ventricular systolic dysfunction, with normal sinus rhythm and a QRS-interval duration of more than 150 ms, received transvenous atriobiventricular pacemakers (with leads in one atrium and each ventricle). This single-blind, randomized, controlled cross-over study compared the responses of the patients during two periods: a 3-month period of inactive pacing (ventricular inhibited pacing at a basic rate of 40 bpm), and a 3-month period of active (atriobiventricular) pacing. The mean distance walked in 6 min was 22% greater with active pacing ($399 \pm 100$ m vs. $326 \pm 134$ m, $P < 0.001$), the quality-of-life score improved by 32% ($P < 0.001$), peak oxygen uptake increased by 8% ($P < 0.03$), hospitalizations decreased by two thirds ($P < 0.05$), and active pacing was preferred by 85% of the patients ($P < 0.001$) (Cazeau *et al.*, 2001).

In the MIRACLE trial, the first parallel-group randomized evaluation of the efficacy of cardiac resynchronization in patients with NYHA class III–IV heart failure and a QRS duration of $>130$ ms, 266 patients received the Medtronic InSync device and were then randomized to resynchronization vs. no resynchronization for 6 months while background medication was maintained. The clinical composite score was defined as the primary endpoint, which characterized patients as improved (if they showed improvement in NYHA class or patient global assessment), unchanged, or worse (if they died, had worsening heart failure leading to hospitalization or discontinuation of treatment, or had worse NYHA class or global assessment). More patients improved (63% vs. 38%) and fewer patients deteriorated (22% vs. 29%) in the group with the activated device as compared to the control group (Packer and Abraham, 2001).

The Comparison of Medical Therapy, Pacing, and Defibrillation in Chronic Heart Failure (COMPANION) trial was a randomized, open-label, three-arm study of patients with New York Heart Association class III or IV heart failure, an ejection fraction of 35% or less, and a QRS duration of >120 ms. The COMPANION study objectives were to determine whether optimal pharmacological therapy used with (1) ventricular resynchronization therapy alone or (2) ventricular resynchronization therapy combined with cardioverter-defibrillator capability is superior to optimal pharmacological therapy alone in reducing combined all-cause mortality and in modifying other endpoints (Bristow *et al.*, 2000). A total of 1520 patients who had advanced heart failure (New York Heart Association class III or IV) due to ischemic or nonischemic cardiomyopathies and a QRS interval of at least 120 ms were randomly assigned in a 1:2:2 ratio to receive optimal pharmacological therapy (diuretics, angiotensin-converting enzyme inhibitors, beta-blockers, and spironolactone) alone or in combination with cardiac resynchronization therapy with either a pacemaker or a pacemaker/defibrillator. The primary composite endpoint was the time to death from or hospitalization for any cause.

Compared to optimal pharmacological therapy alone, cardiac resynchronization therapy with a pacemaker decreased the risk of the primary endpoint (hazard ratio, 0.81; $P = 0.014$), as did cardiac resynchronization therapy with a pacemaker/defibrillator (hazard ratio, 0.80; $P = 0.01$). The risk of the combined endpoint of death from or hospitalization for heart failure was reduced by 34% in the pacemaker group ($P < 0.002$) and by 40% in the pacemaker/defibrillator group ($P < 0.001$ for the comparison with the pharmacological therapy group). A pacemaker reduced the risk of the secondary endpoint of death from any cause by 24% ($P = 0.059$), and a pacemaker/defibrillator reduced the risk by 36% ($P = 0.003$). The authors concluded that for patients with advanced heart failure and a prolonged QRS interval, cardiac resynchronization therapy decreases the combined risk of death from any cause or first hospitalization and, when combined with an implantable defibrillator, significantly reduces mortality (Bristow *et al.*, 2004).

In the Cardiac Resynchronization Heart Failure (CARE-HF) study, patients with New York Heart Association class III or IV heart failure due to left ventricular systolic dysfunction and cardiac dyssynchrony who were receiving standard pharmacological therapy were randomly assigned to receive medical therapy alone or with cardiac resynchronization. The primary endpoint was the time to death from any cause or an unplanned hospitalization for a major cardiovascular event. The principal secondary endpoint was death from any cause. A total of 813 patients were enrolled and followed for a mean of 29.4 months. The primary endpoint was reached by 159 patients in the cardiac resynchronization group, as compared with 224 patients in the medical therapy group (39% vs. 55%; hazard ratio, 0.63; 95% CI, 0.51 to 0.77; $P < 0.001$). There were 82 deaths in the cardiac resynchronization group, as compared with 120 in the medical therapy group (20% vs. 30%; hazard ratio, 0.64; 95% CI, 0.48 to 0.85; $P < 0.002$). Compared with medical therapy, cardiac resynchronization reduced the interventricular mechanical delay, the end-systolic volume index, and the area of the mitral regurgitant jet; increased the left ventricular ejection fraction; and improved symptoms and the quality of life ($P < 0.01$ for all comparisons).

The authors concluded that in patients with heart failure and cardiac dyssynchrony, cardiac resynchronization improves symptoms and the quality of life and reduces complications and the risk of death. These benefits are in addition to those afforded by standard pharmacological therapy. The implantation of a cardiac resynchronization device should be routinely considered in such patients. The beneficial effects of CRT in this group of patients were impressive, considering that these patients were receiving optimal medical therapy with diuretics, beta-blockers, spironolactone, angiotensin-converting enzyme inhibitor, or angiotensin receptor blocker at the time of enrollment. The results showed that for every nine devices implanted, one death and three hospital stays were prevented (Cleland *et al.*, 2005).

## Defibrillator

***Randomized Clinical Trials.*** The publication of the Sudden Cardiac Death Heart Failure Trial (SCD-HeFT) in January 2005 provided a definite answer to the question of comparative survival benefit by defibrillator vs. amiodarone in patients with NYHA class II or III heart failure and an ejection fraction of <35%. The SCD-HeFT investigators randomly assigned 2521 patients with New York Heart Association (NYHA) class II or III CHF and a left ventricular ejection fraction (LVEF) of 35% or less to conventional therapy for CHF plus placebo (847 patients), conventional therapy plus amiodarone (845 patients), or conventional therapy plus a conservatively programmed, shock-only, single-lead ICD (829 patients). Placebo and amiodarone were administered in a double-blind fashion. The primary endpoint was death from any cause. The median LVEF in patients was 25%; 70% were in NYHA class II, and 30% were in class III CHF. The cause of CHF was ischemic in 52% of patients and nonischemic in 48% of patients. The median follow-up was 45.5 months.

There were 244 (29%) deaths in the placebo group, 240 (28%) in the amiodarone group, and 182 (22%) in the ICD group. Compared with placebo, amiodarone was associated with a similar risk of death (hazard ratio, 1.06; 97.5% CI, 0.86 to 1.30; $P = 0.53$), and ICD therapy was associated with a decreased risk of death of 23% (hazard ratio, 0.77; 97.5% CI, 0.62 to 0.96; $P = 0.007$) and an absolute decrease in mortality of 7.2% after 5 years in the overall population. Results did not vary according to either ischemic or nonischemic causes of CHF, but they did vary according to the NYHA class. The authors concluded that in patients with NYHA class II or III CHF and LVEF of 35% or less, amiodarone has no favorable effect on survival, whereas single-lead, shock-only ICD therapy reduces overall mortality by 23%. This study concluded a long debate over the potential benefit of amiodarone in heart failure and the role of the defibrillator (Bardy *et al.*, 2005).

With these results in place, the implantable cardioverter-defibrillator (ICD) has to be considered the major therapeutic tool to prevent sudden arrhythmic death in these patients. Before SCD-HeFT, the Multicenter Automatic Defibrillator Implantation Trial (MADIT) studied whether prophylactic therapy with an implanted cardioverter-defibrillator, as compared with conventional medical therapy, would improve survival in a high-risk group of patients with nonsustained ventricular tachycardia, previous myocardial infarction, and left ventricular dysfunction (estimated 2-year mortality rate of 30%). Over the course of 5 years, 196 patients in New York Heart Association functional class I, II, or III with prior myocardial infarction, a left ventricular ejection fraction of <35% (a documented episode of asymptomatic nonsustained ventricular tachycardia), and inducible, nonsuppressible ventricular tachyarrhythmia on electrophysiological study were randomly assigned to receive an implanted defibrillator ($n = 95$) or conventional medical therapy ($n = 101$). During an average follow-up of 27 months, there were 15 deaths in the defibrillator group and 39 deaths in the conventional therapy group ($P = 0.009$). There was no evidence that amiodarone, beta-blockers, or any other antiarrhythmic therapy had a significant influence on the observed hazard ratio. It was concluded that in patients with a prior myocardial infarction who are at high risk for ventricular tachyarrhythmia, prophylactic therapy with an implanted defibrillator leads to improved survival as compared with conventional medical therapy (Moss *et al.*, 1996).

The AVID investigators (1997) conducted a randomized comparison of defibrillator and antiarrhythmic drugs in patients who had been resuscitated from near-fatal ventricular fibrillation or who had undergone cardioversion from sustained ventricular tachycardia. Patients with ventricular tachycardia also had syncope or other serious cardiac symptoms, along with a left ventricular ejection fraction of 0.40 or less. One group of patients had cardioverter-defibrillator implantation ($n = 507$); the other received class III antiarrhythmic drugs ($n = 509$). Overall survival was greater with the implantable defibrillator, with unadjusted estimates of 89.3% as compared with 82.3% in the antiarrhythmic drug group at 1 year, 81.6% vs. 74.7% at 2 years, and 75.4% vs. 64.1% at 3 years ($P < 0.02$) (AVID, 1997).

In the MUSTT trial, the hypothesis tested was that electrophysiologically guided antiarrhythmic therapy would reduce the risk of sudden death among patients with coronary artery disease, a left ventricular ejection fraction of <40%, and asymptomatic, nonsustained ventricular tachycardia. Patients in whom sustained ventricular tachyarrhythmias were induced by programmed stimulation were randomly assigned to receive either antiarrhythmic therapy, including drugs and implantable defibrillators as indicated by the inducibility during electrophysiological testing, or no intervention if noninducible. Angiotensin-converting enzyme inhibitors and beta-adrenergic blocking agents were administered as tolerated. A total of 704 patients with inducible, sustained ventricular tachyarrhythmias were randomly assigned to different treatment groups. Five-year Kaplan–Meier estimates of the incidence of the primary endpoint of cardiac arrest or death from arrhythmia were 25% among patients receiving electrophysiologically guided therapy and 32% among those assigned to no antiarrhythmic therapy. Neither the rate of cardiac arrest or death from arrhythmia nor the overall mortality rate was lower among the patients assigned to electrophysiologically guided therapy and treated with antiarrhythmic drugs than among the patients assigned to no antiarrhythmic therapy (Buxton *et al.*, 1999).

A follow-up study to MADIT, MADIT II demonstrated a 30% all-cause mortality risk reduction from defibrillator implantation in over 1200 patients from 76 institutions with ischemic heart disease and an ejection fraction of <30%. It examined the prophylactic benefit in coronary artery disease patients with a left ventricular ejection fraction of <30% who had at least one myocardial infarction, but required no further risk stratification. Invasive electrophysiological testing for risk stratification was not required. MADIT II applied a sequential design trial that compared ICD vs. no ICD therapy. Programmed electrical stimulation to test the inducibility of ventricular tachycardia was performed during ICD implantation, and various noninvasive risk markers were tested after randomization. The primary endpoint was total mortality, and secondary objectives were quality-of-life issues as well as the cost-effectiveness ratio. Over the course of 4 years, the MADIT II investigators enrolled 1232 patients with a prior myocardial infarction and a left ventricular ejection fraction of 0.30 or less. Patients were randomly assigned in a 3:2 ratio to receive an implantable defibrillator (742 patients) or conventional medical therapy (490 patients). The clinical characteristics at baseline and the prevalence of medication use at the time of the last follow-up visit were similar in the two treatment groups.

During an average follow-up of 20 months, the mortality rates were 19.8% in the conventional therapy group and 14.2% in the defibrillator group. The hazard ratio for the risk of death from any cause in the defibrillator group as compared with the conventional therapy group was

0.69 (95% CI, 0.51 to 0.93; $P = 0.016$). The effect of defibrillator therapy on survival was similar in subgroup analyses stratified according to age, sex, ejection fraction, New York Heart Association class, and the QRS interval. The investigators concluded that in patients with a prior myocardial infarction and advanced left ventricular dysfunction, prophylactic implantation of a defibrillator improves survival (Moss *et al.*, 2002).

On the other hand, there was no evidence of improved survival among patients with coronary heart disease, a depressed left ventricular ejection fraction, and an abnormal signal-averaged electrocardiogram, in whom a defibrillator was implanted prophylactically at the time of elective coronary bypass surgery (Bigger, 1997). The Defibrillator in Acute Myocardial Infarction Trial (DINAMIT) randomized 674 patients who had recently suffered a myocardial infarction (6 to 40 days after myocardial infarction), had a left ventricular ejection fraction of $\leq$35%, and had impaired cardiac autonomic function (decreased heart rate variability or elevated average heart rate as determined by 24-h ambulatory monitoring) to receive either ICD implantation or no ICD therapy. A percutaneous coronary intervention on the infarct-related artery was performed in only 36% of study patients. During a follow-up period of $30 \pm 13$ months, there was no significant difference in overall mortality between the two treatment groups. However, annual mortality rates were low in both groups: 7.5% for ICD-treated patients and 6.9% for control patients. These results suggested that the prophylactic use of ICD placement within the first month after acute myocardial infarction remains of unproven benefit (Hohnloser *et al.*, 2004).

Despite a steady decline in the risk of death from pump failure, many patients remain at high risk for sudden cardiac death. The incidence of sudden cardiac death in the US alone has been estimated at 184 000 to over 400 000 cases anually. During the past decade, substantial advances have been made in the use of device-based therapy for this population. The role of the implantable cardioverter-defibrillator (ICD) in routine heart failure management continues to evolve (Cesario and Dec, 2006). Implantable cardioverter-defibrillator therapy should not be used for patients with advanced heart failure symptoms (NYHA functional class IV) that remain refractory to optimal medical therapy for whom cardiac transplantation is not an option. However, some of these patients may still be considered for cardiac resynchronization therapy with ICD backup capability. Sweeney *et al.* have shown little improvement in survival after ICD implantation for these patients, most of whom died of progressive pump failure (Sweeney *et al.*, 1995). Furthermore, ICD treatment is contraindicated in the presence of medically intractable ventricular tachycardia or ventricular fibrillation. Implantable cardioverter-defibrillator therapy remains unproven for patients with substantially impaired systolic function and coronary artery disease, who lack evidence of sustained or nonsustained ventricular tachycardia and are scheduled to undergo coronary revascularization.

## Coronary Artery Bypass Surgery

***Randomized Clinical Trials.***   High-risk revascularization may constitute the treatment of choice in the subgroup of advanced heart failure patients with ischemic cardiomyopathy, an ejection fraction of <35%, viable myocardium, and vessels suitable for grafting. To address this issue, the NIH-sponsored Surgical Treatment for Ischemic Heart Failure (STICH) trial with 2800 patients aims to answer two key questions of therapeutic strategy in the management of patients with symptomatic heart failure, left ventricular dysfunction, and coronary artery disease amenable to CABG: (1) Does surgical coronary revascularization in addition to aggressive medical HF management confer long-term mortality, morbidity, quality of life, or cost benefits beyond aggressive medical management alone? (2) Does surgical ventricular shape restoration in combination with CABG improve the outcome compared to coronary revascularization alone or medical therapy alone (Joyce *et al.*, 2003)?

***Non-RCT Evidence.***   To assess the effect of CABG on future risk of death in patients with LV dysfunction and heart failure, mortality and modes of death in 5410 patients with ischemic LV dysfunction who were enrolled in the Studies Of Left Ventricular Dysfunction (SOLVD) trials were retrospectively evaluated. Outcomes of patients with ($n = 1870$; 35%) vs. without ($n = 3540$) a history of prior CABG were compared, and stratification by baseline ejection fraction values (<0.25, 0.25–0.30, and >0.30) was performed. Prior CABG was associated with a 25% reduction in risk of death and a 46% reduction in risk of sudden death independent of EF and severity of heart failure symptoms. It was concluded that in patients with ischemic LV dysfunction, prior CABG is associated with a significant independent reduction in mortality (Veenhuyzen *et al.*, 2001). Different trials have suggested the benefit of revascularization in advanced heart failure if angina (Winkel and Piccione, 1997) or hibernation (Di Carli *et al.*, 1995; Hausmann *et al.*, 1997; Elefteriades *et al.*, 1993; Olson *et al.*, 1993; Mickleborough *et al.*, 1995) is present. If no viable myocardium is present, the prospect of improvement with revascularization is reduced; thus, cardiac transplantation should be considered for appropriate candidates (Dreyfus *et al.*, 1993; Kron *et al.*, 1989; Lansman *et al.*, 1993; Tjan *et al.*, 2000).

## Mitral Valve Surgery

***Non-RCT Evidence.***   Severe mitral regurgitation is a frequent complication of end-stage cardiomyopathy that contributes to heart failure and predicts poor survival. The group at the University of Michigan, Ann Arbor, studied the intermediate-term outcome of mitral reconstruction in 48 patients who had cardiomyopathy with severe mitral regurgitation (63 ± 6 years, EF 16% ± 3%, maximal drug therapy, New York Heart Association class III–IV, refractory 4+ mitral regurgitation). All 48 had undersized flexible annuloplasty rings inserted, 7 had coronary bypass grafts for incidental disease, 11 had prior bypass grafts, and 11 also had tricuspid valve repair. One operative death occurred as a result of right ventricular failure. Postoperative transesophageal echocardiography revealed mild mitral regurgitation in 7 patients and no mitral regurgitation in 41. There were 10 late deaths, 2 to 47 months after mitral valve reconstruction. The 1- and 2-year actuarial survival rates were 82% and 71%. At a mean follow-up of 22 months, the number of hospitalizations for heart failure had decreased, and one patient had heart transplantation. Significantly, the New York Heart Association class improved from 3.9 ± 0.3 before the operation to 2.0 ± 0.6 after the operation. Twenty-four months after the operation, left ventricular volume and sphericity decreased, whereas ejection fraction and cardiac output repeatedly increased (Bolling *et al.*, 1998).

# Left Ventricular Geometry Restoration

***Non-RCT Evidence.*** To evaluate the safety and efficacy of surgical anterior ventricular endocardial restoration (SAVER), which excludes non-contracting segments in the dilated remodeled ventricle after anterior myocardial infarction, an international group of cardiologists and surgeons from 11 centers investigated the role of SAVER in patients after anterior myocardial infarction. From January 1998 to July 1999, a total of 439 patients underwent the procedure and were followed for 18 months. Early outcomes of the procedure and risk factors were investigated. Concomitant procedures included coronary artery bypass grafting in 89% of patients, mitral valve repair in 22%, and MV replacement in 4%. The hospital mortality rate was 6.6%, and few patients required mechanical support devices such as intra-aortic balloon counterpulsation (7.7%), left ventricular assist device (0.5%), or extracorporeal membrane oxygenation (1.3%). Postoperatively, the ejection fraction increased from 29% $\pm$ 10.4% to 39% $\pm$ 12.4%, and the left ventricular end-systolic volume index decreased from 109 $\pm$ 71 mL/m$^2$ to 69 $\pm$ 42 mL/m$^2$ ($p < 0.005$). At 18 months, the survival rate was 89.2%. Time-related survival at 18 months was 84% in the overall group and 88% among the 421 patients who had coronary artery bypass grafting or MV repair (Athanasuleas *et al.*, 2001; Athanasuleas *et al.*, 2004).

The echocardiographic changes and functional outcome from mitral valve repair, combined with partial left ventriculectomy (the Batista procedure), were investigated by the Cleveland Clinic. From May 1996 to August 1997, the operation was performed on 57 patients, primarily (95%) transplant candidates with idiopathic dilated cardiomyopathy. All were NYHA class IV (36.8% had improved to class III by the time of surgery) on medical therapy, including 40% hospitalized on inotropes and three patients on intra-aortic balloon pumps. The mean cardiac index was 2.1 $\pm$ 0.6 L/min/m$^2$ with a wedge pressure of 24 $\pm$ 8 mm Hg. There were two in-hospital mortalities (3.5%). At 3 months, there were significant persistent changes in LV end-diastolic diameter (8.1 $\pm$ 1.0 cm to 6.3 $\pm$ 0.9 cm) and ejection fraction (13.6% $\pm$ 6% to 23% $\pm$ 7.7%). Subjective improvement included a mean change in NYHA functional class from 3.7 to 2.2, and objective changes included improvement in peak oxygen consumption from

10.6 ± 4 mL/kg/min to 15.4 ± 4.5 mL/kg/min. The actuarial survival rate at 1 year was 82.1%; and freedom from death, relisting for transplantation, and need for LVAD support were 58% (McCarthy *et al.*, 2000).

Most recently, the Reconstructive Endoventricular Surgery, Returning Torsion Original Radius Elliptical Shape to the Left Ventricle (RESTORE) study group tested how surgical ventricular restoration affects early and late survival in a registry of 1198 postanterior infarction congestive heart failure patients treated by the international RESTORE team. They applied surgical ventricular restoration to 1198 postinfarction patients between 1998 and 2003. Early and late outcomes were examined, and risk factors were identified. Concomitant procedures included coronary artery bypass grafting in 95% of patients, mitral valve repair in 22%, and mitral valve replacement in 1%.

Overall 30-day mortality after SVR was 5.3% (8.7% with mitral repair vs. 4.0% without repair; $p < 0.001$). Perioperative mechanical support was uncommon ($<9\%$). Global systolic function improved postoperatively. Ejection fraction (EF) increased from 29.6% ± 11.0% preoperatively to 39.5% ± 12.3% postoperatively ($p < 0.001$). The left ventricular end-systolic volume index (LVESVI) decreased from 80.4 ± 51.4 mL/m$^2$ preoperatively to 56.6 ± 34.3 mL/m$^2$ postoperatively ($p < 0.001$). Overall 5-year survival was 68.6% ± 2.8%. Logistic regression analysis identified EF of ≤30%, LVESVI of ≥80 mL/m$^2$, advanced New York Heart Association (NYHA) functional class, and age of ≥75 years as risk factors for death. Five-year freedom from hospital readmission for CHF was 78%. Preoperatively, 67% of patients were NYHA functional class III or IV; and postoperatively, 85% were class I or II. Based on these results, the group concluded that surgical ventricular restoration improves ventricular function and is a highly effective therapy in the treatment of ischemic cardiomyopathy with an excellent 5-year outcome (Athanasuleas *et al.*, 2004).

## Cardiac Transplantation

***Non-RCT Evidence.***   In the context of contemporary medical and surgical therapy, there is growing recognition that the relative role of cardiac transplantation may need to be redefined (Stevenson *et al.*, 1991; Levine *et al.*, 1996; Kao *et al.*, 1994; Frigerio *et al.*, 1997; St. John Kolar, 2000).

Based on the assumption that its goal is to prolong life (Hunt *et al.*, 1976) while improving its quality (O'Brien *et al.*, 1987; Marzo *et al.*, 1992; Grady *et al.*, 1998) and in the absence of randomized clinical trial proof of its benefit, data from early studies, recent observational cohort studies (Hosenpud *et al.*, 1999; Hosenpud *et al.*, 2001), and more recent effective therapies in advanced heart failure have to be reassessed to characterize patients with those clinical profiles who may now be considered "too well" for cardiac transplantation (Hunt, 2000).

These profiles likely include patients with low risk according to the Heart Failure Survival Score (Aaronson and Mancini, 1999; Deng *et al*, 2000); peak $VO_2$ >14–18 mL/kg/min without other indications; left ventricular EF <20% alone, history of NYHA class III/IV symptoms alone; history of ventricular arrhythmias alone; patients with advanced heart failure in whom angiotensin-converting enzyme inhibitor, beta-blockade, or spironolactone therapy has not been attempted; and patients who have not been subjected to a structured cardiac transplantation evaluation in a designated cardiac transplantation center.

## Advanced Heart Failure Treatment Algorithm

*Defining Clinical Profiles of Patients Too Well for Transplantation.*
Referral to a designated cardiac transplantation center for evaluation usually takes place when the treating cardiologist/internist has exhausted all lifestyle and medical options without success, in the setting of decompensation and progression of advanced heart failure, a phase known to be associated with a high risk of death. A structured management algorithm (Fig. 2) needs to be applied in order to recompensate the patient, initiate neurohormonal blockade and lifestyle changes, or — if recompensation cannot be achieved — evaluate cardiac transplantation with the option of mechanical circulatory support device (MCSD) bridging. All patients who can be recompensated and who tolerate neurohormonal blockade should be considered too well for cardiac transplantation at that time. This definition is facilitated by an allocation algorithm based on medical urgency and not on waiting time, because the team does not need to make an extrapolation of the likely clinical course of the patient over the next 6–12 months. The

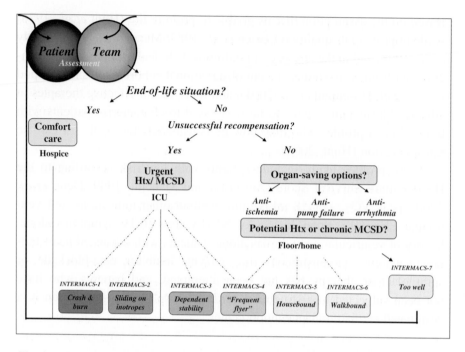

**Fig. 2.** The selection algorithm starts with the encounter between patient and team, and is followed by a stepwise evaluation of important issues including the following: (1) Is an end-of-life situation present? (2) Can the patient be recompensated? (3) After neuro-hormonal blockade initiation, are there organ-saving options including revascularization, contractility enhancement, and antiarrhythmia therapy? (4) Is the patient a suitable candidate for heart replacement options, including mechanical circulatory support and heart transplantation?

evaluation may serve to designate a patient as a "potential transplant candidate", who could be placed on a national "potential transplant candidate list". This algorithm combines the psychological benefit for the patient of being accepted by the program with ongoing access to a diversity of advanced heart failure treatment modalities, not committing to transplantation as the only therapeutic option (Deng *et al.*, 2002).

If the initial evaluation reveals hemodynamic instability (therefore, completing cardiac transplant evaluation and listing), follow-up may still lead to stabilization without transplantation, thus enabling delisting in individual cases. If at initial evaluation, refractory hemodynamic instability is accompanied by advanced multiorgan dysfunction, then comfort care has to be considered. The initial assessment is not a complete cardiac transplantation evaluation, but rather an approach to address the following main questions: How severe is the heart failure condition? Are there reversible causes? Are there risk factors limiting the overall prognosis?

The recompensation phase, either with or without right heart catheter monitoring, aims to acutely optimize volume status, contractility, afterload, heart rate, gas exchange, urine output, and potentially reversible precipitating factors. The neurohormonal blockade, initated after recompensation is accomplished, aims at downtitration of the maladaptive activation of the neurohormonal systems by administration of angiotensin-converting enzyme inhibitors, beta-blockers, and aldosterone antagonists.

In the COPERNICUS trial, a subgroup of more advanced heart failure patients was included, and classified as recent or recurrent cardiac decompensation or severely depressed cardiac function, characterized by the presence of pulmonary rales, ascites, or edema at randomization; three or more hospitalizations for heart failure within the previous year; the need for intravenous positive inotropic agents or an intravenous vasodilator drug within 14 days; or an ejection fraction of <15%. In patients who were likely to receive a cardiac transplant and had symptomatic hypotension or severe renal dysfunction, it was recommended that, rather than starting carvedilol during acute decompensation, measures should first be taken to stabilize their clinical condition (particularly with respect to their volume status) and then initiate adrenergic blockade. It was pointed out that expertise in the care of patients with advanced heart failure is important in this management process (Packer *et al.*, 1999).

The EFICAT trial examined the question of whether or not patients considered as transplantation candidates and thus excluded from participation in the COPERNICUS trial could be safely administered carvedilol. The primary endpoint was the absolute change from baseline to latest available LV ejection fraction measurement determined by radionuclide ventriculography between carvedilol and placebo. The trial prospectively randomized 118 patients with CHF of ischemic ($n = 44$) or nonischemic ($n = 74$) etiology, a mean age of $53.3 \pm 9.8$ years, and a mean LVEF at baseline of $19.9\% \pm 6.6\%$. The mean absolute change of LVEF from baseline was $6.0\% \pm 9.3\%$ in the carvedilol group vs. $0.7\% \pm 7.1\%$ in the placebo-treated patients ($p < 0.008$). Serious adverse events were experienced by

33/60 patients (13 deaths) on placebo and 29/58 patients (9 deaths) on carvedilol. It was concluded that carvedilol is an efficacious and safe drug in euvolemic patients considered for the cardiac transplantation waiting list (Angermann *et al.*, 2001).

***Structured Prognostication Algorithm in a Designated Transplant Center as Prerequisite.*** Beyond recompensation and neurohormonal blockade, prognostication is an integral part of the management algorithm (Fig. 2). Based on the groundbreaking work of Mancini and coworkers (Mancini *et al.*, 1991), the UCLA team assessed the role of peak oxygen uptake in the re-evaluation of candidates awaiting heart transplantation. All ambulatory transplant candidates with an initial peak oxygen uptake of <14 mL/kg per min were identified. Of 107 such patients listed, 68 survived without early deterioration or transplantation to undergo repeat exercise. In 38 of these 68 patients, peak oxygen uptake increased by ≥2 mL/kg per min to a level of ≥12 mL/kg per min after 6 ± 5 months, together with an increase in anaerobic threshold, peak oxygen pulse, and exercise heart rate reserve, and a decrease in heart rate at rest. Increased peak oxygen uptake was accompanied by stable clinical status without congestion in 31 of 38 patients, and these 31 were taken off the active waiting list. At 2 years, their actuarial survival rate was 100% and the survival rate without relisting for transplantation was 85%. The authors concluded that an algorithm with scheduled re-evaluation of exercise capacity and clinical status allows identification of patients who are "too well" during follow-up. They estimated that 29% of ambulatory transplant candidates can be removed from the waiting list with excellent early survival despite low peak oxygen uptake on initial testing, thus allowing to defer transplantation in favor of more compromised candidates (Stevenson *et al.*, 1995).

In order to refine risk stratification in ambulatory cardiac transplantation candidates and estimate their survival probability without transplantation (and thus the potential benefit from transplantation), the group at the University of Pennsylvania and Columbia University developed the first independently validated prognostication tool, entailing a high-risk, medium-risk, and low-risk stratum. Event-free (death or urgent transplantation) survival rates at 1 year for the low-, medium-, and high-risk HFSS strata were 93%±2%, 72%±5%, and 43%±7%, respectively. Event-free survival rates for the medium- and high-risk strata were much worse than expected after cardiac transplantation; the low-risk stratum had an event-free survival rate that was better than with transplantation. Based on this excellent prognostication tool, patients with HFSS low risk would be considered too well for cardiac transplantation (Aaronson *et al.*, 1997). Risk stratification of hospital-bound cardiac transplantation candidates who are inotrope- or left ventricular assist device-dependent can be improved by the inclusion of further parameters (Smits *et al.*, 2003b).

***Clinical Profiles of Patients Too Well for Transplantation.*** In summary, according to the available evidence summarized above, patients with the following clinical profiles should be considered too well for cardiac transplantation (Deng *et al.*, 2002):

- patients with low-risk HFSS;
- patients with a peak $VO_2$ >14–18 mL/kg/min without other indications;
- patients with a left ventricular EF <20% alone;
- patients with a history of NYHA class III/IV symptoms alone;
- patients with a history of ventricular arrhythmias alone;
- patients with advanced heart failure (class IV symptoms, ejection fraction <25%) in whom angiotensin-converting enzyme inhibitor, beta-blockade, or spironolactone therapy has not been attempted; and
- patients who have not been subjected to a structured cardiac transplantation evaluation in a designated cardiac transplantation center.

***Implications for Listing and Allocation Rules.*** To formalize the staged approach towards cardiac transplantation listing, a national potential transplant candidate list based on a systematic screening process in a designated transplant center should be considered. This would facilitate placement on the (urgency-driven) waiting list should deterioration subsequently occur. The potential transplant candidate list would emphasize to the patient the temporary nature of the evaluation process, which is often not adequately appreciated in current transplant practice.

In response to a debate on the fairness of the organ allocation system in the US, the US Department of Health and Human Services published a regulation termed the "Organ Procurement and Transplantation Network:

Final Rule" (Federal Register, 1998) to assure that the allocation of scarce organs will be based on common medical criteria, not accidents of geography. The stated principles favor the establishment of more effective federal oversight, increase of public access to information, implementation of consistent medical listing criteria, emphasis on medical need, and reduction of geographic disparities in waiting times. In line with these data, allocation systems are moving towards a system that favors medical urgency over waiting time (Gibbons *et al.*, 2000). Within this framework, patients who are in a less urgent medical condition with respect to their heart failure severity should be considered too well for cardiac transplantation.

# DEFINITION OF MECHANICAL CIRCULATORY SUPPORT

## General Definition

Mechanical circulatory support devices (MCSDs) are defined as mechanical pumps assisting or replacing the left, right, or both ventricles of the heart to pump blood. While the term left ventricular assist device (LVAD) or left ventricular assist system (LVAS) indicates left ventricular support, the broader term MCSD has been adopted to include left ventricular, right ventricular, and biventricular devices, the latter including biventricular assist devices as well as complete heart replacement devices.

## Specific Forms

Over the last two decades, mechanical circulatory support devices (MCSDs) have been developed at a rapid pace with the goal of supporting patients with advanced heart failure as a bridge to cardiac transplantation (BTT), a bridge to recovery (BTR), and an alternative to transplantation (ATT). Their clinical impact is rapidly increasing after the publication of the first randomized trial demonstrating their positive impact on survival and quality of life (Rose *et al.*, 2001). The current generation of devices provides a differentiated spectrum of circulatory support, ranging from short to intermediate and long-term duration. Also, partial left ventricular support, more complete left ventricular support, right ventricular support, and biventricular support options can be tailored to the hemodynamic needs

of the patient. On a technical level, the device positions range from paracorporeal pumps (intracorporeal pumps with transcutaneous drivelines) to
completely implantable systems.

# EVOLUTION OF MECHANICAL CIRCULATORY SUPPORT

**Ted L
(born 1943)**

**The heart
pump**

**The Heart Pump**

On April 1, 2004, I was rushed to Columbia Presbyterian
Hospital and almost checked out before I checked in. I was
one very sick fellow. Dr Donna Mancini, the head of the
heart transplant unit, and Dr Yoshifumi Naka, one of the
specialists in heart surgery, told my wife that I was too sick
for a transplant and that the only course of action was to
implant a heart assist device in my chest: an LVAD (left
ventricular assist device). It would take over for my heart's
main pumping chamber, the left ventricle. Dr Naka did this
on April 13, 2004.

The LVAD was implanted in my chest and was very
obvious to anyone within 15 feet of me. First, it was physically intimidating. It was just under the skin of my chest
and weighed 5 pounds. It was 5 inches in diameter, 2 inches
thick, and had an external tube coming out of my chest for
the electrical wires to the motor and as an exhaust for the
pump. Most notable was the sound and feel of the pump.
With each heartbeat, it went "wish, wish, wish". Besides
hearing the exhaust, I could hear and feel the pump with
each beat of my heart. What fantastic state-of-the-art equipment! Each day, the nurses meticulously cleansed the opening and put new bandages over the wound to make sure that
I did not get infected. I became amazed at just how hard
the heart works every moment of every day.

Once I recovered and had completed my physical therapy, the doctors discharged me on May 26, 2004 — 56
days after arriving. Over the next 14 months, with the help
of the heart pump, I recovered all my bodily functions and
went on to get myself in the best physical shape I had
been in for a decade or so. I worked out 3 days a week

at the Cornell Cardiac Fitness Center on stationary bicycles, treadmills, and rowing machines. I kept this up until the day I got my call for a new heart. I basically got myself into better shape than I had been in the previous 10–15 years through exercise, carefully sticking to the prescribed diet, and keeping myself mentally and physically active.

Before leaving the hospital, both my wife and I were trained in the use of the LVAD. Trina became an expert in cleansing and changing my bandages, and she followed my exercises and dietary activities each day. I began calling my wife Dr L. When I first came home and was just recuperating around the apartment, the set of batteries would run the pump for about 7 $1/2$ hours, but as I became more active this dropped to about 5 hours. When I was going to bed at night, I used a 25-foot extension cord from my power unit that limited my movements to the bed, the chair, and the bathroom. The power unit charged my four sets of batteries each night while I slept.

It is quite an experience to carry an implanted 5-pound pump, two external batteries weighing 10 pounds, and a computer regulating the pump and sending messages about the state of its operation. I also had to carry with me a beeper for instant communications with the hospital and a cell phone to call anyone.

Since the pump continually needed new batteries and could possibly malfunction, I carried an extra set of batteries, an extra computer, and a hand pump. The LVAD, if necessary, could be operated with a hand pump should something happen to the electrical system; however, that would be the ultimate emergency.

The biggest concern was that the batteries would run out of juice before I could get home and get to my backup batteries. Most people leave home each morning with the idea that if plans change, they will adapt. But if I was stuck somewhere and was unable to get home to replace and recharge my batteries, I would be in severe trouble, having to rely on the hand pump.

Learning how to take a shower properly became a challenge. No water could ever get into the exhaust tube, or the electrical motor could short-circuit and stop. Not good, as they say. After cutting up plastic shower curtains and using tape, my wife and I realized that it wouldn't work. The tape always came loose. After much trial and error, I settled on large sheets of tegaderm bandages — totally adhesive-backed and water-repellent. Before you knew it, I was enjoying 20-minute showers without any concern.

I will never forget the first time my wife and I went to the opera. We found our places, the lights went dim, and all noises stopped, with one exception: my heart pump kept going "wish, wish, wish". People to the left, right, behind, and in front of us began to wonder what that irritating noise was. One fellow turned around and said, "Would you turn off whatever it is that's making the noise?"

In the summer of 2004, there were bomb scares by terrorists at several buildings in New York City. One was my favorite haunt, the Citicorp Center building, because the Barnes & Noble bookstore was located there — my home away from home while I was on the LVAD. Two policemen were stationed at every door, and you should have seen their reaction to my equipment. Carrying two black boxes in a shoulder holster and a black box on my belt got their attention. Eventually, they came to know me and asked how I was coming along. They became quite interested in the heart pump, as they had never heard of such a thing.

The highlight of my life on the LVAD came at a charitable dance at Mt. Sinai Hospital. My wife's firm had taken a table and we were invited to attend. I told Trina that I would try to get out on the dance floor, but was not sure how long I would last. We started with a waltz, but before you knew it the band was doing more upbeat rhythms. We began jitterbugging and I was able to keep up. Meanwhile, back at the table, my wife's associates began asking themselves, "Tell me again, who is it that is waiting for a heart transplant?"

> Many people have asked me how I withstood the waiting, never knowing when the call would come. My answer to that was this: I set a schedule each day and stuck to it, just as if I were in college and had classes to attend. I filled each day reading books, studying about medications and transplantation, took courses on geopolitics, went to New York University School of Continuing and Professional Studies for a certificate in foundation management, volunteered at the New York Organ Donor Network, and made sure to meet and talk to friends about my heart pump.

## Early History

Early descriptions of mechanical support of the human circulation are documented at least back to the early 19th century. The experimental application of mechanical support in animal models was reported in the 1930s. Major interest in mechanical support of the human circulation would await the advent of open heart surgery in the 1950s (Kirklin, 2006). The basic pump design has changed little over this development period, but the power delivery and control have moved from large bedside consoles to wearable components, enabling patient autonomy in an outpatient setting (Schmid *et al.*, 1999). This has brought about substantial improvements in patients' quality of life (Dew *et al.*, 1999) and reductions in resource use (Gelijns *et al.*, 1997).

Smaller, inexpensive, and less obtrusive blood pumps are undergoing development, and some are being tested in clinical trials (Katsumata and Westaby, 1998; Wieselthaler *et al.*, 2000; Goldstein *et al.*, 2005). However, while the potential benefits are encouraging, these designs still have to prove their durability, reliability, and physiological suitability for chronic applications (DeBakey, 2005). An excellent monograph with overviews of the current MCSD-device types was recently published by the International Society of Heart and Lung Transplantation (Frazier and Kirklin, 2006). Other excellent monographs on MCSDs have been published over the last decade (Goldstein and Oz, 2000; Rose and Stevenson, 1998).

## Recent Regulatory Approval Processes in the US

Following the initiative by the US National Heart, Lung, and Blood Institute in the 1970s to develop long-term artificial heart devices (Hogness and VanAntwerp, 1991), two electrically powered pumps emerged from this initiative and completed trials sponsored by the Food and Drug Administration for evaluating safety and efficacy. In 1998, they received certification for commercial application: the Heart-Mate® VE (ThermoCardio Systems, Woburn, MA) (Poirier, 1999) and the Novacor® N100 PC (World Heart Corporation, Oakland, CA) (Portner *et al.*, 1989; Robbins and Oyer, 1999). In September 2006, the ABIOCOR total artificial heart (Abiomed, Inc., Danvers, MA) received Humanitarian Device Exemption (HDE) from the FDA.

## INDIVIDUAL MECHANICAL CIRCULATORY SUPPORT DEVICES (see Appendix 2 for contacts)

| | |
|---|---|
| **Eric G (born 1950)** **Description of HeartMate I device** | It sounds simple and I suppose it is. Then, there's the reality: the realization that for my immediate (and possibly longer-term) future, I have a leash. In my chest is a titanium drum about 4 inches in diameter and about 2 inches thick. It's attached via tubing to my heart and my aorta. Then, there's that tube sticking up out of my belly that connects to an air vent and the controller unit, which in turn connects to the power for this device. During the day, I have batteries that have to be charged and ready 24/7. Even to walk down the block to see my neighbors, I need a hand pump just in case the batteries die, a cable breaks, or a controller fails; if I don't manually pump the device in these scary scenarios, I will die. The controller is the brain behind the pump's ability to keep me alive. It is directly and securely attached to the tube that is sticking out of my belly. It is always with me. On the positive side, it isn't terribly large (perhaps $4.5'' \times 5'' \times 1''$) and it weighs practically nothing. The controller requires two power connections. |

In order to maximize living with an LVAD, the developers gave the unit two ways to be powered. During the day, the unit uses two rechargable batteries. Remove one or the other without replacing it quickly, and an alarm will sound: the system will admonish you. There are two power sources, even though one might be strong enough; there's no "safety" with just one power source. The first time you hear the alarm, you will panic, although you know what it means (change the battery a little faster). Really, is it just the battery or have I accidentally ended my life? Just the battery, whew.

At night, my leash is electric. A power base unit (PBU) is plugged into the wall. It has two cords that plug into the two cords on my controller. By changing one battery to AC and then the second battery to the AC, a continuity of power is maintained and no alarms sound. I have a range of about 20 feet at my disposal. Luckily, we worked out how to include both the bed and the bath inside that length.

But wait, there is no battery! What if the power fails tonight? Storms can happen at any time, a tree could fall and snap the power lines; through no fault of my own, I would be dead. However, the base unit has a safety battery built in. If the unit stops improperly, alarms sound and an internal battery that isn't obvious from the outside takes over, thus giving me precious minutes to reattach batteries. The rechargable batteries last only 4–6 hours; even with several sets, the batteries last for just 20—24 hours. Therefore, as another safety measure, there's a massive battery pack (almost the weight of a car battery) that is good for 24 hours.

Characteristics of currently available MCSDs are summarized in Table 1.

## Thoratec

*Company History.* Thoratec® Corporation (www.thoratec.com) was founded in California in March 1976. The company currently markets the

**Table 1.** Characteristics of currently available MCSDs.

| Type | Ventricle | Flow | Pump position | Implant # |
|---|---|---|---|---|
| AbioCor | Total heart | Pulsatile | Intrathoracic | >10 |
| Abiomed BVS 5000 | Left & right | Pulsatile | Paracorporeal | >3000 |
| Abiomed AB 5000 | Left & right | Pulsatile | Intracorporeal | >30 |
| BerlinHeart INCOR | Left | Nonpulsatile | Intra-abdominal | >250 |
| BerlinHeart EXCOR | Left & right | Pulsatile | Paracorporeal | >30 |
| CardioWest | Total heart | Pulsatile | Intrathoracic | >200 |
| CorAide (Arrow) | Left | Nonpulsatile | Intra-abdominal | >2 |
| DuraHeart (Terumo) | Left | Nonpulsatile | Intra-abdominal | Preclinical |
| EVAHEART | Left | Nonpulsatile | Intra-abdominal | Preclinical |
| HeartWare | Left | Nonpulsatile | Intra-abdominal | 1 |
| Jarvik 2000 | Left | Nonpulsatile | Intra-abdominal | >100 |
| LionHeart | Left | Pulsatile | Intra-addominal | >25 |
| MEDOS | Left & right | Pulsatile | Paracorporeal | >200 |
| MicroMed DeBakey | Left | Nonpulsatile | Intra-abdominal | >380 |
| Thoratec HeartMate I | Left | Pulsatile | Intra-abdominal | >4100 |
| Thoratec HeartMate II | Left | Nonpulsatile | Intra-abdominal | >50 |
| Thoratec HeartMate III | Left | Nonpulsatile | Intra-abdominal | Preclinical |
| Thoratec TLC-II | Left & right | Pulsatile | Paracorporeal | >2800 |
| Thoratec IVAD | Left & right | Pulsatile | Intra-abdominal | >30 |
| VentrAssist | Left | Nonpulsatile | Intra-abdominal | >60 |
| WorldHeart Novacor | Left | Pulsatile | Intra-abdominal | >1700 |
| WorldHeart Novacor II | Left | Pulsatile | Intra-abdominal | Preclinical |
| WorldHeart Novacor Rotary | Left | Nonpulsatile | Intra-abdominal | >1 |

Thoratec® MCSD and the HeartMate® MCSD in the United States and internationally for use as a bridge to heart transplant. Additionally, the Thoratec MCSD System is marketed for use in the recovery of the heart after open heart surgery, and the HeartMate MCSD is marketed internationally as an alternative to medical therapy. On February 14, 2001, Thoratec completed a merger with Thermo Cardiosystems Inc., originally founded in Massachusetts in 1988.

***Thoratec MCSD.*** The Thoratec® VAD System — now also called the paracorporeal VAD System — is currently (i.e. as of 2006) the only device approved by the US Food and Drug Administration (FDA) that can provide left, right, or biventricular support for both bridge to heart transplant and recovery of the heart after open heart surgery. Thoratec is also pursuing additional indications for the Thoratec MCSD System, and is developing other circulatory support products for patients suffering from heart failure.

As of July 2006, the Thoratec MCSD System has been used in more than 2800 patients worldwide, ranging in age from 6 to 77 years and in weight from 37 to 317 pounds (17 to 144 kg) (Fig. 3).

***Thoratec IVAD.*** The Thoratec IVAD (implantable ventricular assist device) is now FDA-approved for use in bridge-to-transplantation and postcardiotomy-recovery patients who are unable to be weaned from cardiopulmonary bypass. The IVAD is the only currently approved implantable cardiac assist device that can provide left, right, or biventricular support. It has been approved for use in Europe for over a year. The IVAD's size facilitates BiVAD implants and enables it to accommodate patients, including those who were previously unable to receive an implantable, pulsatile device. The IVAD is based on the Thoratec® VAD System, which has been implanted in over 2800 patients worldwide.

In developing the IVAD, Thoratec obtained extensive surgeon input to deliver an implantable VAD and surgical accessories designed to facilitate implantation ease. With the use of the IVAD "sizer", the IVAD pump pocket is created. The reusable "sizer" can be used not only to help determine the proper pocket size and position for the IVAD, but also to assist in selecting the appropriately sized cannulae for the patient. Flared cannula ends and an adapted valve housing design allow IVAD cannulae to slide onto the IVAD pump. The collet system reduces the possibility of using

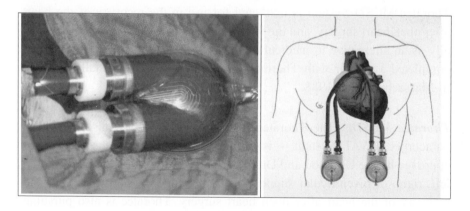

**Fig. 3.** The Thoratec MCSD System.

incompatible components together. The IVAD Cannula Connector Wrench facilitates the securing of the cannula connectors onto the pump. Percutaneous line tunneling is facilitated with the IVAD Percutaneous Line Tunneler. The tunneler is used for creating the subcutaneous tunneling path and for passing the pump's percutaneous line through the abdomen and out the exit site. In order to accommodate a wide range of patient sizes, two percutaneous line tunnelers of different lengths and curvatures are available.

As of September 2003, a total of 30 patients with advanced heart failure have been supported with the Thoratec IVAD for bridge-to-transplantation or postcardiotomy ventricular failure in Europe and the United States. Sixty-eight percent were successfully treated through transplantation or ventricular recovery, with many of these patients discharged to their homes through the use of the TLC-II® Portable VAD Driver. The initial IVAD results indicate that the device can successfully treat a wide array of patients with a low incidence of many serious, adverse events that are commonly associated with VAD use, such as embolic stroke and systemic infection (Fig. 4).

*HeartMate I MCSD.* The HeartMate I MCSD is an implantable heart assist device that is designed to perform substantially all or part of the pumping function of the left ventricle of the natural heart for patients suffering from cardiovascular disease. Two systems have been commercialized

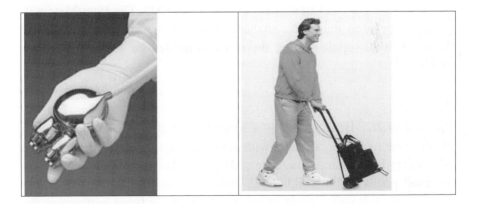

**Fig. 4.** The Thoratec IVAD.

for patients requiring cardiac support: an implantable pneumatic MCSD (HeartMate® IP) that is powered by an external electrically driven air pump, and an electric MCSD (HeartMate® VE) that is driven by an implanted electric motor and powered by a lightweight battery pack worn by the patient.

In 1994, the FDA granted approval for the commercial sale of the Heart-Mate IP for use as a bridge to transplant. The HeartMate VE was granted the same approval by the FDA in September 1998. With these approvals, both systems became available for sale to cardiac centers throughout the United States. In August 1998, the HeartMate IP received Canadian approval, permitting the sale of both the air-driven and electric versions throughout Canada. The HeartMate IP received the European Conformity Mark in April 1994, and the HeartMate VE received the same marking in August 1995. In late 1995, the FDA approved the protocol for conducting clinical trials of the HeartMate VE MCSD as an alternative to medical therapy in the REMATCH trial; and in May 1998, the first patient was implanted with it as part of this trial. The HeartMate VE MCSD is being used in Europe as both a bridge to transplant and as an alternative to medical therapy.

As of July 2006, over 4100 patients worldwide have been supported with the HeartMate MCSD. The use of the HeartMate as a destination therapy was approved by the FDA in November 2002. The overall costs for use of the HeartMate as a destination therapy are estimated to be similar to the costs for a heart transplant, or about $160 000. The HeartMate will probably be used much like dialysis treatment to support patients with kidney failure, supplementing the heart as needed on a long-term basis (Fig. 5).

*HeartMate II.*   HeartMate II is a second-generation MCSD that features a miniature rotary blood pump with axial bearings. Because of their small size, rotary blood pumps may potentially be used to provide cardiac support in small adults and in children. In 2000, the clinical trial for HeartMate II was initiated, with a team of cardiac surgeons in Israel performing the first human implant. Clinical trials are underway in Europe and the US (Fig. 6).

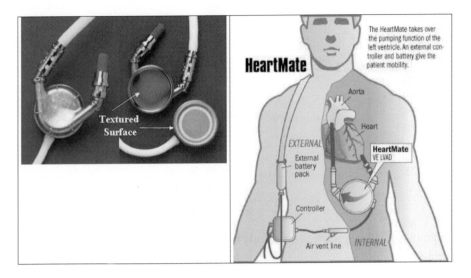

**Fig. 5.** The HeartMate I MCSD.

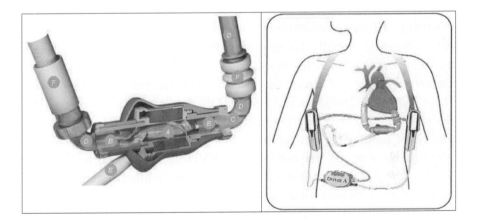

**Fig. 6.** The HeartMate II MCSD.

***HeartMate III.*** Thoratec is developing another advanced HeartMate system, HeartMate® III, designed to meet the needs of a wider range of patients, offer extended durability and longevity, and further improve patients' quality of life. HeartMate III is a third-generation heart assist system featuring a miniature centrifugal pump and state-of-the-art magnetic

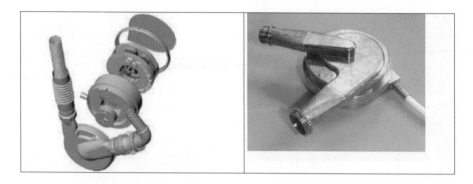

**Fig. 7.** The HeartMate III MCSD.

technology. This system is currently being evaluated in an ongoing animal trial (Fig. 7).

## WorldHeart

***Company History.*** WorldHeart (www.worldheart.com) is a medical device business initially based on the HeartSaver® MCSD and related technologies developed by the Cardiovascular Devices Division of the University of Ottawa Heart Institute. In 1989, the University of Ottawa Heart Institute's Cardiovascular Devices Division (CVD) began conducting research into and developing a fully implantable ventricular assist device capable of prolonging life and maintaining an acceptable quality of life at a reasonable cost. By the end of 1996, CVD had developed its artificial heart — the EMCSD — and had proven that this unified system resolved each of these technical barriers.

In May 1996, WorldHeart acquired exclusive worldwide rights to the EMCSD and related technologies developed by CVD, with the EMCSD providing the basis for WorldHeart's HeartSaver. On June 30, 2000, World-Heart completed the acquisition of Novacor®, the Oakland, CA, ventricular assist device operation previously owned by Edwards Lifesciences Inc. of Irvine, CA. This acquisition brought together the manufacturing and clinical experience of Novacor in the current generation of pulsatile ventricular assist devices with the next generation of fully implantable pulsatile MCSDs, HeartSaver.

***HeartSaver MCSD.*** WorldHeart's initial product was a unique, patented heart assist device fully implantable in the chest alongside the natural heart to provide long-term support of pulsatile blood flow in people suffering from advanced heart failure. The HeartSaver is intended for long-term use; leaves no permanent openings in the skin or tissue; and can be remotely powered, monitored, and controlled using patented transcutaneous energy transfer and proprietary biotelemetry technologies. Recipients are expected to leave the hospital and resume relatively normal day-to-day activities. In 2005, however, World Heart Inc. discontinued the development of the HeartSaver.

***Novacor MCSD.*** The Novacor® MCSD was developed at Stanford University and used in the first successful MCSD bridge to transplant in 1984 (Portner *et al.*, 1989). The pump drive unit is implanted below the diaphragm, anterior to the posterior rectus sheath and connected in parallel to the natural circulation, taking blood from the left ventricle and returning it to the ascending aorta. Since this model (N100 PC) was released in Europe as a commercial product, clinicians in participating centers were not bound by the constraints of an investigational protocol and predefined implantation criteria; therefore, selection practices between different centers varied greatly, with a large percentage of patients moribund at the time of implantation.

In order to promote an evidence-based perspective in mechanically supported advanced heart failure patients, the Novacor European Registry was initiated in 1997 by clinicians (European Cardiology Advisory Board) active in the use of mechanical circulatory support (Deng *et al.*, 2001a). The Novacor has been in use for more than 15 years, and is considered the industry standard for durability and reliability. As of July 2006, more than 1700 implants have been done at over 90 centers worldwide, out of which 95 patients were supported for >1 year and 2 patients for >4 years. It was the first MCSD technology to be approved in Romania and pass the Drug & Food Council in Japan in June 2001. The Novacor is approved in Europe without restriction, and in the US and Canada for the BTT indication (Fig. 8).

***Novacor II MCSD.*** Evolving from the original Novacor technology, the Novacor II next-generation MCSD currently under development is a

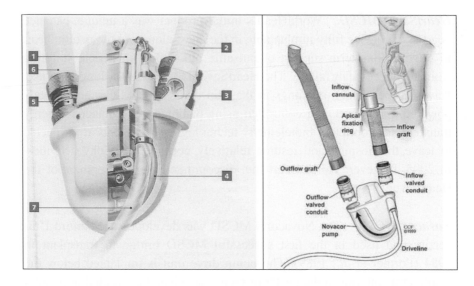

**Fig. 8.** The Novacor MCSD.

miniaturized, bearingless, pulsatile ventricular assist system. Half the size of the first-generation pulsatile system, it retains the physiology pumping mechanism while reducing complexity. It can be fully implantable without the need for a volume compensator. The Novacor II contains no wearing elements (Golding *et al.*, 2006) (Fig. 9).

***Novacor Rotary MCSD.***    The Novacor Rotary VAD is a next-generation rotary blood pump intended for destination therapy. With blood-lubricated bearings, the Novacor Rotary VAD is a compact, centrifugal pump with an impeller that is completely magnetically levitated (MagLev™). Full magnetic levitation eliminates wear mechanisms within the pump. It also permits greater clearances and more optimized blood flow around the impeller, while eliminating dependence on the patient's blood for suspension. The Novacor Rotary VAD's levitation technology employs a unique combination of passive and single-axis active control. The Novacor Rotary VAD is not currently available. The clinical feasibility trial began in March 2006.

Like the current Novacor® LVAS, the Novacor Rotary VAD is implanted within the abdomen. Blood enters the pump through an inflow

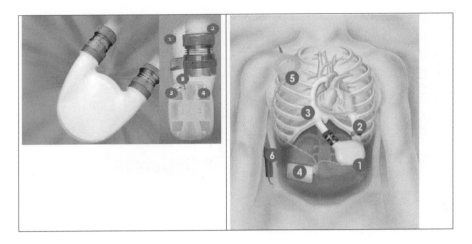

**Fig. 9.** The Novacor II MCSD.

conduit connected to the recipient's left ventricle. The pump then ejects blood through an outflow conduit into the arterial system, thereby supporting the systemic circulation. The physiological control system, currently under development, will allow the device to be self-regulating, automatically adjusting the rotor speed in response to the recipient's changing circulatory requirements. In the initial configuration shown, a percutaneous (through the skin) lead will connect the implanted pump to an external controller and rechargable power pack. This represents the simplest system with the fewest implanted components. Ultimately, the system could be made available in a fully implantable configuration, in which the controller and a standby battery pack are implanted. A transcutaneous (across the skin) energy transfer system (TETS) would conduct power from an external battery pack to the implanted system (Fig. 10).

## MicroMed

***Company History.*** MicroMed originated in 1984 (www.micromedtech.com). In 1984, Dr Michael DeBakey and Dr George Noon performed heart transplant surgery on NASA–Johnson Space Center engineer David Saucier, following a severe heart attack. Six months later, Saucier returned to work with the desire to apply spacecraft technology to help

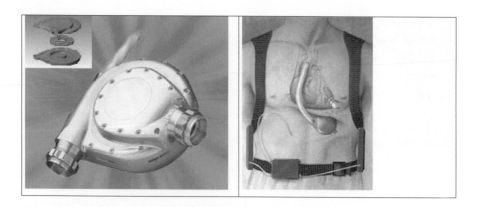

**Fig. 10.** The Novacor Rotary MCSD.

people with diseased hearts. In 1987, informal meetings were initiated to design a low-cost, low-power implantable ventricular assist device. NASA began formal funding of the development of the device 4 years later, bringing space technology to earth-bound applications.

***MicroMed DeBakey MCSD.*** The MicroMed DeBakey® MCSD is a miniaturized heart pump designed to provide increased blood flow (up to 10 L/min) from the left ventricle of the heart throughout the body for patients with end-stage heart failure. About 1/10 the size of competitive pulsatile MCSD products on the market and weighing less than 4 ounces, the MicroMed DeBakey MCSD® measures $1'' \times 3''$. This smaller size gives treatment hope to those with smaller body types, such as petite women and children, because larger devices cannot be implanted in them. The small size of the device and flexible percutaneous cable also enable lower infection rates. The MicroMed DeBakey MCSD® was projected to be 1/3 less expensive than currently marketed pulsatile MCSDs, making the process more affordable to a wider group of patients. The device's potential for decreased rates of hemolysis and thromboembolic complications improves its safety. The device only contains one moving part, the inducer/impeller. Third-party studies project that the mechanical durability will last in excess of 5 years. The MicroMed DeBakey MCSD® is virtually silent compared to other devices, improving patient comfort while on the device. Additionally, the portable controller and battery pack enables patient mobility to preserve quality of life.

In 1996, MicroMed received an exclusive license from NASA to use this rotary blood pump for cardiovascular applications. MicroMed then began the development of the critical support systems that would allow the device to be approved by regulatory agencies and to be utilized in life-saving applications in humans. European clinical trials of the MicroMed DeBakey MCSD began in November 1998, and CE Mark certification was awarded in May 2001. US clinical trials began in June 2000; and in April 2001, the FDA expanded the clinical trial parameters to 20 clinical sites and 178 patients. As of July 2006, over 380 patients at 14 heart centers in 7 countries have been implanted with the device (Fig. 11).

## Jarvik Heart

*Company History.* Jarvik Heart, Inc. (www.jarvikheart.com), and the Texas Heart Institute have been developing the Jarvik 2000 for more than 10 years.

*Jarvik 2000 MCSD.* The Jarvik 2000 continuous flow pump MCSD is a nonpulsatile device developed by Robert Jarvik, one of the pioneers in the development of heart assist technologies. The Jarvik device is much simpler and more compact than pulsatile devices, operating at 25 000 rpm. About the size of a C battery, the Jarvik® 2000 MCSD is a valveless,

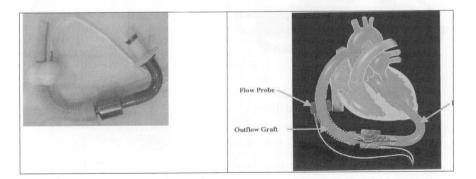

**Fig. 11.** The MicroMed DeBakey® MCSD.

electrically powered miniature axial flow pump that fits directly into the left ventricle and pushes oxygenated blood throughout the body.

The FDA has granted the Texas Heart Institute and St. Luke's Episcopal Hospital an initial Investigational Device Exemption for the implantation of the Jarvik 2000 as a bridge to transplant in a limited number of patients. While the Jarvik 2000 was initially developed for use as a bridge to transplant, Jarvik is in discussions with the FDA to determine the steps necessary to allow the device to be approved as a destination therapy. As of July 2006, over 100 patients have been implanted with this device (Fig. 12).

## Arrow LionHeart

*Company* History.    Arrow International, Inc. manufactures the Arrow LionHeart™ MCSD, the result of an 8-year collaboration between Arrow International (www.arrowintl.com) and the Department of Surgery's Section of Artificial Organs at Pennsylvania State University's Hershey Medical Center. Essential research in the area of sustained mechanical circulatory support that helped to define and develop the Arrow Lion-Heart™ MCSD has been ongoing at Pennsylvania State University for over 30 years.

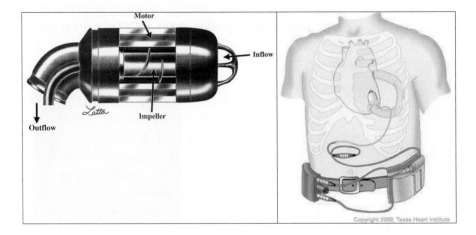

**Fig. 12.** The Jarvik MCSD.

***LionHeart MCSD.*** The Arrow LionHeart™ MCSD, manufactured by Arrow International, Inc., was designed to be used as a long-term option for patients with progressive, irreversible end-stage (NYHA class IV) congestive heart failure, for whom heart transplantation is not an option. The Arrow LionHeart™ MCSD was not intended as a bridge to transplant or as a bridge to recovery of ventricular function. The LionHeart™ is fully implantable. The MCSD devices that are currently available require percutaneous drivelines and external tethers to a power source. In the Arrow LionHeart™ MCSD, these lines and tethers are eliminated through the use of a transcutaneous energy transmission system. Power is supplied in the Arrow LionHeart™ MCSD through transcutaneous energy, which charges implanted batteries in patients and allows patients to be completely untethered for approximately 20 minutes. This represents a significant advance in mechanical circulatory assist technology. A fully automated control algorithm automatically responds to changes in the recipient's condition.

The Arrow LionHeart™ MCSD optimizes the amount of blood that can be pumped to meet the patient's needs. The modular design of the Arrow LionHeart™ MCSD allows for the exchange of discrete subsystems that require replacement or upgrading over time. The blood pump is electrically powered and is implanted in the preperitoneal space, beneath the left costal margin. The blood pump features a motor, a pusher plate mechanism, a smooth blood sac, and two tilting disk valves for unidirectional flow. The blood pump is connected to the native circulation via inlet and outlet cannulae. The motor controller and internal coil control the operation of the blood pump. The blood pump and electronic motor controller are powered by either external sources or rechargable batteries located in the motor controller. External power is received transcutaneously by the internal coil, and sent to the motor controller and blood pump for continuous operation. The internal coil is placed in the subcutaneous tissue of the chest wall.

The compliance chamber and access port serve as a variable gas volume accumulator. The compliance chamber provides gas to evacuated chambers of the blood pump during its operation. This compliance chamber is periodically replenished via the access port with room air. The compliance chamber is placed in the left pleural space. The access port is passed through the intercostal space and located in the subcutaneous tissue over the left anterior chest wall.

The first human implant of the Arrow LionHeart™ MCSD occurred on October 26, 1999, at the Heart and Diabetes Center in Bad Oeynhausen, Germany. In February 2001, Arrow received an Investigational Device Exemption from the FDA to begin a seven-patient, phase I human clinical trial in the United States for its Arrow LionHeart™ system. The lead investigator for this pilot study is Dr Walter Pae of Penn State's Hershey Medical Center. All seven patients have been enrolled in the initial phase of the study. In December 2001, the FDA approved the addition of seven more phase I implants of the LionHeart™ in the US These additional implants began in late January or February of 2002, following hospital approvals of amended patient section requirements and screening of potential patients, as part of an ongoing European clinical investigation sponsored by Arrow to demonstrate the safety and performance of the LionHeart™ MCSD for the purpose of obtaining a European Conformity Mark (CE), which was obtained in 2003. As per July 2006, a total of 26 patients have been implanted with the Arrow LionHeart™ MCSD (Fig. 13).

## CardioWest

*Company History.*   SynCardia Systems, Inc. (www.syncardia.com), is the manufacturer and distributor of the CardioWest temporary Total Artificial Heart (TAH-t). The CardioWest heart is a descendant of the Jarvik-7-70

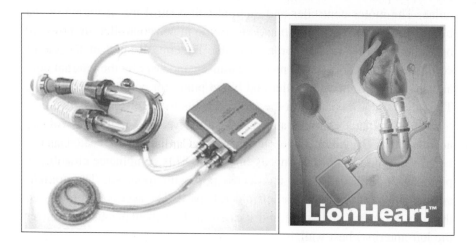

**Fig. 13.**  The LionHeart MCSD.

heart, which was developed at the University of Utah by Drs Jarvik, Kolff, Olsen, and others. In 1982, Barney Clark received the first artificial heart as a permanent replacement and survived on the device for 112 days. In 1985, at the University Medical Center, Tucson, AZ, heart surgeon Dr Jack G. Copeland and colleagues became the first in the world to use an artificial heart, the Jarvik-7-100, as a successful bridge to transplantation. The Jarvik 7-70, a smaller TAH, was designed to fit into smaller patients, and quickly became the preferred TAH because of its size and adequate cardiac output. A total of 175 patients were implanted with the Jarvik-7 and Jarvik-7-70 before the FDA withdrew the IDE from its sponsor, Symbion Corp., in January 1990.

In 1991, CardioWest, Inc (Tucson, AZ), was formed by Drs Don Olsen and Jack Copeland to continue the TAH technology and conduct a new FDA IDE trial of the TAH as a bridge-to-transplantation device. In 1998, CE approval was obtained for the CardioWest C-70 TAH-t. In order to commercialize the CardioWest TAH-t and complete the FDA IDE trial, SynCardia Systems, Inc., was formed in 2001 and acquired all assets of CardioWest, Inc., in 2002. In 2004, the CardioWest TAH-t received FDA approval as a bridge-to-transplantation device.

*CardioWest TAH-t.* The CardioWest TAH-t is a biventricular pulsatile pump that replaces the failing heart and serves as a bridge to transplantation. The CardioWest TAH-t has prosthetic ventricles made of polyurethane and four Medtronic-Hall mechanical valves. Blood and air are separated by a seamless, four-layer, polyurethane diaphragm, which is pushed down by blood during diastole and is displaced forward by compressed air during systole to propel blood out of the ventricles. The TAH-t can provide flows of up to 9.5 L/min or more; typically, it is operated with flows of 6–8 L/min. The Circulatory Support System (CSS) Console, along with the WCOMDU software program, operates the CardioWest TAH-t in the hospital while patients await transplantation. In Europe, SynCardia Systems, Inc., has CE approval to use the Berlin Heart EXCOR TAH-t Portable Driver on TAH-t patients who are stable in the hospital or who are discharged home while awaiting a donor heart. By the end of 2006, the CardioWest TAH-t had been implanted in 635 patients for a total duration of over 100 patient-years. The CardioWest TAH-t is the only FDA-approved artificial heart used as a temporary device for bridge to transplantation (Copeland *et al.*, 2004) (Fig. 14).

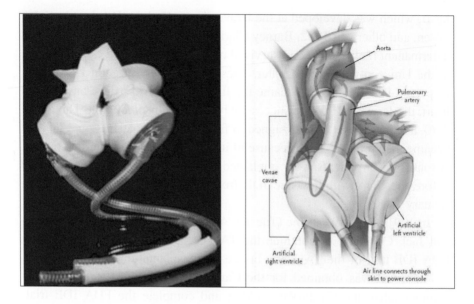

**Fig. 14.**  The CardioWest MCSD.

## Abiomed

***Company History.***   The cardiac assist and heart replacement products developed by Abiomed (www.abiomed.com) are designed to complement and/or simulate the heart's natural pumping action. Abiomed's first cardiovascular product, the BVS® 5000 Bi-ventricular Support System, is now the most widely used advanced cardiac assist system worldwide. The quest for an artificial heart started with the advent of successful heart surgery to remove shell fragments from soldiers during World War II.

***AbioMed BVS 5000.***   Abiomed's BVS® 5000 cardiac support system provides a patient's failing heart with full circulatory assistance while allowing the heart to rest, heal, and recover its function. The BVS 5000 has been approved in the FDA's rigorous PMA process as a bridge-to-recovery device for the treatment of all patients with potentially reversible heart failure. It is now the most widely used advanced cardiac assist system in the world. It is installed in 600 leading medical centers worldwide. The BVS 5000 is most frequently used in patients whose hearts

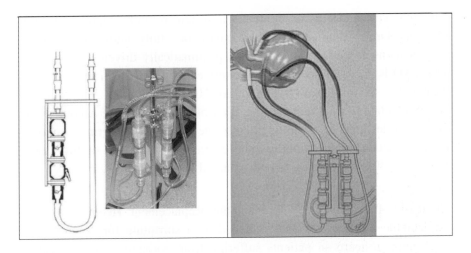

**Fig. 15a.** The Abiomed BVS 5000 MCSD.

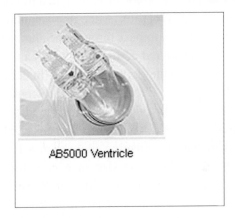

AB5000 Ventricle

**Fig. 15b.** The Abiomed AB 5000 MCSD.

do not immediately recover their function following heart surgery. As of July 2006, more than 3000 systems have been implanted worldwide (Fig. 15a).

***Abiomed AB 5000.*** Abiomed's AB® 5000 cardiac support system also provides a patient's failing heart with full circulatory assistance while allowing the heart to rest, heal, and recover its function. The Abiomed

AB 5000 ventricular assist device is a system recently approved by the Food and Drug Administration that consists of a fully automatic, vacuum-assisted console and a paracorporeal, pneumatically driven blood pump. The VAD is designed for short- or intermediate-term use. The console is designed to support the BVS 5000 or AB 5000 blood pumps. The cannulas and implantation are similar to the BVS 5000 system. The Abiomed AB 5000 was designed to be an upgrade to the BVS 5000 in terms of patient mobility, blood pump durability, and overall versatility. As of July 2006, more than 30 systems have been implanted worldwide (Fig. 15b).

*AbioCor.* The AbioCor™ Implantable Replacement Heart is a fully implantable prosthetic system intended as a substitute for severely diseased human hearts in patients suffering from coronary heart disease or some form of end-stage congestive heart failure. When these patients are at imminent risk of death, the AbioCor is designed to both extend life and provide a reasonable quality of life. After implantation, the device does not require any tubes or wires to pass through the skin. The power to drive the prosthetic heart is transmitted across the intact skin, thus avoiding skin penetration, which may provide opportunities for infection.

The AbioCor Implantable Replacement Heart consists of two blood-pumping chambers. The right pump supplies blood to the lungs, while the left pump provides blood to other vital organs of the body. Each of the two pumps is capable of delivering more than 8 L of blood per min. The replacement heart is about the size of a grapefruit and is quiet. A stethoscope is required to listen to the heart sounds. The pumps and valves are made from Angioflex™, a proprietary Abiomed material. An internal controller regulates the power delivered to the prosthetic heart. Without penetrating the skin, an external unit transmits power to the internal unit. A rechargable internal battery allows the patient to be completely free of the external power transmission unit for some period of time monitored by the internal system. The AbioCor system is designed to increase or decrease its pump rate in response to bodily needs. The AbioCor also includes an active monitoring system that provides detailed performance feedback, and alarms in the event of irregularities.

As of mid-November 2001, a total of 273 patient-days were accumulated with the AbioCor, with no significant problems observed (except

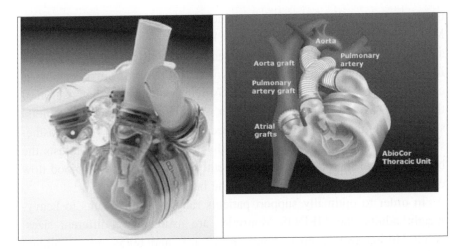

**Fig. 16.** The AbioCor MCSD.

for the incident with the first patient). All patients who received the implants had a 30-day estimated survival of less than 30% prior to receiving their implant. As of July 2006, fourteen patients have received AbioCor implants, and the first patient has had the device in place for over 130 days. As part of the Humanitarian Device Exemption (HDE) program, the US FDA has approved the AbioCor for destination implantation (www.fda.gov/bbs/topics/NEWS/2006/NEW01443) (Fig. 16).

## MEDOS

*Company History.* MEDOS is a German medical device company that has developed a unique multifunctional approach to MCSDs (www.medos-ag.de).

*MEDOS MCSD.* The MEDOS MCSD System is a mechanical assist device for short- and medium-term heart assist. The MEDOS ventricles were developed according to a construction-size concept. It allows high flexibility with the application of the system as a univentricular and biventricular assist device for the complete patient spectrum, ranging from infant to adult. The MEDOS driving unit was developed especially for the use of the MEDOS Ventricle, which is the main component of the MEDOS System. This blood pump is known for excellent flow features and biocompatibility, and was developed in line with the latest know-how in construction techniques and hemodynamics. Pressured air or vacuum is created by the MEDOS VAD Driving System, which shifts the position of the double-layered membrane in such a way that the volume on the blood side is rhythmically enlarged or reduced. The three-leaflet valve prosthesis of polyurethane, developed especially for this application, adjusts the bloodstream of the pump; the consequently emerging pulsatile blood flow corresponds to the natural support of the heart.

In order to optimally support patients ranging from infants to heavyweight adults, the MEDOS Ventricles are available in different sizes: Adult HiFlux (80/72 mL), Adult (80/72 mL and 60/54 mL), Children (25/22.5 mL), and Infants (10/9 mL). The MEDOS VAD Cannulas are especially adjusted to the various pump sizes, and guarantee optimal flow conditions and a high degree of flexibility. As per July 2006, the MEDOS System has been used in more than 350 applications in 84 hospitals worldwide as a bridge to recovery as well as a bridge to transplant in the age

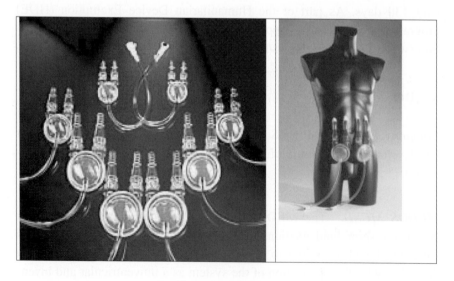

**Fig. 17.** The MEDOS MCSD.

range of 4 days to 76 years and weight range of 3 kg to 135 kg in left ventricular, right ventricular, and biventricular applications (Fig. 17).

## Ventracor

*Company History.* Ventracor is an Australian company producing the mechanical circulatory support device VentrAssist™ Left Ventricular Assist Device (LVAD) (www.ventracor.com).

*VentrAssist.* The VentrAssist™ is a new third-generation implantable heart device primarily designed as an alternative to heart transplantation for people with cardiac failure. It may also be used for patients waiting for heart transplants as a bridge to transplant or as a bridge to recovery. It is a blood pump that connects to the left ventricle of the diseased heart to help the ailing heart's pumping function and to assist in restoring a better quality of life. VentrAssist™ has only one moving part: a hydrodynamically suspended impeller with a fully redundant backup motor drive, controller, and processor. It has been designed not to have any wearing parts or cause blood damage. It weighs 298 g (10 oz) and measures 60 mm (2.5 inches) in diameter, making it suitable for both children and adults. The implanted parts of the VentrAssist™ device use materials that are fully biocompatible, including titanium alloys with diamond-like carbon coating on blood-contacting surfaces. Its components are light, strong, nontoxic, and highly resistant to degradation within the body.

As per July 2006, Ventracor is the only company with a third-generation LVAD in clinical trials in the USA. In Europe, enrollment targets under the CE Mark Trial have all been met, and Ventracor expects to obtain CE market approval for the commencement of commercial sales in Europe in early 2007. In the US, the Food and Drug Administration (FDA) requires separate clinical trials for bridge to transplant (BTT) and destination therapy (DT). The US Feasibility Trial is aimed at obtaining initial safety data in order to satisfy the regulatory requirements to proceed to the US Bridge to Transplant Pivotal Trial and the US Destination Therapy Trial, which may be run concurrently. Ventracor is currently conducting a five-center, 10-patient US feasibility trial (Fig. 18).

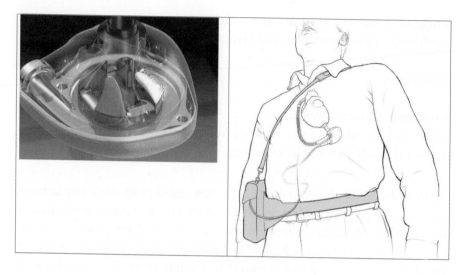

**Fig. 18.** The Ventracor MCSD.

# BerlinHeart

***Company History.*** BerlinHeart is a German company producing the MCSD BerlinHeart and INCOR (www.berlinheart.com). BerlinHeart AG develops, produces, and trades innovative devices for the mechanical support of the heart. Its products — INCOR®, EXCOR®, and EXCOR® Pediatric — cover the whole range of medical indication for all ages, from the newborn to the adult. As a result, the international BerlinHeart AG is the market leader in Germany and Europe. The claim is to develop trend-setting solutions with the utmost precision and reliability. The short period of innovation and the technological characteristics of its products are unique. Since the foundation of the wholly owned subsidiary BerlinHeart, Inc., in October 2005, the company is also represented in the US.

***INCOR® MCSD.*** The INCOR® MCSD is an implantable left ventricle assist device. Its global uniqueness lies in the free-floating, active magnetic bearing of the axial impeller. INCOR® has been specially conceived to deal with increasingly long-term applications within the destination therapy framework, so that it is in a position to take over the work of the left ventricle without any wear to the parts and on a permanent basis. Naturally,

INCOR® is also used in bridge-to-transplant and bridge-to-recovery programs. In addition to the implantable pump, the INCOR® system also includes a small external control unit and rechargable batteries that help the patient to enjoy almost unrestricted mobility. Further external components are a laptop, through which the pump can be started up, monitored, and adjusted; a power supply unit; and a battery charger.

The blood coming from the heart flows into the INCOR® axial flow pump and first passes the inducer, which guides the laminar flow onto the actual impeller. The impeller is suspended by a magnetic bearing and floats free of contact with other parts. It is responsible for the actual pumping, operating at speeds between 5000 and 10 000 rotations per min. The stationary diffuser behind the rotor has specially aligned blades, which reduce the rotational effects of the blood flow and add additional pressure to assist the transport of the blood from the outflow cannula to the aorta. The necessary power to drive the pump is supplied through a cable inserted under the skin on the patient's right side. This cable is connected to a small control unit that monitors and regulates the whole system. A main power pack and a backup power pack are attached to the control unit and supply INCOR® with sufficient electrical current. INCOR® generates a steady blood flow which, in combination with the residual activity of the native left ventricle, leads to reduced pulsatility for the patient. The blood contact surfaces of INCOR® are coated with Carmeda® BioActive Surface.

INCOR® is the only axial system worldwide to be equipped with an active magnetic bearing that allows for a freely floating impeller. The INCOR® impeller is axially active and radially passive without producing any actual physical contact. There is no direct mechanical contact between it — as the only movable part in the INCOR® pump — and its static components. This prevents any mechanical friction and, therefore, produces no frictional heat. This means no wear and tear at all to the parts and, consequently, a potentially infinite product life span for the INCOR® heart support system.

The company designed the blades of the internal components using numerical simulations of laser measurements in a fluid dynamics model, which suggests a significant reduction in the rate of hemolysis. The INCOR® motor is extremely efficient (>90%), and therefore has an exceedingly low energy consumption. Any warming of the pump in operation is so minimal that no denaturation of proteins occurs. Both these factors stand in stark contrast to mechanical bearings, which generate at least local heat (in accordance with the laws of physics) and cause possible thrombal problems through blood protein denaturation. The extremely precise sensors linked to the magnetic bearing supply the patient and the user with a wealth of important data about flow rates and pump performance. These values are also utilized by the pulsality control. This prevents any suction through the pump in the left ventricle by detecting the residual pulsality linked with it. The pump then automatically reduces its rotation speed and allows a renewed filling of the ventricle. The originally selected pump performance is then restored slowly and in a controlled way.

Because of its small size, the INCOR® pump is easily implantable. The installation of a separate pump pack is not necessary. An additional special feature is the new snap-in fasteners, which ensure a safe, quick, and uncomplicated connection between pump and cannulas. The silicone sheath prevents an ingrowing of the surrounding tissue. The percutaneous pump cable connects the INCOR® pump with the small external power pack. It is completely encased in silicone. At the place where the cable enters the skin, there is also a polyester velour coating to guarantee safe healing (Fig. 19). INCOR® was first used in clinical studies in June 2002, and received CE mark approval in March 2003. As of January 2007, the INCOR® LVAD has been used in 313 patients in 15 countries.

***EXCOR® MCSD.***   The EXCOR® ventricular assist device can be used to support one or both ventricles. The blood pump consists of a transparent

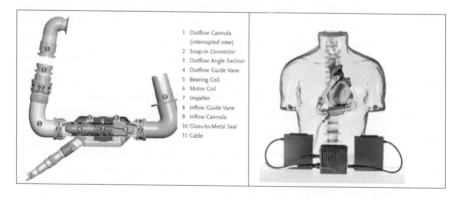

1 Outflow Cannula (interrupted view)
2 Snap-in Connector
3 Outflow Angle Section
4 Outflow Guide Vane
5 Bearing Coil
6 Motor Coil
7 Impeller
8 Inflow Guide Vane
9 Inflow Cannula
10 Glass-to-Metal Seal
11 Cable

**Fig. 19.** The INCOR MCSD.

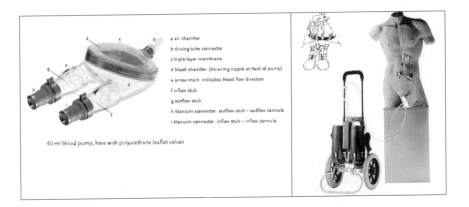

**Fig. 20.** The EXCOR MCSD.

polyurethane housing that is divided into one air chamber and one blood chamber by a three-layer membrane. Graphite between the membranes helps to minimize friction. The membrane on the blood side merges without a seam into the surface of the housing. A specially produced CARMEDA® coating is plated on the slick, flow-optimized blood contact surface. Inflow and outflow sockets, which are made of polyurethane and bear titan connectors for the connection of the cannulas, lead from the blood chamber to the inflow or outflow cannulas. On the air side of the membrane lays the connection for the pneumatic driving tube. Deairing is effected through the deairing socket. Mechanical valves in the sockets ensure an adjusted blood flow. The blood pumps are available with two different types of valves: a tilting disc, which is approved and reliable for long-term applications; and a polyurethane valve, which operates soundless (Fig. 20). EXCOR® was first used in June 1988. As of January 2007, it has been used in 26 countries in 1600 patients, of which 237 were pediatric patients. In North America, it has been used in 74 patients in 26 clinics since 2000.

## Terumo

***Company History.*** Terumo Heart, Inc. (Ann Arbor, MI), is a wholly owned US subsidiary of Terumo Corp. (Tokyo, Japan), producing a third-generation centrifugal pump called DuraHeart™ LVAS.

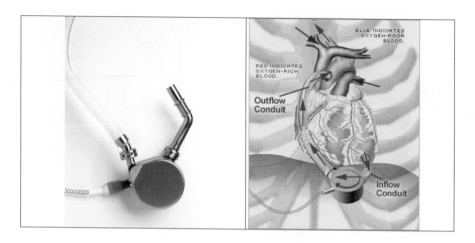

**Fig. 21.** The DuraHeart MCSD.

***DuraHeart.*** DuraHeart™ (Terumo Heart, Inc., Ann Arbor, MI) is a third-generation LVAD comprising a centrifugal blood pump with a magnetically levitated impeller. The pump consists of a titanium blood chamber containing an impeller, and two titanium compartments housing an electro-magnetic bearing mechanism and a brushless DC motor. The motor is magnetically coupled to the impeller without a mechanical shaft. The impeller rotates inside the blood chamber without material wear. The blood-contacting surfaces of the pump are modified with a heparin immobilization technique to enhance blood compatibility. The pump was first implanted in Bad Oeynhausen, Germany, for the European multicenter clinical trial. As of January 2007, twenty-nine devices have been implanted with a mean duration of 165 days. Eleven patients were supported for more than 6 months, and 4 for more than 1 year (Golding *et al.*, 2006) (Fig. 21).

## CorAide

***Company History.*** Arrow International, in collaboration with the Cleveland Clinic Foundation, produces the CorAide™ MCSD (www.arrowintl.com).

***Company History.*** The Arrow CorAide (Cleveland Clinic, Learner Research Institute, Cleveland, OH) is a third-generation centrifugal titanium pump. Problems with rotor balancing and thrombus deposition led

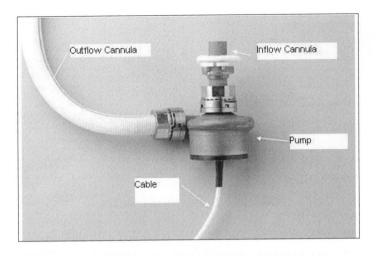

**Fig. 22.** The CorAide MCSD.

to significant design revision to a more conventional radial design, but with a continuation of the rotor suspension method, the blood-lubricated journal bearing, and the inverted contact-free motor. The Arrow-patented apical cuff clamp allows for positioning and fixation of the apical cannula to optimize flow into the biocompatible coated pump. The first clinical trial was initiated in Europe in 2003; but after the first implanted device was replaced with another bridge device, the clinical trial was suspended. Hemolysis by the journal-bearing clearance dimensions and the effect of that on the critical thickness of the lubricating thin film were the major cause. In February 2005, the European Bridge-to-Transplant Clinical Trial was restarted. As of July 2006, 21 implants have been done; patients were supported for 23–400 + days. (Golding *et al.*, 2006) (Fig. 22).

## EvaHeart

***Company History.*** EVAHEART is a Japanese company (www.evaheart-usa.com) producing the EVAHEART Left Ventricular Assist Device MCSD.

***EVAHEART MCSD.*** The EVAHEART Left Ventricular Assist Device is a third-generation centrifugal pump. The pump has a unique thromboresistant coating (2-methacryloyloxyethyl phosphorylcholine) over its

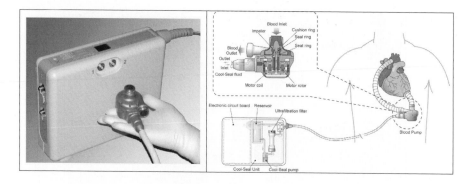

**Fig. 23.** The EVAHEART MCSD.

blood-contacting surfaces. The impeller is cooled with fluid that is pumped by way of a percutaneous channel from an external device. Electric power to the motor stator creates a rotating magnetic field, which is coupled inactively to the permanent magnet that is bonded to the pump shaft. A pilot bridge-to-transplant clinical trial was initiated in Japan in 2005. Three patients were implanted with the device, and all survived the 98- to 164-day support (Golding *et al.*, 2006) (Fig. 23).

## HeartWare

***Company History.*** HeartWare's head office is located in Sydney, Australia. HeartWare's technology is based on a proprietary miniaturization platform, which allows the development of smaller devices that are designed for long-term use and may be implantable by minimally invasive techniques.

***Heartware MCSD.*** HeartWare's left ventricular assist device (HVAD™) system is the company's first product to undergo human implantation. The device can generate up to 10 L/min flow, and is designed for use in a wide range of patients because it has a diameter of 4 cm and a height of less than 2 cm with an integrated inflow conduit. The small size of the HVAD™ pump allows intrapericardial placement, which reduces surgical trauma and facilitates the implant procedure. A unique wide-bladed impeller integrates magnets within the impeller blades, which reduces the pump height and

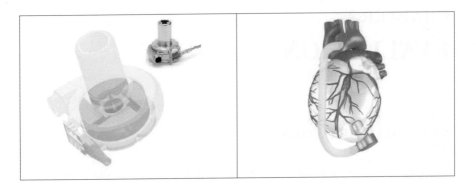

**Fig. 24.** The HeartWare MCSD.

permits the use of redundant motors in the pump housing for added safety. The impeller is the only moving part, and is suspended by a proprietary hybrid magnetic and hydrodynamic bearing system. The HVAD$^{TM}$ pump contains no sensors, mechanical bearings, or points of physical contact within the pump housing. These design features allow the HVAD$^{TM}$ pump to be smaller, quieter, and more durable than otherwise possible.

HeartWare is currently running a combined European and Australian bridge-to-transplant clinical trial aimed at achieving CE mark and TGA approval for the HVAD$^{TM}$ system. Implants are conducted at a minimum of five centers, including Vienna General Hospital (Austria), Royal Perth Hospital (Australia), St Vincent's Hospital (Australia), Harefield Hospital (UK), and Hannover Medical Center (Germany). Trials began in March 2006, when the first implant was conducted at Vienna General Hospital, Austria. As of January 2007, seven patients have undergone implantation of the HVAD$^{TM}$ pump and are awaiting transplantation. HeartWare plans to begin a bridge-to-transplant clinical trial in the United States towards the end of 2007, subject to FDA approval. A destination therapy trial will commence after initiation of the US bridge-to-transplant trial (Fig. 24).

# CHAPTER 2

# EVALUATION

## REFERRAL NETWORK

| | |
|---|---|
| **Eric G (born 1950)**<br><br>**Decision by family for LVAD** | It wasn't exactly like I had a choice in the matter, the matter being the actual use of the equipment. I had a heart attack one Saturday afternoon in the fall of 2004. Although I appeared to those around me as if I had my wits about me, the fact is that I have no recollection of anything that happened over a 2-week period. The memory lapse spans from the moment I passed out at home, while waiting for the paramedics to take me to the hospital, until 2 weeks later, when I woke up in a coronary care unit in one of New York's most prestigious hospitals. My wife and children made the decision for me and I'm going to have to live with it for the rest of my life. |
| **Janice (wife of Eric G, born 1950)**<br><br>**Referral for MCSD** | I first heard the word LVAD when we were at Mountainside Hospital, where my husband was taken by EMTs after he passed out at our home. The on-call cardiologist came out and told us that this hospital had done all they could for him, but they were just not equipped to provide any more assistance. His heart attack was much more serious than we thought. My husband was sitting up, talking to our children and seemingly stable. He was fooling us. The staff ensured us that he was absolutely **not** stable. He was about as critical as one could get.<br><br>The doctor called Columbia Presbyterian Hospital and had him transported there because it is one of the premier transplant hospitals. They also had this device that might be able to help my husband, something called an LVAD. Two things in that statement terrified |

me: "transplant", a term I was familiar with; and "LVAD", a term unknown to me, which was even scarier. My husband would end up needing both of these things. The LVAD would come first and would be a bridge to an eventual heart transplant.

| | |
|---|---|
| **Betty** (wife of **Abraham M**, born 1940) **Referral for MCSD** | Our story begins on the morning of July 22, 2004. When my husband awoke very early, we had breakfast and he went back to bed. When he reawoke, he complained of feeling chilly; he said that he was cold. My daughter called and I told her, "I don't know what's happening with daddy, he says that he has the chills." She advised me to call an ambulance. My husband did not want us to fuss. My daughter and son-in-law ran over to appraise the situation. A short while later, Abe was taken to South Nassau Hospital with my son-in-law. While we waited for him to be transported to Columbia Presbyterian Hospital, we went through a large pallet of feelings.<br><br>Finally, under the directions of Dr Simon Maybaum, Abe was transferred to Columbia. We all knew that Columbia was our only hope. As excited, happy, tense, and nervous as we were, the sight of two ambulances surprised us. You may wonder and ask why two as we did, and the answer that we were given was just in case something broke down. We can't even begin to tell you how nervous we were at a time like this. However, the kindness and the gentle way of the cardiac staff at South Nassau Hospital and the ambulance drivers gave us strength. The sight of the two ambulances was an assurance that my husband was in good hands. |

| | |
|---|---|
| **Deborah** (mother of **Joel L**, born 1969) **Referral for MCSD** | You had asked quite some time ago for both Joel and I, and also his father and sister, to send you our thoughts about the LVAD. I had avoided this, as the emotions generated by putting onto paper those terrible months in 2002 were more than I could bear. But after reading Candy's book (Moose, 2005), I realized that we too had a story that should be shared.<br><br>From the moment I received the phone call from Dr Shuster on Monday, February 11, 2002, all color went |

out of my life and I saw the world in shades of gray. Joel had myocarditis, he said, and I was savvy enough to know that this meant Joel would need a heart transplant if he had any chance to survive at all. How did I know this so immediately, Joel's father had often asked. Probably from an article in *Women's Day* or *Ladies' Home Journal* about the courage of a family whose son got viral myocarditis. I can't be sure of the publication.

I was sitting at work at Beth Israel Deaconess Medical Center in Boston when the call came in. I immediately called my boss in the OR to tell him that I was leaving for an indefinite time, called Joel's father to tell him the news, and then walked out of my office, never to return again as an employee. I can't remember if I drove to my apartment in my own car or if I took a cab home. I remember throwing clothes in a bag, feeding my cat and leaving a key and a note for my neighbor to look after my cat, and then off I went to Stamford.

It was snowing heavily that day, the first snowstorm of 2002, and the road conditions were poor. At various points during the trip, I thought about pulling into a train station to take the train, but I knew I could not tolerate waiting for connections, and so I ignored the nearly white-out conditions and speeded along Route 95. I think I made it in record time even with the storm, arriving in Stamford just about 3 hours later.

Joel was in intensive care at Stamford Hospital when I arrived. He was upbeat, joking as he always was, and was busy watching the Winter Olympics. His major topic of discussion was whether the poster boy of those games, a speed skater, was going to win all that was predicted by the media.

Signs of Joel being ill? Some shortness of breath and the inability to urinate. Wow, maybe the doctor had over-called this one and all would be right in a few days. Joel was scheduled for an angiogram the next morning, and the results of this would tell us what the next step would be. Maybe this was only endocarditis with damage to one of the valves. Maybe he only needed a valve replacement, and he would be up on his bike again and back to normal. I prayed for this diagnosis, but foolishly worried about the sound that a mechanical valve makes and how that would impact on Joel's psyche. How naive I was!

The angiogram the next morning showed the worst-case scenario: Joel had myocarditis and needed to be transported to Columbia Presbyterian Hospital ASAP. Ironically, I had worked at CPMC in clinical pathology from 1965–1968, and his father had graduated from P&S in 1968. We met there while he was a medical student and I was working in the third-year medical students' clinical pathology laboratory on the medical floor. Now, all these years later, this was a sort of unwelcome homecoming for us.

Joel was transported by ambulance and his father, sister Alicia, and I drove to NYC after picking up a change of clothing. We had not been to the Medical Center in well over 20 years and had no idea of how it had changed. We instinctively went to Admitting Emergency on Broadway and 168th St., only to be told that he was in Cardiac Intensive Care of Milstein, a building that certainly did not exist during our tenure at CPMC. We ran down 168th St. to Fort Washington, and somehow made our way to the fifth floor of Milstein and Joel's cubicle. Gathered around him were interns, residents, medical students, and nurses.

Just a few days before, I had been given an article from the NY Times on "The Practice of Medicine" written by a young resident from Harvard. She had gone into great detail about how medical students learn to put in a central line and how painful this was to the patients. There, in the middle of this gaggle of medical personnel, was my son, crying out while a student/intern/resident was trying to put in a central line. "Stop!" I screamed. "You will not practice on my son!" I was quickly grabbed and pulled from the room, and was told that Joel was in grave condition and that this procedure was necessary to save his life. Soon after this, my niece who is a physician in NYC arrived at the hospital. She had been called from Stamford, told of Joel's condition, and she had alerted doctors she knew at CPMC that he was going there.

## Advanced Heart Failure Referral Network Logistics

Advanced heart failure (AHF) therapy with MCSD is currently being practiced in less than 200 selected hospitals out of over 3000 in the USA alone. In order to provide equitable and high-quality access to MCSD therapy, a referral network has to be in place. This network, which requires a structure similar to the referral network for heart transplantation, includes the local general practitioner, internist, and cardiologist; the local and regional hospital; and the tertiary care center. The referral is often initiated by the local or regional colleagues who are taking care of a patient at a stage of the advanced heart failure syndrome that is not sufficiently responsive to medical therapy. Upon contacting the tertiary care center, patient history information is shared between the two hospitals. If the patient is deemed likely to benefit from the evaluation for mechanical circulatory support and heart transplantation, then the transfer is initiated.

***Advanced Heart Failure Transfer Decision Making.***    The decision of a local center to ask for the transfer of a patient to a center providing MCSD therapy is followed by an evaluation and decision of the accepting MCSD center. This evaluation is critically important. A transfer should be in the interest of a patient who has a higher chance of longevity and good quality of life with MCSD therapy, but not for a patient who is likely too well or too ill for MCSD therapy.

***Tertiary Center Outreach Team.***    The MCSD center may organize an outreach team on call. This team can perform the evaluation in the transfer-requesting hospital. This approach is advantageous for (1) the patient, minimizing unnecessary transfers; (2) the transferring hospital, maximizing educational decision-making experience; and (3) the MCSD center; minimizing medically unnecessary resource consumption and maximizing networking in the region.

***Decision-Making Algorithm.***    The decision-making algorithm is initiated when the patient is referred for evaluation to an established heart failure/MCSD center (Crespo Leiro and Paniagua Martin, 2004; McMurray and Pfeffer, 2005; Nieminen *et al.*, 2005; Grady *et al.*, 2004). Referral to a designated center takes place when the treating cardiologist or internist has exhausted all lifestyle and medical options without success in the setting of decompensation and progression of AHF, a phase known to be associated with a high risk of death. Any time during the management, there may arise a situation in which a patient may not benefit from any of the modern therapies because of multiorgan failure or other coconditions, thus leading to patient preference for comfort care facilitating a humane form of death instead of prolonged suffering (Bramstedt and Nash, 2005; Hauptman and Havranek, 2005). A structured management algorithm should be applied to recompensate the patient and to initiate a neurohormonal blockade and lifestyle changes; or if recompensation cannot be achieved and the patient is not a suitable candidate for cardiac transplantation, destination MCSD therapy should be considered (Miller and Lietz, 2006).

In 2005, the International Society for Heart and Lung Transplantation (ISHLT) organized a consensus conference to provide clinical evidence and expert opinion–based guidelines for the consideration of MCSD implantation (Mehra *et al.*, 2006). Care must be taken in MCSD centers to adhere to evidence-based destination MCSD implantation guidelines and not to inadvertently drift to other patient selection criteria, such as patients who are less sick or patients who are sicker than the original REMATCH cohort and thus would have a survival/QoL-benefit that would be difficult to predict (Deng *et al.*, 2005a).

## INITIAL ENCOUNTER

| | |
|---|---|
| **Ed S (born 1956)** **Referral for MCSD** | I am a recipient of the HeartMate LVAD. I was diagnosed with cardiomyopathy in March 2000, and was told that I had an ejection fraction of 18%. I had caught a flu virus along with the rest of my family on New Year's Eve 1999. The rest of the family recovered, but I started to have the symptoms of congestive heart failure shortly after the new year. I was treated using drug therapy and functioned quite well for 5 years, save for a few hospitalizations with bronchitis, etc. |
| | In June 2004, I was in the best physical shape I had been in for quite a while. I was swimming laps, working |

out on exercise machines, and doing quite a bit of walking and biking. In July, I went on vacation with my wife and 6-year-old son. I had a slight congestion sensation in my lungs. Within 2 weeks, I was laying on a couch for 2 weeks, not able to eat and only able to take sips of water without feeling bloated. To compound the problem, I knew of at least six people who were going through an intestinal virus of sorts, so I just assumed that I was going through the same things that they were experiencing. But, my liver and kidneys weren't functioning properly due to a lack of proper blood flow.

I have been a patient at Columbia Presbyterian Hospital since being recommended by my local cardiologist in 2001. I was admitted to the hospital on August 8, 2004, in serious condition. I responded to the intravenous medication, and after a month went home on the automatic pump system. I got sicker day by day, and after 10 days was readmitted back to the hospital, coughing constantly, damn near 24 hours a day, and unable to sleep for 3 days at a clip. I walked into the CCU and was admitted. They told me they don't get many patients who walk into the CCU. Ha! Shortly after I arrived, the doctors who examined me said that I was in dire need of an LVAD and that I was on the heart transplant list.

## Initial Presentation

*Arrival.*   Upon arrival at the tertiary care center, the patient is evaluated regarding his/her acute condition and MCSD candidacy. Depending on his/her vital signs, the patient is admitted (preferably after direct transfer, and not via the Columbia University Medical Center Emergency Room or other major centers) to the intensive care unit or the floor. Acute evaluation and recompensation along the lines of published expert and institutional guidelines are initiated. At the same time, the host hospital's left ventricular assist device (LVAD) team starts the specific MCSD evaluation for BTT, BTR, and ATT indications.

*Point Person.* From the patient's perspective, it is very important that the initial team introduces themselves with their respective roles (preferably with their official business cards containing their names, titles, roles, and contact information) and that the patient and family have the chance to identify one reliable communication partner from the initial encounter onwards.

*Team Tasks.* At initial presentation, it is important that

- the team gains a basic impression of the patient as a person and the severity of his/her condition;
- the patient and his/her relatives gain a basic impression of the nature of the management and care program in the center; and
- the cornerstone of a long-term working relationship is founded.

Patients are evaluated for MCSD implantation and/or transplantation after referral by their local cardiologist or by a cardiologist at the tertiary care center. When the referral comes from a physician outside the center, an initial telephone screening is performed. This preliminary screening includes the following:

- Patient age
- Cardiac diagnosis and functional status
- Current treatment regimen
- Presence of coexisting conditions, which constitute absolute contraindications
- Feasibility of inpatient versus outpatient evaluation
- Brief review of patient insurance and general financial resources

The telephone screening is done by one of the heart failure/MCSD/ transplant cardiologists or transplant surgeons, or by the senior MCSD/ transplant coordinator. A determination is then made on whether admission to the hospital is required or whether arrangements for outpatient evaluation should be made. In some instances, patients are initially seen in the heart failure clinic or heart transplant clinic before the decision is made to submit the patient to formal evaluation for MCSD implantation/transplantation.

Once it is determined that a patient is potentially an appropriate candidate for MCSD implantation/transplantation, a complete pretransplant evaluation is performed on an inpatient or outpatient basis. For patients who are unstable and require hospitalization for management of their medical condition, the entire workup is performed as an inpatient. For ambulatory patients, the majority of the workup is done as an outpatient. For stable outpatients who require continuous anticoagulation (i.e. history of emboli, prosthetic valves), right heart catheterization is performed in the hospital on heparin.

## TESTS

### General Rationale for Standardized Testing

One group of tests aims at answering the following questions: How severe is the heart failure condition? How is the survival prognosis within this stage of heart failure? Are there any unexploited evidence-based treatment options? The other group of tests aims at answering these questions: If there is an expected benefit from MCSD implantation derived from the cardiac condition, are there any risk factors related to (1) other disease conditions or (2) psychosocial risk factors that would diminish the anticipated benefit? Which of these conditions are reversible? These tests are summarized in the Table below (Table 2), and are included in the evaluation.

### Specific Tests

The tests follow a standardized scheme similar to the evaluation scheme for heart transplantation (Table 2). They are based on the rationale to detect any of the conditions that constitute potential indications and contraindications for MCSD implantation (see chapter 3).

## GENERAL INDICATIONS/CONTRAINDICATIONS

### MCSD Risk Prediction

*Columbia MCSD Risk Score.*   The group at Columbia University previously calculated a risk factor summation score that successfully predicted survival after the insertion of a left ventricular assist device (Oz *et al.*,

**Table 2.**  MCSD evaluation tests (adapted from Deng and Naka, 2002).

| | |
|---|---|
| **History** | Specific emphasis on duration and severity of heart failure symptoms, medication, allergies, infectious diseases |
| **Physical** | Specific emphasis on heart failure impact and end-organ dysfunction assessment |
| **Laboratory** | Creatinine, BUN, electrolytes, liver panel, lipid panel, CA, $PO_4$, total protein, albumine, uric acid, CBC with differential and platelet count, thyroid panel, ANA, ESR, RPR, iron binding, PTT, PT |
| | Blood type |
| | IgG and IgM antibodies against CMV, HSV, HIV, VZV, HbsAg, HCV, toxoplasmosis, other titers when indicated |
| | Prostate-specific antigen (males $>50$ years), mammogram and pap smear (females $>40$ years) |
| | Screening against a panel of donor antigens (PRA) and HLA phenotype |
| | 24-h urine for creatinine clearance and total protein, urinalysis, urine culture |
| | Baseline bacterial and fungal cultures if indicated |
| **Cardiac** | 12-lead electrocardiogram, 24-h Holter monitor, Signal-averaged EKG |
| | Echocardiogram |
| | Thallium scan if indicated |
| | Exercise stress test with oxygen uptake measurements |
| | Right and left heart catheterization |
| | Myocardial biopsy on selected cases where etiology of heart failure is in question |
| **Vascular** | Transcranial Doppler |
| | Peripheral vascular studies |
| | Carotid Doppler $>55$ years |
| **Renal** | IV pyelogram if indicated |
| **Pulmonary** | Chest X-ray |
| | Pulmonary function tests |
| | Chest CT $>65$ years (thoracic aorta) |
| **Gastrointestinal** | Abdominal ultrasound $>55$ years |
| | Upper GI series if indicated |
| | Barium enema if indicated |
| | Liver biopsy if indicated |
| **Metabolic** | Bone densitometry |
| **Neurologic** | Screening evaluation |
| **Psychiatric** | Screening evaluation |
| **Dental** | Complete dental evaluation |
| **Cardiothor surg** | Evaluation |
| **Physical therapy** | Evaluation |
| **Social work** | Patient attitude and family support, medical insurance and general financial resources |
| **TX coordinator** | Education |

1995). Most recently, they validated the previous score by using a single center's clinical experience to determine the emerging risk factors for mortality after device insertion. The clinical records of 130 consecutive patients who received the HeartMate VE left ventricular assist device (Thoratec Corp; Pleasanton, CA) at our institution between June 1996 and March 2001 as a bridge to transplantation were reviewed. Univariate and multivariable analyses were performed to determine the predictors of operative mortality after device insertion. Using the relative risks for each identified variable, a new risk factor summation score was devised. The new and old scores were then compared by using linear regression analyses to determine whether the revised score improved statistical accuracy.

Overall operative mortality was 25% ($n = 33$). The old score successfully predicted operative mortality in the current patient population (operative mortality of 38% for a score of $>5$ vs. 13% for a score of $\leq 5$). However, the revised score improved risk discrimination (operative mortality of 46% for a score of $>5$ vs. 12% for a score of $\leq 5$). Statistical accuracy was comparable between scores, but the relationship between observed and predicted outcomes was improved with the revised score. The authors concluded that the changing demographic profile and management of patients presenting for mechanical circulatory support have led to a change in the predictors of mortality after device insertion. Periodic remodeling and recalibration of risk indices help to accurately predict the outcomes in high-risk patient groups and identify emerging risk factors for mortality (Rao *et al.*, 2003).

***The St. Louis University Experience.***    To more fully identify the factors influencing survival to transplant, the group at St. Louis University in Missouri reviewed the preoperative and postoperative VAD courses of 105 bridge-to-transplant patients. Sixty-four parameters (34 pre-VAD, 30 post-VAD), including hemodynamics, complications, and evaluations of major organ functions, were examined and analyzed. Thirty-three (31%) patients died on VADs and 72 (69%) were transplanted. There were two posttransplant operative deaths (3%). By univariate analysis, 23 of 64 factors were significant. These 23 factors were entered into a stepwise logistic regression analysis to identify the predictors of survival to transplant.

Four factors — pre-VAD intubation ($p < 0.005$), CPB time during VAD insertion ($p < 0.0001$), mean pulmonary artery pressure (first postoperative day after VAD) ($p < 0.0002$), and highest post-VAD creatinine ($p < 0.01$) — were independent predictors of transplantation. Other than the need for intubation, pre-VAD variables were of little value in predicting survival to transplant. Problems during VAD insertion (long CPB time) and post-VAD renal insufficiency were independent predictors. Severe complications that developed during the interval of VAD support, including cerebrovascular accident, bleeding, and infection, were surprisingly not predictors of transplantation (McBride *et al.*, 2001).

***Predicting Organ Dysfunction/Recovery.*** The testing of end-organ dysfunction recovery potential in AHF patients evaluated for long-term MCSD implantation needs to be done within a comprehensive multidisciplinary approach (Cadeiras *et al.*, 2005). Predictive tools are limited, and there is not yet enough means and evidence to accurately assess the likelihood of end-organ dysfunction recovery. Heart failure has been widely studied and identified as a systemic inflammatory syndrome, in which certain chemokines such as interleukin-6 and TNF-$\beta$ have been involved in cardiac remodeling and disease progression (Gwechenberger *et al.*, 2004).

On top of the chronic activation of the neurohormonal/immune system by AHF, MCSD implantation leads to chronic modulation of immune/inflammatory cascades, causing persistent platelet activation and reactivity as well as endothelial activation (Houel *et al.*, 2004) that can hypothetically be linked to the elevated incidence of infections and coagulopathies. These may contribute to the fact that although there is an improvement in survival after MCSD implantation in transplant-ineligible patients, morbidity from infections and coagulopathies is still unacceptably high (Park *et al.*, 2005; Deng *et al.*, 2005a).

***Clinical Scores.*** Current modes of assessment of end-organ reserve capacity for advanced end-organ dysfunction are not well established. The use of general clinical predictive scores has been useful in multiple clinical settings, but their applicability in the MCSD destination therapy population has not been studied. To determine which patients have higher risk within the heart failure population, the Heart Failure Survival Score (HFSS) was developed and validated before neurohormonal blockade was definitively established as a mainstay therapy for AHF. However, HFSS remains useful to identify those patients most severely compromised (Koelling *et al.*, 2004).

The Columbia University Risk Score for MCSD outcomes was designed and validated to predict preoperative risk based on simple organ-function parameters (Rao *et al.*, 2003). Indeed, classical risk tools have been repeatedly validated for the risk prediction of multiorgan failure. EuroSCORE is helpful to predict in-hospital postoperative length of stay and specific major postoperative complications after cardiac surgery (Toumpoulis *et al.*, 2005). In post–coronary-artery-bypass-graft (CABG) patients, the likelihood of renal outcome is related to medical conditions such as the need for emergency surgery, the development of acute renal failure (ARF) during stay in ICU, the need for mechanical ventilation, and the number of other failed organ systems (Ostermann and Chang, 2005). From this standpoint, the use of risk scores offers the possibility for more objective measurement reports and comparisons.

A clinical risk score to predict the occurrence of ARF after open heart surgery was recently developed at the Cleveland Clinic, and may be adopted for planning future clinical trials of acute renal failure in MCSD patients (Thakar *et al.*, 2005). Most challenging, novel approaches using functional proteomics from urine samples have been used to identify early biomarker patterns for ischemic renal injury in patients undergoing cardiopulmonary bypass. Using surface-enhanced laser desorption/ionization time-of-flight mass spectrometry (SELDI-ToF-MS), it was demonstrated that protein biomarkers sensitively predict acute renal injury following cardiopulmonary bypass (Nguyen *et al.*, 2005). In order to assess the reversibility or irreversibility of pulmonary dysfunction and the feasibility of weaning mechanical ventilation in old and very sick patients, known preoperative predictors of extubation failure may be assessed in this population. The prognostic system Acute Physiology and Chronic Health Evaluation II (APACHE II) evaluates aspects regarding hospital mortality and weaning outcome after long-term mechanical ventilation, and can be useful to predict the weaning outcome (Schonhofer *et al.*, 2004).

***Laboratory Parameter Scores.***    In patients with systemic inflammatory response syndrome and multiple organ dysfunction syndrome, changes in prothrombotic/antithrombotic molecules and endothelial activation have been related to mortality. It is also known that exogenous supplementation of activated protein C improves survival, and that elevated baseline protein C levels are related to better outcomes during sepsis (Liaw *et al.*, 2004). This observation brings up the hypothesis that this phenotype characterizes a high-risk population for MCSD implantation.

Changes in leukocyte biology during sepsis have been related to prognosis. The expression of human leukocyte antigen (HLA)-DR on monocytes is proposed as a major feature of sepsis-induced immunodepression probably mediated by transcriptional CIITA-regulated genes (Pachot *et al.*, 2005), and delayed neutrophil apoptosis might sustain inflammation during sepsis and relate to a worse outcome. Gene expression profiling analysis has yielded changes in a large number of genes involved in inflammation, metabolism, signaling, mitochondrial function, and apoptosis, and a number of genes have been identified as suitable targets responsible for the regulation of neutrophil apoptosis (O'Neill *et al.*, 2004).

Validated risk scores have been developed to predict mortality in end-stage liver disease patients waiting for liver transplantation. The use of the MELD score and modifications might be useful to improve the selection of MCSD patients with cirrhosis (Ruf *et al.*, 2005). Serial evaluation of hepatic regeneration by serum levels of alpha-fetoprotein has been studied in patients after acetaminophen intoxication, and might be a useful variable for risk prediction (Schmidt and Dalhoff, 2005). Diffuse cerebral dysfunction is often present in sepsis, which is potentially reversible. It can be triggered by the septic process itself and can be complicated by mechanisms dependent on concomitant organ dysfunctions. Specific electroencephalographic patterns might be related to septic encephalopathy, which is known to worsen the prognosis of critically ill patients (Consales and De Gaudio, 2005).

Translational research is gaining relevance in risk evaluation. Variations in end-organ dysfunction capacity of recovery and susceptibility to infection can be explained by polymorphisms of genes encoding proteins involved in the innate immune response, the inflammatory cascade, coagulation, and fibrinolysis (Texereau *et al.*, 2004; D'Aiuto *et al.*, 2005; Wang, 2005). High-throughput biology using microarray analysis can lead to the development of newer diagnostic and therapeutic tools, as already tested in airway smooth muscle and edema fluid from acute lung injury (Olman *et al.*, 2004; Henger *et al.*, 2004), sepsis, nephropathies, and transplantation (Deng *et al.*, 2003b), evaluating multiple genes and complex pathways (Sharma *et al.*, 2005) using modern bioinformatics approaches as reverse engineering that can predict key "hubs" in gene networks (Basso *et al.*, 2005).

## ISHLT: Consensus Guidelines 2006 for MCSD Therapy

The indications and contraindications for MCSD therapy differ with respect to the intention-to-treat, bridge-to-transplantation, bridge-to-recovery, or destination MCSD. However, there is a general consensus about which patients have severe enough heart failure and do not have a prohibitively high risk for the procedure to likely benefit from MCSD implantation. This consensus was recently published by the International Society for Heart and Lung Transplantation (Mehra *et al.*, 2006). In the decision-making process prior to MCSD implantation, other cardiac, noncardiac, and technical factors must be considered. The indication as a bridge to heart transplantation may change to bridge to recovery (weaning) or destination therapy, balancing possible advantages and disadvantages. The recommendation for MCSD therapy is based on the comparison of short- and long-term survival and quality-of-life outcomes with conventional therapy.

At present, device development, clinical trial design, regulatory approval, and reimbursement decisions for the clinical application of mechanical cardiac support devices continue to be considered in the context of these clinical indications. Although understandable from a historical perspective, these arbitrary divisions are inconsistent with the clinical realities of advanced heart failure therapy. By narrowly focusing on transplant eligibility at a static point in the clinical course, the current guidelines impede the broader application of ventricular assist device technology to the growing population of patients who may benefit from this therapy (Felker and Rogers, 2006). The following consensus recommendations of the ISHLT — which are structured according to evidence-based medicine criteria of the AHA/ACC (see Appendix 1) — must not be viewed in isolation, but rather in their cumulative effect on outcomes in a given patient.

# Age

*Class I Recommendation.* In patients older than 60 years, a thorough evaluation for the presence of other clinical risk factors should be done (Level of Evidence: C). Age should not itself be considered a contraindication to mechanical circulatory support (Level of Evidence: C).

*Background.* An inverse relationship is generally reported between the age of >60–65 years and the outcome, although encouraging results have now been obtained in selected patients up to 70 years (Deng *et al.*, 2001a; Aaronson *et al.*, 2003; Miller, 2003; Deng *et al.*, 2004; Jurmann *et al.*, 2004; Topkara *et al.*, 2005).

# Body Size

*Class I Recommendation.* The use of pulsatile intracorporeal devices (e.g. HeartMate XVE, Thoratec Corporation, Pleasanton, CA; Novacor LVS, WorldHeart Corporation, Oakland, CA) should be limited to patients with a body surface area (BSA) of >1.5 m². For smaller individuals, the use of paracorporeal or axial flow devices should be considered (Level of Evidence: C).

*Background.* The large size of intracorporeal pulsatile devices requires adequate thoracic and abdominal capacity. This limitation is overcome by the availability of paracorporeal small-sized pulsatile devices or by the use of intracorporeal/intraventricular axial flow devices (Williams and Oz, 2001; Frazier and Delgado, 2003).

# Renal Function

*Class I Recommendation.* All patients evaluated for MCSD therapy should have creatinine and BUN measured. Patients with a creatinine of > 3.0 mg/dL are at higher risk. Patients with serum creatinine above this value may be considered MCSD candidates if renal failure is acute and renal recovery is likely (e.g. acute renal failure in young patients with previously normal renal function) (Level of Evidence: C).

*Class III Recommendation.*    Patients dependent on chronic dialysis should not be considered as MCSD candidates (Level of Evidence: C).

*Background.*    Renal dysfunction is a strong determinant of unsuccessful MCSD support, but in many cases it recovers after adequate circulatory support (McBride *et al.*, 2001; Williams and Oz, 2001; Aaronson *et al.*, 2003; Miller, 2003; Granfeldt *et al.*, 2003; Rao *et al.*, 2003; Dembitsky *et al.*, 2004). Besides clinically established parameters such as serum creatinine and BUN (Novis *et al.*, 1994; Brandt *et al.*, 1996), preoperative creatinine clearance has been shown to correlate with postoperative outcomes (Aronson and Blumenthal, 1998). The Acute Physiology and Chronic Health Evaluation (APACHE) II score has been used in perioperative renal dysfunction risk assessment (Parker *et al.*, 1998).

## Pulmonary Function

*Class I Recommendation.*    All patients evaluated for MCSD therapy should have chest X-rays and pulmonary function tests done, if feasible. Mechanical ventilation in the absence of significant pre-existing pulmonary dysfunction or inflammatory infiltrates is a risk factor, but should not be considered an absolute contraindication to VAD support. A lung CT scan should be considered in selected patients to rule out undiagnosed conditions on chest X-ray (Level of Evidence: C).

*Class III Recommendation.*    Patients with severe pulmonary dysfunction contraindicating heart transplantation (e.g. FEV1 < 1) should not be considered MCSD candidates (Level of Evidence: C).

*Background.*    Mechanical ventilation in cardiogenic shock is a severe risk factor for poor postimplant outcome. Recent pulmonary embolism or inflammatory parenchymal infiltrates can lead to the development of infectious foci that are difficult to treat under mechanical circulation (Williams and Oz, 2001; Aaronson *et al.*, 2003; Miller, 2003; Rao *et al.*, 2003).

## Hepatic Function

*Class I Recommendation.*    All patients evaluated for MCSD therapy should have their liver function assessed. Patients with alanine aminotransferase (ALT) or aspartate aminotransferase (AST) greater than three times the control are at higher risk. Biventricular support may be considered the first option in the case of hepatic dysfunction associated with RV failure (Level of Evidence: C).

*Class III Recommendation.*    Patients with cirrhosis and portal hypertension should be excluded from MCSD implantation (Level of Evidence: C).

*Background.*    Elevated serum bilirubin and deficiency in clotting factors have a serious adverse impact on postimplant outcomes. However, because hepatic dysfunction is often a consequence of RV failure, it is a strong predictor of the necessity of biventricular support (McBride *et al.*, 2001; Williams and Oz, 2001; Aaronson *et al.*, 2003; Miller, 2003; Rao *et al.*, 2003; Dembitsky *et al.*, 2004). The prognostic Model for End-Stage Liver Disease (MELD) is gaining increasing importance. This score includes the logs of bilirubin (mg/dL), creatinine (mg/dL), and INR, and the cause of the underlying disease (Christensen, 2004; Suman *et al.*, 2004). Besides bilirubin, liver enzyme levels predict survival after MCSD implantation as a bridge to transplantation (Reinhartz *et al.*, 1998; Masai *et al.*, 2002).

## Coagulation Disorders

*Class I Recommendation.*    All patients evaluated for MCSD therapy should have complete routine coagulation tests performed. Patients with a spontaneous INR of >2.5 are at increased risk of bleeding complications (Level of Evidence: C).

*Class III Recommendation.*    Patients with heparin-induced thrombocytopenia are generally not considered MCSD candidates (Level of Evidence: C).

*Background.*    Most clinical decisions are currently guided by measurement of the INR. However, as coagulation control is crucial, measurements such as activated protein C (APC), thrombomodulin, and endothelial cell protein C receptor may provide more precise guidance in the near future (Liaw *et al.*, 2004).

## Infectious Diseases and Inflammatory Activation

*Class I Recommendation.* All patients evaluated for MCSD therapy should have a thorough screening for infectious foci. Any ongoing infection should be identified and adequately treated before MCSD implantation. In particular, all conditions that might enhance the risk of fungal infection should be considered and properly managed (Level of Evidence: C).

*Class III Recommendation.* Patients with an acute systemic infection should not be considered as MCSD candidates (Level of Evidence: C).

*Background.* Fungal infection deserves special attention, as MCSD patients are more prone to fungal infection and less responsive to medical treatment (Nurozler *et al.*, 2001; Barbone *et al.*, 2004).

## Arrhythmias

*Class I Recommendation.* Biventricular support for recurrent sustained ventricular tachycardia or ventricular fibrillation should be considered only in the presence of an untreatable arrhythmogenic pathological substrate (e.g. giant cell myocarditis). Otherwise, appropriate medical antiarrhythmic therapy, antibradycardia pacing, ICD implantation, or VT ablation can generally adequately control bradyarrhythmias or tachyarrhythmias during LVAD support (Level of Evidence: C).

*Background.* Ventricular tachycardia and ventricular fibrillation may resolve after adequate LVAD support, except in the case of underlying proarrhythmic pathology. During MCSD support, tachyarrhythmias or bradyarrhythmias are generally tolerated in the presence of normal pulmonary resistance because of Fontan-like circulation, and the necessity for biventricular support is unusual (Oz *et al.*, 1994; Swartz *et al.*, 1999; Aaronson *et al.*, 2003; Miller, 2003.) In rare situations, the implantation/use of either antibradycardia pacing or antitachycardia devices may be necessary (Deng *et al.*, 1999b).

## Right Ventricular Function

*Class I Recommendation.* Evaluation of the reversibility of pulmonary hypertension and RV performance should be performed prior to MCSD implantation. In the case of irreversible pulmonary hypertension, RV failure, or multiorgan dysfunction, biventricular support should be considered. Patients older than 65 years with biventricular failure are at the highest risk for RV failure; thus, they should be considered with great caution as MCSD candidates (Level of Evidence: C).

*Background.* RV failure constitutes one of the most powerful predictors of adverse post-MCSD outcomes (Deng *et al.*, 2004; Deng *et al.*, 2005a). The functional status of the right ventricle and its relationship to the pulmonary circulation are of utmost importance in the decision-making process for MCSD implantation and in the differential indication between the use of an LVAD or a biventricular assist device (BVAD) (Williams and Oz, 2001; Ochiai *et al.*, 2002; Aaronson *et al.*, 2003; Miller, 2003; Kucuker *et al.*, 2004; Morgan *et al.*, 2004). Low RV systolic pressure, coupled with elevated RA pressure and low systolic stroke volume, indicates severe RV impairment with poor reversibility (Morgan *et al.*, 2004).

## Valvular Diseases

*Class I Recommendation.* When using a completely unloading pulsatile MCSD, such as the Novacor, HeartMate I, or Thoratec, the aortic valve should be sutured or replaced with a bioprosthesis when more than mild aortic insufficiency is present. The replacement of a mechanical prosthesis with a bioprothesis should also be considered (Level of Evidence: C). Anticoagulation therapy is strongly advised when a prosthetic valve is present (Level of Evidence: C). Severe mitral stenosis should be treated and, if weaning from MCSDs is foreseen, significant mitral insufficiency should also be corrected (Level of Evidence: C).

*Background.* More than minimal aortic insufficiency can rapidly evolve to moderate/severe grades, due to continuously elevated pressure in the aortic root created by the pump and not counteracted by phasic LV pressure rise.

Mitral stenosis can reduce native ventricular filling and limit the output of the device. Mitral insufficiency does not interfere with MCSD function, but can adversely affect future weaning and explantation. Severe tricuspid regurgitation should always be considered as an adjunctive mechanism of worsening RV function in LVAD patients (Holman *et al.*, 1994). The presence of any prosthetic valve is potentially thrombogenic (Swartz *et al.*, 1999; Tisol *et al.*, 2001; Rao *et al.*, 2003; Barbone *et al.*, 2002; Park *et al.*, 2004). A consensus does not exist yet on whether and how severe tricuspid regurgitation should be treated.

### Neurological Function

*Class I Recommendation.*   A thorough neurological examination should be performed to determine potential neurological risk factors and contraindications for MCSD implantation. Specifically, poststroke motor deficits should be assessed in order to determine the ability of the patient to cope with the device. In emergency cases with uncertain neurological recovery, a short-term MCSD such as a paracorporeal centrifugal pump should be adopted, allowing for recovery and full evaluation of long-term MCSD candidacy. A recent or evolving stroke is considered at least a temporary contraindication (Level of Evidence: C).

*Background.*   Knowledge about the neurological status of patients referred for mechanical assistance on an emergency basis is crucial to determine the appropriateness of the procedure (Williams and Oz, 2001; Aaronson *et al.*, 2003; Miller, 2003).

### Nutritional Status

*Class IIb Recommendation.*   Cachexia should be considered as a strong risk factor for MCSD implantation (Level of Evidence: C).

*Background.*   Cardiac cachexia is a syndrome characterized by a striking weight loss, leading to a body mass index (BMI) of $<21$ kg/m$^2$ in males and $<19$ kg/m$^2$ in females. Heart failure patients may be characterized by the presence of anorexia, early satiety, weight loss, weakness, anemia, and edema. These features occur to a variable extent in different patients, and may change in severity during the course of a patient's illness. The cachexia syndrome in advanced heart failure patients with low $VO_2$ peak is a strong independent indicator of dismal prognosis (Anker *et al.*, 1997).

## *Multiorgan Failure*

*Class III Recommendation.*    Multiorgan failure should be considered as a strong contraindication to MCSD implantation (Level of Evidence: C).

*Background.*    Multiorgan failure is defined as a multiple, progressive end-organ dysfunction with critical, unmanagable impairment of vital functions linked to the central nervous system, kidney, liver, and lung. It is almost invariably associated with a poor post-MCSD implantation outcome (Stevenson *et al.*, 2001; Deng *et al.*, 2005a).

## *Malignancies*

*Class IIb Recommendation.*    Patients with potentially curable tumors may undergo MCSD implantation as a potential bridge to heart transplantation (Level of Evidence: C).

*Background.*    Whereas active malignancies are an absolute contraindication to heart transplantation, in selected cases mechanical support can be utilized either to extend life expectancy so as to allow proper oncological treatment before transplantation (Williams and Oz, 2001) or as a destination therapy.

## *Psychiatric Conditions*

*Class I Recommendation.*    A thorough psychiatric examination should be performed to determine potential psychiatric risk factors and contraindications for MCSD implantation. Specifically, patients with a significant psychiatric history, alcoholism, or drug addiction should be referred to a psychiatrist and/or therapist as early as possible to ensure that proper treatment is initiated or optimized (Level of Evidence: C).

*Class III Recommendation.*    Active psychiatric disease is a contraindication for MCSD implantation, as many psychiatric conditions can lead to noncompliance (Level of Evidence: C).

*Background.*  The patient's psychiatric history should be explored in detail. Any history of depression, anxiety, or suicide attempts should be documented (Dew *et al.*, 2001a; Dew *et al.*, 2001b). Patients with a positive psychiatric history or concerning symptoms should be referred to a psychiatrist and/or therapist as early as possible to ensure that proper treatment is initiated or optimized. Methods of coping with stress and illness should be discussed to enable the transplant team to adjust the care for each patient's needs. Standardized testing such as the Minnesota Living with Heart Failure Questionnaire or the Sickness Impact Profile should be administered if possible, as this may give more objective information regarding patient coping skills.

Patients and their care providers should be referred to available support groups (Dew *et al.*, 2001a; Dew *et al.*, 2001b; Grady *et al.*, 2002; Grady *et al.*, 2003; Savage, 2003). An assessment should be done to determine if the patient has a history of substance abuse, specifically a history of tobacco, alcohol, or drug abuse. If the patient is already involved in a recovery program, the continuation of this should be highly encouraged. If the patient is not presently in a recovery or drug rehabilitation program, this should be mandated. Referral to a substance abuse expert should be made as an adjunct to therapy.

## Nursing Care Aspects of Nutritional Status

The impact of inadequate nutrition is crucial for MCSD implantation outcome (Butler *et al.*, 2005). Cachexia is a strong independent risk factor in patients undergoing MCSD placement as a bridge to transplant (Mustafa and Leverve, 2001). Additionally, implantation of an intracorporeal pump such as the Thoratec HeartMate® or Novacor LVS can cause problems with persistent ileus and early satiety, which further limit the ability to improve nutrition.

It is recommended that a thorough nutritional evaluation be undertaken preoperatively (Baudouin and Evans, 2003; Sabol, 2004; Thoratec, 2004). The main goals of a preoperative nutritional plan are to promote surgical wound healing, optimize immune function, and improve the macronutrient and micronutrient substrates (Baudouin and Evans, 2003). The restoration and maintenance of protein stores also facilitate anticoagulation management with warfarin for patients on LVADs that require anticoagulation. The following should be included in a preop work-up:

### Nutritional Assessment

1. A thorough history should be taken of dietary habits and current assessment of bowel motility. This should be documented for patients who have a history of previous abdominal surgery or malabsorption syndromes (Sabol, 2004).
2. Prealbumin, albumin, and transferrin should be measured with weekly follow-ups until nutritional goals are reached (Sabol, 2004).
3. Work-up for diabetes (Hb $A_{1C}$) and tight control of blood sugar are recommended (DiNardo *et al.*, 2004; Van den Berghe *et al.*, 2001).

### Optimization of Nutritional Status

1. Consider formal nutritional consultation for patients who are significantly cachectic, obese, or diabetic, or who have significant renal dysfunction.
2. Include micronutrient supplements such as multivitamin, folate, zinc sulfate, and vitamin C (the latter to facilitate wound healing) (Sabol, 2004).
3. Institute enteral feedings preoperatively in selected cases (Mustafa and Leverve, 2001; Baudouin and Evans, 2003).

### Other Considerations

1. Measure C-reactive protein preoperatively and at postoperative intervals to monitor changes in inflammatory response (Mustafa and Leverve, 2001).

2. Use indirect calorimetry or other metabolic studies to better define caloric needs (Sabol, 2004).
3. Institute parenteral nutrition if the enteral route is not feasible (Thoratec, 2004).
4. Continue follow-ups with formal nutritional consultants as indicated.

## Social, Family, Religious, and Personal Issue Assessments

In order to help determine whether patients receiving MCSD therapy have adequate family/social support, a detailed psychosocial evaluation should be completed. This should be performed by social workers familiar with VAD therapy and the heart transplant process. The patient and his or her family/social support should be involved in the evaluation, although the patient may be too ill to be an active part of this process. Demographic information should be obtained, including distance from home to transplant center and emergency contacts. The names of the patient's family and social supports should be obtained. Documentation of the primary support person should be established (Andrus *et al.*, 2003). An evaluation of patient and family support understanding of past medical history and the present medical situation should be obtained (Gordon and Shore, 2000). This assessment may provide insight into past history of compliance. The primary language and educational level should be established in order to guide teaching. Perceptions about VAD therapy and transplant should be explored. The data gathered will yield important information that will identify potential barriers and transfer to educational goals for possible discharge to home.

Marital status and personal relationships should be assessed, including the length and quality of the relationship (Gordon and Shore, 2000; Richenbacher and Seemuth, 2001). This evaluation should also include a discussion on how difficult situations or problems were handled in the past. Additional family/support systems should be established, as the primary caregiver may need assistance (Grady *et al.*, 2002; Grady *et al.*, 2003).

The patient's cultural background and religious beliefs should be obtained. Beliefs/background may provide another source of social support and may also alert the team of a patient's wishes not to undergo particular treatments. A complete assessment of the patient's financial situation should also be performed. Insurance and prescription coverage or charity care initiatives must be thoroughly established in order to determine if the patient has adequate financial support to undergo VAD therapy and heart transplantation (Gordon and Shore, 2000). End-of-life issues should be discussed with the patient and his/her social support prior to VAD implantation. An advanced directive and/or healthcare proxy should be completed if possible. The assessment of patient and social support should be ongoing, as stressors may change the dynamics and willingness of family/friends to provide continued support. This should be done on a monthly or as-needed basis (Gordon and Shore, 2000).

## BRIDGE-TO-TRANSPLANTATION MECHANICAL CIRCULATORY SUPPORT

| | |
|---|---|
| **Jill (partner of Robert R, born 1947)** <br><br> **Heart transplant is coming up** | After some "dry runs", he got his new heart. In true Rob's fashion, he drove himself to his own transplant. We had just 2 hours to get from our home in Pennsylvania to the hospital, and the low-battery alarm went off as we crossed the George Washington Bridge. He wouldn't stop for me to reach over and change them. "Great", I thought, "he is going to die before we get there." But we made it, and to this day I am in awe of his courage that night. I asked him how he could be so calm, and his answer was, "I am an engineer, Jill. It is very logical. I see the problem, I know what has to be done, and I'm going to do it." |

### Indications for MCSD Implantation as a Bridge to Heart Transplantation

The indications for bridge-to-transplantation (BTT) MCSD therapy are similar to the evaluation scheme for heart transplantation. BTT MCSD therapy is often recommended when the clinical progression of a patient listed for heart transplantation requires additional positive inotropes and an upgrade of medical urgency status. In this situation, the team faces the challenge of deciding between two recommendations to the patient: continue optimal medical therapy as a bridge to transplant, or switch to the more invasive but also more powerful mechanical circulatory support as a bridge to transplantantion. The current ISHLT guidelines, published in 2006, recommend the following strategy (Mehra *et al.*, 2006).

***Class I Recommendation.***    MCSD therapy should be considered when the patient on the heart transplantation waiting list requires incremental increases of inotropic or diuretic drug doses or additional parenteral agents, or when deterioration in status (including signs of end-organ dysfunction) occurs despite these changes (Level of Evidence: C).

*Background.*    The use of inotropic therapy — specifically the use of dopamine, dobutamine, and phosphodiesterase inhibitors (milrinone and enoximone) — should be reserved for patients with refractory symptoms of heart failure and impending organ dysfunction as a consequence of the heart failure syndrome, typically for a low-output state. It has become increasingly clear that the use of dobutamine and milrinone/enoximone has long-term adverse effects on survival (Cuffe *et al.*, 2002). However, it is also clear that these drugs are in the short term effective in improving hemodynamics, leading to a reversal of end-organ dysfunction. It is not clear if the elective move toward MCSD therapy in a stable heart transplant candidate awaiting transplantation on chronic inotropic therapy is indicated.

***Class I Recommendation.***    Weaning from inotropes should be attempted when stable clinical conditions are achieved, but repeated withdrawal should be avoided if dependence is well established (Level of Evidence: C).

*Background.*    Most patients treated with inotropic and/or vasodilator drugs respond with an improvement in symptoms and the resolution of the end-organ effects of the low cardiac output state, specifically improvements in renal or liver function. The failure to achieve these goals may be an indication for mechanical circulatory support. For patients responsive to inotropic therapy, a period of slow weaning from inotropes is mandatory to reduce the risk of long-term inotropic therapy. Failure to wean from inotropes may be defined as (1) a recurrence of symptoms (shortness of breath refractory to diuretics, hypotension, and/or hypoperfusion); and/or (2) a declining urinary output and a progressive rise in the BUN and creatinine.

*Class IIa Recommendation.* MCSD therapy should be considered as a useful strategy to bridge patients to heart transplantation for patients who are not considered as transplant candidates due to the degree and persistence of pulmonary hypertension despite inotropic therapy (Level of Evidence: C).

*Background.* High pulmonary vascular resistance, which limits heart transplantation indication, may persist under inotropic therapy. Complete unloading of the left ventricle by MCSD implantation may lead to a reversal of high-resistance pulmonary hypertension, thus allowing heart transplantation.

*Class IIa Recommendation.* In challenging clinical cases where it is hard to discriminate between HF progression and the unfavorable effect of medical therapy, it is reasonable to perform right heart hemodynamic assessment to verify a patient's volume status and cardiac output in order to tailor inotropic drug doses if prolonged administration is being considered (Level of Evidence: C). It is reasonable to consider right heart hemodynamic assessment to demonstrate or establish an association of clinical and biochemical markers with measured hemodynamic deterioration following the withdrawal of inotropic therapy (Level of Evidence: C).

## BRIDGE-TO-RECOVERY MECHANICAL CIRCULATORY SUPPORT

The indications for bridge-to-recovery MCSD therapy are based on the concept of an acute, severe, and likely reversible cause of myocardial dysfunction in the presence of an otherwise well-maintained biological situation. Typical situations include acute inflammatory (myocarditis, post-cardiotomy low-output syndrome) or ischemic insults (large heart attacks) to the myocardium in a patient who is otherwise in good health. Currently, there are no validated predictors of recovery.

The group at Duke University examined a large national clinical database to assess trends in the incidence of post–cardiac surgery shock requiring VAD implantation, survival rates, and risk factors of mortality. They identified patients undergoing MCSD implantation after cardiac surgery at US hospitals participating in the Society of Thoracic Surgeons' National Cardiac Database during the years 1995–2004. Baseline characteristics and operative outcomes were analyzed in 2.5-year increments. Logistic regression modeling was performed to provide risk-adjusted operative mortality and morbidity rates. A total of 5735 patients had an MCSD placed during the 10-year period (0.3% cardiac surgeries).

The overall survival rate to discharge following MCSD placement was 54.1%. Risk-adjusted mortality declined from 58.1% during the earliest period of the study (January 1995–June 1997) to 39.1% during the latest period of the study (July 2002–December 2004) ($P < 0.0001$). Likewise, risk-adjusted combined mortality/morbidity decreased from 3.1% to 60.6% over the same time periods ($P < 0.0001$). Perioperative characteristics associated with increased mortality were urgency of procedure, reoperation, renal failure, myocardial infarction, aortic stenosis, female gender, race, peripheral vascular disease, NYHA class IV, cardiogenic shock, left main coronary stenosis, and valve procedure (c-index = 0.756). The authors concluded that, after adjustment for the clinical characteristics of patients requiring mechanical circulatory support, the rates of survival to hospital discharge have improved dramatically. Insertion of an MCSD for post–cardiac surgery shock is an important therapeutic intervention that has saved the lives of the majority of these patients (Hernandez *et al.*, in press).

## DESTINATION MECHANICAL CIRCULATORY SUPPORT

### Evaluation for Destination Mechanical Circulatory Support

*Center Infrastructure.* Mechanical circulatory support therapy, specifically alternative-to-transplantation (ATT) or destination MCSD implantation, requires a sophisticated infrastructure within an established heart failure/heart transplantation center. Within this context, it has been shown that early referral for evaluation improves survival (Morris *et al.*, 2005). This infrastructural requirement — as reflected by the US Joint Commission on Accreditation of Healthcare Organizations (http://www.jcaho.org) — states that destination MCSD centers need to fulfill certain eligibility criteria to obtain certification for mechanical support implantation, including having Medicare; having an approved heart failure facility; having a faculty that is an active, continuous member of the national audited registry, which requires submission of health data on all MCSD implantations with destination intention from the date of implantation through the remainder of the patient's life; and actively practicing at a heart transplant facility or currently approved MCSD treatment center. These considerations are important not only to optimize the benefit from MCSD implantation for the patient population, but also to maintain an optimal cost:benefit ratio. The cost of long-term MCSD implantation is commensurate with other life-saving organ transplantation procedures (Digiorgi *et al.*, 2005).

## Current Destination MCSD Indications

Indications for destination or lifetime MCSD therapy are based on the concept of a chronic, severe, irreversible cause of myocardial dysfunction in the presence of an established contraindication to cardiac transplantation, but an otherwise overall maintained medium-term life expectancy. The ISHLT guidelines recommend the following criteria (Mehra *et al.*, 2006).

*Class I Recommendation.*   Elective MCSD implantation as destination therapy should be considered in nontransplant candidates who are dependent on the chronic administration of intravenous inotropes to maintain a stable state (Level of Evidence: B).

*Class III Recommendation.*   Metastatic tumors should be considered as an absolute contraindication to mechanical support (Level of Evidence: C).

*Class IIb Recommendation.*   Despite the presence of a malignancy when a life expectancy of greater than 2 years is foreseeable, mechanical assistance may be considered as a destination therapy (Level of Evidence: C).

*Background.* Elective MCSD therapy has been performed with LVAD implantation in patients with severe functional impairment despite maximum medical therapy (including inotropic support), but with a relatively stable status. This definition excludes patients receiving ventilatory support, ultrafiltration, or percutaneous mechanical support, or patients showing signs of progressive end-organ damage or multiorgan failure due to heart failure. However, there is very little information available to help determine the optimal time for the recommendation of elective device therapy as a bridge to transplantation.

Most of the experiences with MCSD have been gained from the implantation of devices in patients who were critically ill in the ICU. The listed relevant issues for MCSD implantation as a bridge to heart transplant also apply to patients considered for destination therapy. In order to define the nontransplant patient population that will benefit the most from elective LVAD (left ventricular assist device) therapy, it is important to determine the prognosis of patients with advanced, refractory heart failure. The best description of survival in this population is the analysis of the Randomized Evaluation of Mechanical Assistance for the Treatment of Congestive Heart Failure (REMATCH) clinical trial, where patients were randomized to either medical therapy or the placement of a Thoratec Heart-Mate® I LVAD. The survival rates for patients on chronic inotropic therapy ($n = 91$) were only 39% and 24% vs. 60% and 49% in the LVAD group at 6 months and 12 months, respectively. In contrast, in patients with refractory heart failure who did not require chronic inotropic therapy ($n = 38$), survival at 6 months and 12 months was 67% and 40%, respectively.

Thus, the REMATCH data support the premise that patients with refractory heart failure not on inotropic therapy have a similar survival to patients receiving LVAD support (Stevenson *et al.*, 2004). These data relate to an older population (average age 68 years) than that of heart transplant candidates with severe heart failure symptoms (NYHA functional class IV), and provide the evidence to generate recommendations on LVAD therapy as a destination therapy.

## Columbia University Medical Center Criteria for Destination MCSD Implantation (July 2003)

### Inclusion Criteria for First Device Implant

1. Inotrope-dependent
   a. Failed first weaning attempt
2. Tolerating maximum medical therapy with $VO_2 < 10$ (if not able to tolerate beta-blockers, then $VO_2 < 12$)

### Exclusion Criteria for First Device Implant

1. Renal dysfunction
   a. Cr >3.0
   b. Dependent on dialysis, including continuous venous-venous hemodialysis
2. Hepatic failure
   a. INR >2.5
   b. ALT, AST >3X control
3. BMI <18 and >35, or BSA ≤1.5
4. FEV1 <1 without intrinsic lung disease
5. PVR >8 wood units (WU)
6. Severe right ventricular dysfunction with expectation for right ventricular support
7. Neuro Mini-Mental exam score of <20
8. High surgical risks (i.e. ascending aorta calcification), ≥ two cardiac surgeries
9. Previous neurological event with significant residual shunt
10. Comorbidity with life expectancy of <2 years (i.e. malignancy)
11. Acute condition (gastrointestinal bleeding, infection, etc.)
12. Severe peripheral vascular disease
13. Heparin-induced thrombocytopenia (HIT)

### Inclusion Criteria to Replace Pump

1. Young age
2. Acute device malfunction in fully functional patient

3. Patient with a curable disease
4. High potential for recovery
5. Expected survival of >2 years

### Exclusion Criteria to Replace Pump

1. Infected patient unable to withstand another surgery
2. Multisystem organ failure
3. Irreversible neurological dysfunction
4. Development of comorbidity that would limit survival of <2 years
5. Poor support system
6. Other high surgical risks

## DIFFERENTIAL INDICATIONS BY MCSD TYPE

### Advanced Heart Failure: Phenotype and Support Duration as Major Criteria

For bridge-to-recovery and bridge-to-transplant indications, left ventricular or biventricular assist devices that have the potential of full support and unloading of the left or left/right ventricle and that can be placed intracorporeally or paracorporeally/extracorporeally are being used. The intracorporeal position is advantageous for patients with a typical waiting time in the range of months, because it allows for a potentially more complete reversal of secondary organ dysfunction and a higher quality of life. For destination indications, only left ventricular (not biventricular) assist devices that have the potential of either full or partial support and that can be placed intracorporeally are being used.

The vision of the entire community is to have a completely implantable MCSD available. The future perspective on MCSD design is discussed in chapter 6. These differential MCSD recommendations are widely overlapping. For example, the discussion on whether AHF does better with complete unloading (pulsatile MCSD: HeartMate I/Novacor) or partial unloading (low-pulsatile MCSD: DeBakey/HeartMate II/Jarvik 2000) is unresolved (Klotz *et al.*, 2004). The recommendation also depends on institutional availability and on the surgeon's team's experience.

## Uncertainty Principle of Destination vs. Bridging Intention

Guidelines for destination MCSD indicators are based on the REMATCH experience (Rose *et al.*, 2001). The current criteria at Columbia are sum-marized above. Mechanical cardiac support with ventricular assist devices is an established therapy for a variety of clinical scenarios, including postcardiotomy shock, bridge to transplant, and destination therapy. At present, device development, clinical trial design, regulatory approval, and reimbursement decisions for the clinical application of mechanical cardiac support devices continue to be considered in the context of these clinical indications. Although understandable from a historical perspective, these arbitrary divisions are inconsistent with the clinical realities of advanced heart failure therapy. By narrowly focusing on transplant eligibility at a static point in the clinical course, the current guidelines impede the broader application of ventricular assist device technology to the growing popula-tion of patients who may benefit from this therapy (Felker and Rogers, 2006).

## TEAM RECOMMENDATION

| | |
|---|---|
| **Daughter of Eric G (born 1950)** <br><br> **Evaluation and preparation for MCSD** | My mother, my younger sister, and I waited with baited breath as the seconds ticked by to hear of any news or changes. Nothing was stable anymore. If my father, the most constant, indestructible force in my life, could be unconscious and in such critical condition, then everything was up for grabs. The world as I knew it was about to change, but his world … his world was about to be flipped left, right, and upside down. <br><br> All I really heard when the doctors talked about the LVAD was that my dad would have to be attached to a machine. Oh my God. Oh my God. The tears poured out. Hooked up to a machine? My dad was 54, in great shape, and incredibly active. What kind of life could he possibly have now? Oh my God, please, no, no, no. My father had been unconscious for days now, after what should have been a fatal heart attack. It was overwhelming to me that |

he had no idea what was going on. I hoped that he was having wonderful dreams because when or if he woke up, it would be into the middle of a nightmare. I just wanted him to sit up and ask, "What's for dinner?" (This, by the way, was what my father said to the doctors while he was on the stretcher having his first heart attack, a mild one though it was, 15 years ago. Yup, always the funny guy.)

| | |
|---|---|
| **Daughter of Eric G (born 1950)** **Preoperative consent for MCSD** | The doctors asked for our consent to put my father on the LVAD "just in case". They were going to try and do a bypass, but they wouldn't be able to discern what needed to be done until they opened him up. They sort of explained what the LVAD was, but we all had such faith in my dad's strength that we believed it wouldn't be necessary. However, when the doctors saw his heart, they had no choice. I felt so bad for him. I pitied him. I was so upset for him, or rather for his upcoming struggle. |

It took some time (and sleep) to give me a bit of clarity on the matter. I realized that if he did have to live with the LVAD, well, at least he'd be living — the most important thing, after all. My dad is so inventive and a relentless fighter; I knew he'd figure out a way to deal with the LVAD, both physically and emotionally. In fact, being a computer whiz, he'd probably think it was kind of cool. For the battery packs that he would have to wear if he wanted to be mobile, I imagined him concocting some sort of harness/sling to better carry the weight. And you know what? When my father woke up after the LVAD had given him another chance at life, that's exactly what he did.

## Consensus Processes in the Team

Upon completion of the evaluation, the team has a discussion and comes to a decision on the recommendation that they think is in the best interest of the patient referred for MCSD evaluation. Often, this recommendation requires a multidisciplinary dialog to assess the relative weight of arguments against or in favor of MCSD implantation. A frequently encountered situation is the temptation to accept a patient with borderline elevated risk for MCSD implantation.

The formalization of risk scoring and repeated periodic outcome analyses are critically important to guide this consensus process in the team. At Columbia, we have formalized the process in our heart transplantation conference (Fridays, 7–9 AM) for BTT and BTR candidates, and also in our MCSD conference (Mondays, 8–9 AM) for ATT candidates. In this process, a standardized evaluation form (see Appendix 6) is presented by the patient's advocate, usually the heart failure/heart transplant cardiologist taking care of the patient. This presentation is then followed by a team discussion, a review of scientific evidence applicable to the patient's case, and a team recommendation.

These discussions are sometimes very controversial and may take 15–60 minutes in the 40-person multidisciplinary team. The review process starts from a comprehensive description of the clinical scenario, followed by an evaluation of the psychiatric assessment and recommendations, social evaluation, and financial aspects. Special situations are discussed with specialty leaders (i.e. infectious disease, renal, liver, hematology/oncology). After the discussion, the decision on whether or not the patient should be included as a candidate is made; if so, priority status is determined after team consensus.

## Urgency of MCSD Recommendation (Based on Heart Failure Risk)

To better identify the urgency of the MCSD implant recommendation as well as to risk-stratify patients and estimate their survival benefit from MCSD implantation, the classification scheme proposed by the US Interagency Registry for Mechanical Circulatory Support (INTERMACS) aggregates patients failing medical treatment into seven distinct levels.

*Level 1.* "Crash and burn" indicates that the patient needs a definitive intervention within hours. Patients have refractory life-threatening hypotension with critical organ hypoperfusion.

***Level 2.*** "Sliding on inotropes" patients are those that require a definitive intervention within days, and include those patients with declining function despite intravenous support.

***Level 3.*** "Dependent stability" patients require a definitive intervention electively over a period of weeks. These are patients whose clinical status is stable under inotropic support, but the drugs cannot be discontinued.

***Level 4.*** "Frequent flyer" identifies a subgroup of patients who require a definitive intervention electively over a period of months as long as treatment episodes restore a stable baseline, including nutritional status.

***Level 5.*** "Housebound" denotes patients who are limited to day-to-day living activities predominantly within their house. The time of implantation in these patients is variable and depends on the maintenance of nutrition, organ function, and activity level.

***Level 6.*** Patients are labeled as "walking wounded". The time expected to require MCSD implantation is also variable and depends on the maintenance of nutrition, organ function, and activity level as in Level 5; but patients are comfortable with daily living activities and out-of-house general activities.

***Level 7.*** Patients are stable under medical therapy, with only a mild limitation of clinical activities. Therefore, transplantation or circulatory support may not be indicated.

***Modifier Factors.*** In addition to the levels of classification, the modifier factors "arrhythmia" (refractory/repetitive ventricular tachycardia or fibrillation) and "angina" can denote additional stages for each condition (Stevenson, 2006).

A brief summary of management levels based on the US Interagency Registry for Mechanical Circulatory Support (INTERMACS) is provided below (Table 3).

**Table 3.** Management levels based on the US Interagency Registry for Mechanical Circulatory Support (INTERMACS) (adapted source: Stevenson, 2006).

| Level | Short name | Condition | Site of care | Inotropic support | Time frame |
|---|---|---|---|---|---|
| 1 | Crash and burn | Unstable, uncontrolled | ICU | Yes | Hours |
| 2 | Sliding on inotropes | Unstable, uncontrolled | ICU | Yes | Days |
| 3 | Dependent stability | Unstable, controlled | ICU/Telemetry | Yes | Weeks |
| 4 | Frequent flyer | Stable, controlled | Telemetry/Home | No/Yes | Variable |
| 5 | Housebound | Stable, self-controlled | Home | No/Yes | Variable |
| 6 | Walking wounded | Stable, self-controlled | Home | No | Variable |
| 7 | | Stable, self-controlled | Home | No | Reassess |

# PATIENT DECISION

**Eric G (born 1950)**

**Accepting the LVAD decision**

Somewhere in the fog of semiconsciousness, my family and the medical staff repetitiously explained to me what had happened and the medical treatment that had been given to me. But I don't recall any of it. I do recall being aware of wires and "stuff", perhaps even that something had been implanted in my system to supplant my failed heart. The fact that my heart was so damaged that I now needed a transplant was somehow just part of the scheme. No terror, no panic, no shock, just acceptance: it is what it is. An term unknown to me before this point in time — LVAD — is now my primary focus in life.

**Betty (wife of Abraham M, born 1940)**

**Meeting the LVAD**

The next day, Dr Oz came and sat with my husband and the family, and explained everything to us. He brought an LVAD with him to show my husband what would be going into his body. He went over how the LVAD works, and he made sure to allow my husband to discuss anything that was on his mind. He made him feel how heavy the LVAD was, and he explained that he would have this 3-pound machine in his body. I remember one specific question that Dr Oz asked my husband: "Are you afraid?" Abe answered, "No, you have to trust the doctors and the technology that the LVAD will work." Dr Oz went on to explain to my husband that the LVAD makes a sound and that he wouldn't be able to play poker, because when the machine works harder and faster, you can hear it.

| | |
|---|---|
| **Ed S (born 1956)** **MCSD decision** | It was a pretty tough decision. The doctors and my family told me that it was the next logical step, a necessity. But I was the one who had to have the operation. And the thought of having my rib cage cracked open, having the doctors tap into my heart and aorta to install a 4-lb titanium pump in my chest cavity, was not appealing. I felt like I was a science experiment, and it sparked a bit of fear in me to say the least!<br><br>My doctor, Dr Rachel Bijou, was on her weekend off. I waited until she got back, because I wanted to hear her opinion as to whether I should have the pump installed and where I stood as far as options went. I took a leap of faith and agreed to the operation. The doctors here at Columbia Presbyterian have not steered me wrong, and I have a lot of faith in them. |
| **Ed S (born 1956)** **Evaluation and patient decision** | While I was waiting to have the pump installed, I wasn't lucky enough to have someone who had had an LVAD installed and had recovered come in to see me so as to show me that it worked and that it wasn't as bad as I perceived it to be. I have gone to see a lot of patients awaiting the operation while I've been waiting here in the hospital for my transplant, and they usually light up with a little hope when they see someone walking around and functioning quite well with the pump.<br><br>If you saw me, you'd say that I don't even appear to be sick, which wasn't the case 7 months ago. The way I feel now, I don't think the recovery from the transplant will be as bad as the LVAD because the pump has allowed me to become a lot healthier than I was before. I'm glad I decided to go through with the process because there wasn't much hope any other way. |

**Deborah (mother of Joel L, born 1969)**

**MCSD decision**

Dr Oz was the cardiothoracic surgeon on call that day, and he arrived, examined Joel, and explained Joel's condition of heart failure to us and to Joel. He explained that if Joel continued to fail and a heart was not available, then an LVAD could be implanted in him to augment his failing heart and hopefully keep him alive until a donor could be found. He asked for my permission to use the device and I could not give it. Joel was an adult. He needed to decide for himself if he wanted such a device put in him. He was the one to determine what his quality of life would be like, and whether this was what he could live with. To me, this was all too surreal and I could not deal with such a choice.

Dr Oz spoke with Joel, showed him pictures of the device, and told him that in all probability he would be up and walking with the device; if a heart was not immediately available, Joel could still go home with the device and maybe even go to work. Talk about naiveté. Joel called my niece Gail in and they discussed this. Gail felt strongly that this was Joel's only chance and she told him this, but emphasized that it was ultimately his choice. Within a very short time, his breathing became so labored that he asked for the device to be implanted. Much later, I discussed this time with Joel only to find out that he has no memory of any of this.

**Carl K (born 1939)**

**LVAD experience**

My experience with the LVAD, which was implanted in September 2004, was rather unique. My wife and I did not have an opportunity to familiarize ourselves with the device I was to receive or the surgical procedure involved. I was in the hospital as a result of a PICC-line infection that developed 2 days after its insertion, which was to have a dobutamine drip administered to help my heart failure. While in the hospital on intravenous antibiotics, I began experiencing what I perceived to be fainting spells, but fortunately an episode of rapid and repeated attacks of tachycardia occurred while a doctor on rounds and my wife were in my room.

I remember waking up with approximately 15 people around me and a nurse with paddles both under and above my heart while I was being transported to the intensive care unit. Apparently, I was saved by my defibrillator/pacemaker. My condition was so critical that Dr Naka recommended I have immediate surgery to implant an LVAD as soon as I was stabilized. While its function was explained to me, I really did not take it all in, nor did my wife, and we only discovered the true nature and size of the device after it was implanted.

Our first real exposure to it was when an LVAD nurse came to my room with a tote bag and placed what appeared to be a beating canteen with a snorkel hose on top of my blanket. My first reaction was, "That's inside of me? Take it away!" My wife and I were in a state of shock. Whether or not we would have consented to its installation had we known how it operated and the care required to keep it running is an unanswered question.

The device improved my condition tremendously. For the first time in months, I could walk for extended periods without being out of breath. I could eventually taste my food and generally felt better than I had in at least 3 years. However, the recovery period from the surgery was quite painful. The LVAD was to remain implanted until such time as I could receive a heart transplant, for which I had previously qualified and was at Level 1B.

I subsequently found, while waiting for a new heart, that my wife was very troubled by the device and the possibility that we would lose the electrical power necessary to run the pump. In fact, a problem occurred after about 3 months of usage. I discovered that the manufacturer or distributor of the LVAD had shipped us the wrong strength of solution used for cleaning the vent site in my side. The antiseptic given to me was 3% strength, but it should have been 40%. I attribute this error to the development of a Serratia infection at the site, which could not be cured until I got a new heart.

The LVAD ran effectively for approximately 9 months, when it started to develop warning signals and began to fail.

I was changing batteries every $2\frac{1}{2}$ hours and the alarm (gold wrench) was always on. After many trips back and forth to Columbia Presbyterian, it was determined that I could not be sustained on the LVAD as an outpatient, and I was connected to a pneumatic device to keep the pump operating. Since I was then hospitalized, my transplant status was elevated to 1A, and amazingly after 2 weeks a new heart became available for me.

All in all, I would say that the experience with the LVAD was not the best nor was it the worst that I have ever had.

**Elaine (wife of Carl K, born 1939)**

**Wife's perspective on husband's LVAD**

Carl and I both have living wills and healthcare proxies. I am his proxy. When he was coded and the crash cart came, everyone in the hospital who knew us met me in the waiting area. Our transplant coordinator at the time, Kim Hammond, sat with me along with a chaplain (after sending a priest and a rabbi away). At the time, it wasn't clear if Carl would pull through.

The next day, I was in touch with the transplant coordinator at Robert Wood Johnson in NJ who was advising me not to let an LVAD be implanted and to transport Carl by ambulance to Robert Wood Johnson. In fact, Carl may not remember this, but they brought him a phone outside the operating room and he said it was too late; I know that he wouldn't have wanted to be anywhere but Columbia because he always says "it's the best in the world." So, I went to sit in the cardiac/thoracic ICU and was given a pamphlet with a "happy-face little clock", which is supposed to represent an LVAD — you don't get the big binder of material until the surgery is over. I watched the nurse assigned to him after surgery operate this console and about 27 different bags and bottles going into his neck, groin, chest — every orifice. And I thought, "What have I done? He's on a respirator, so I can't ask him!"

You can ask Rosie about my "training". She'll remember because I was the worst person she ever had to teach. In fact, I refused to learn and said that Carl had to go to a nursing home. I asked what would even happen if there was no one to train, and was told that that had been factored in without even asking me. After a tremendous scene with a nurse named Eileen and Rosie, I stayed away for 3 days.

The day I came back to the hospital, Dr Drusin suggested to Carl to "go on battery and take your wife for a walk." So with the aid of a walker, we crawled around the hospital corridors and I thought, "Isn't this just great!" Carl said he would fake that I knew how to operate the hand pump when I told him he would have to die if the time came that he needed to be hand pumped, as long as I would just agree to change his dressing. So, he took his "test" and we were cleared for discharge (but we really didn't know how to do anything complicated, like changing the controller).

I'll leave out my attempt to hire a public advocate and have the pump removed and my one session of psychotherapy, since I'm sure that you wouldn't want to include this in any paper you write. I was asked to talk to the wife of another patient getting an LVAD, Marjorie HG, and I thought, "What the hell am I supposed to say to her that's positive?" In hindsight, she did much better than I did living with the LVAD, and we intend to stay in touch.

Skipping to the day I brought Carl home and thereafter, I was constantly afraid of the device. Taking a shower was the worst, as was helping him put the batteries in that shower kit pouch. Once when he was in the shower, the nozzle came undone and I heard a tremendous sucking noise, and I was sure we were going to end up in the emergency room because water had gone in it, but it didn't. I bought him a police radio dispatcher belt so he could wear the batteries around his waist, but then his pants fell down, so he stuck with the shoulder holster.

The LVAD to lay people is kind of freakish. People who see Carl now comment on how disturbed they were by the noise the pump made (his hair stylist, tailor, dentist, dermatologist, etc.), and carrying a tote bag with the emergency equipment is a bit much. Once, Carl was at a restaurant and had to change batteries, but realized he had uncharged batteries in the bag, so not knowing how long he had before he was in real trouble, he had to race home. I don't know what would have happened if he was more than a half hour away and don't want to know.

I could go on and on, but I guess you get the drift. I am not an LVAD fan and I would never have one implanted in me. I know they say "never say never", but here it is: Never. Never. Never.

All's well that ends well!

## Patient Decision

In our experience at Columbia, it has been essential that the team's recommendation to the patient is presented as one of at least two options, albeit the team's preferred option. It is also essential that the timeline of the team's expectation for a patient's decision is clearly voiced. Sometimes, there is only a narrow time window of a few days to proceed with the MCSD implantation before the patient becomes too sick. Upon being presented with the team's recommendation or alternative recommendations, the patient — after consulting with family and friends, and often after seeking alternative second opinions — then makes a decision regarding his/her preferred treatment choices.

## Team Behavior If Patient Declines Team Recommendation

Occasionally, a patient will decline MCSD implantation, even though the team recommendation in favor of it is unanimously clear. Importantly, this decision may be influenced by the experience of living with an MCSD as communicated by other patients. This is the reason why this monograph includes vignettes on patients' and relatives' experiences of how living with an MCSD feels. If a patient, after receiving the team's recommendation and complementary information of first-hand experience, declines this option, it is essential that the opinion be respected and the patient not pushed. The patient as the ultimate decision maker on his/her behalf must feel comfortable and accepted by the team, whatever his/her decision is.

# CHAPTER 3
# MANAGEMENT

## PREOPERATIVE SITUATION

**Betty (wife of Abraham M, born 1940)**

**Evaluation for MCSD**

When we arrived at Columbia Presbyterian Hospital, Dr Farr was covering for Dr Simon Maybaum. She made sure she spoke to the whole family. Dr Farr advised us that the committee would decide if Abe would be a candidate for the LVAD. The next day, we were called and told that he was going to be operated on, and that I needed to get there as soon as possible to sign the release form for him to be operated on. We were very happy that they had approved him for the LVAD. We did not know that this was a last resort.

Dr Naka did not want to operate because he thought that there was another factor to Abe's condition, and he was correct. Abe had an infection, so they put the LVAD operation on hold and the group began taking care of Abe to get rid of the infection. Within a few days, he was taken off the respirator and started to come back to himself. He was stable and moved to a regular room. On August 5, we found out that he would have the LVAD operation the next day.

**Deborah (mother of Joel L, born 1969)**

**Preoperative situation**

I was called into his room to say goodbye to him and he was quickly sedated, intubated, and rushed off to the OR. Then the waiting began. We as a family waited on the fifth floor. After many hours, we got pillows and blankets and laid on the floor, trying to sleep. Some time in the early morning, Dr Argenziano (the surgeon who had implanted the LVAD) came to tell us that he was out of surgery, all had gone well, and we could see him briefly in the CTICU. I don't think any of the three of us was prepared for what we were about to see.

115

## Standardized Preparation for MCSD Surgery

When a patient decides to go by the team's decision to have an MCSD implanted, surgery is scheduled. A standardized preparation for the implant surgery is initiated.

The challenge in the preoperative situation is that, on the one hand, conditions that would increase the MCSD implantation procedure risk should be identified and reversed; but on the other hand, heart failure-related conditions that can only be reversed by MCSD implantation should give rise to more urgent MCSD implantation to avoid irreversible multiorgan failure.

Table 4 summarizes the preoperative goals (viewed by organ system) and the associated interventions to maximize the benefit from MCSD implantation.

**Table 4.** Preoperative goals (viewed by organ system) and associated interventions.

| Organ system | Goal | Intervention |
|---|---|---|
| Cardiovascular system | Optimize cardiac output | Tailor inotopes, vasodilators, IABP |
| Respiratory system | Optimize gas exchange | Reverse infections + pulmonary edema; practice with incentive spirometer |
| Renal system | Achieve euvolemia + best possible renal function | Tailure diuretics and nesiritide; minimize nephrotoxic agents |
| Hematology system | Optimize RBC + clotting system | Reverse gastrointestinal bleeding, bone marrow depression, anticoagulation |
| Immune system | Optimize immunocompetence | Treat infection |
| Gastrointestinal system | Optimize nutrition + bowel movements | Offer tailored nutrition + fiber-rich diet |
| Nervous system | Optimize coordination | Offer physical therapy + rehabilitation exercises |
| Psychology | Maximize patients' understanding + consent to MCSD | Offer information (e.g. this book), counseling, support group |
| Metabolism | Optimize hormonal homeostasis | Fine-tune diabetes management |
| Muscle and skeletal system | Optimize strength + flexibility | Offer physical therapy + rehabilitation exercises |

# Pre-MCSD Management

***Experienced Team Setting.***   The period that precedes MCSD implantation is characterized by an intensive follow-up, reassurance, and re-evalution activities. The functionality of all the different organ systems should be assessed, and the optimal timing for MCSD implantation should be identified. Recently, the ISHLT published the first of a monograph series focused on mechanical circulatory support (Frazier and Kirklin, 2006). It can be accessed at www.ishlt.org. It provides general knowledge of MCSD practice.

The key principal component of an MCSD program is the development of a multidisciplinary, experienced team for the evaluation and management of end-stage heart failure, including the selection for cardiac transplantation, home monitoring, and provision of end-of-life care. Team members comprise cardiologists; cardiac surgeons; anesthesiologists; perfusionists; nurses; and other healthcare professionals who have been properly trained and equipped to perform MCSD implantation and all subsequent follow-up device management, patient training, and long-term care. Other components include a formal plan to evaluate, select, and follow patients with MCSDs for destination MCSD therapy; as well as a mandatory collection of detailed information regarding patient selection, baseline risk, and perioperative and long-term outcomes (including specific adverse events and quality-of-life information at regular intervals, and the necessary outpatient facilities for chronic care of MCSD patients and surveillance of MCSD malfunction) (Deng *et al.*, 2003c).

***Staged Approach.***   MCSD implantation should only be considered if a patient develops recurrent heart failure despite having received the standard therapies known to improve outcome and clinical status (Stevenson and Shekar, 2005; Hunt *et al.*, 2005). These therapies include aggressive adherence to a low-salt regimen; avoidance of drugs that may promote the development of a congestive status (i.e. NSAIDs); and use of neurohormonal blockade (including ACE inhibitors, beta-blockers, and aldosterone antagonists), with diuretics being used to reduce fluid overload as needed, bearing in mind that diuretics by themselves have been demonstrated to activate neurohormones. The addition of nitrates with or without hydralazine and the use of resynchronization devices in patients meeting the selection criteria should also be considered. The use of inodilators (like dobutamine or milrinone) with defibrillator backup in ambulatory patients may be helpful to improve the deleterious effect of low cardiac output on end-organ function.

***Appropriate Candidate Selection.***   Of utmost importance is the identification of suitable candidates and the timing for MCSD implantation. The Columbia University MCSD risk score incorporates five variables that are weighed according to the relative risk they impose, namely ventilatory support, postcardiotomy status, previous LVAD surgery, CVP >16, and PT >16 (Rao *et al.*, 2003). The predicted operative mortality rate is 46% for a score of >5 and 12% for a score of ≤5. Several other scoring systems utilizing univariate or multivariate models have been described to predict the outcomes of cardiothoracic surgery and might be useful to improve the risk assessment, but have not been validated within the MCSD context.

***Anemia Management.***   Anemia is often seen in congestive heart failure. It is associated with increased mortality and morbidity and increased hospitalizations. Compared with nonanemic patients, the presence of anemia is also associated with worse cardiac clinical status, more severe systolic and diastolic dysfunction, a higher brain natriuretic peptide level, increased extracellular and plasma volume, a more rapid deterioration of renal function, a lower quality of life, and increased medical costs. The correction of the anemia with subcutaneous erythropoietin or darbepoetin in conjunction with oral and intravenous iron has been associated with an improvement in clinical status, number of hospitalizations, cardiac and renal function, and quality of life. The use of angiotensin-converting enzyme inhibitor and angiotensin receptor blockers in CHF may also inhibit the bone marrow response to EPO, and the hemodilution caused by CHF may cause a low hemoglobin level. Renal failure, cardiac failure, and anemia interact to cause or worsen the cardio-renal anemia syndrome. Adequate treatment of all three conditions slows down the progression of both CHF and chronic kidney insufficiency.

*Preoperative Management of Acute Decompensation in Advanced Heart Failure.* Worsening heart failure may require life-saving organ support in order to prevent or reverse organ failure, including the following:

- Intra-aortic balloon pump (IABP)
- Respirator therapy
- Continuous venovenous hemofiltration (CVVH)
- Blood/platelet transfusions
- Complex antimicrobial therapy

## INTRAOPERATIVE SITUATION

| Betty (wife of Abraham M, born 1940) MCSD surgery | The next morning, Friday, August 6, Abe was taken in and was given an LVAD. Dr Naka and Dr Oz performed the operation. In the middle of the night, they retook Abe into the OR because he was getting blood clots near his lungs. Dr Naka performed the operation, after which Abe started doing better. A few days later, Abe had arrhythmias and needed to be given the paddles. Had he not had the LVAD … well, let's just say thank God he had the LVAD prior to the arrhythmias. |
|---|---|

Intraoperatively, a standardized interdisciplinary anesthesiological and cardiosurgical approach is applied. With respect to the detailed techniques, we refer to excellent textbooks on cardiac anesthesia and cardiac surgery (Kirklin and Barratt-Boyes, 1992). Challenges during the preoperative anesthesia induction period include the avoidance of abrupt and excessive hypotension. Sometimes, the institution of preoperative IABP support is necessary to allow for a safe transition to long-term MCSD support.

During the intraoperative period, major challenges include the surgical treatment of adhesions related to previous surgical interventions that increase the surgical time and risk of bleeding complications. The heart-lung machine weaning period constitutes the major challenge after completion of the surgical implantation. Specifically, persistent pulmonary hypertension requires a proactive, pre-emptive institution of pulmonary vasodilators (including inhaled nitric oxide) (MacDonald *et al.*, 1998) and/or positive inotropes (including milrinone and dobutamine).

## POSTOPERATIVE SITUATION

| | |
|---|---|
| **Jill (partner of Robert R, born 1947)** **MCSD surgery** | I cannot begin to tell you how difficult it was waiting all that time for Robert to be conscious enough for me to tell him that he had 8 lbs of titanium in his chest, and the best way I could describe it was that it looked like a water pump from an old car! Those were anxious days in more ways than one. Would he be angry? Would he be outraged? What would he be? As it turned out, he took the news quite well. I was much impressed and greatly relieved. |
| **Betty (wife of Abraham M, born 1940)** **Post-MCSD recovery** | After that, he began to improve. One day, we asked Dr Maybaum how he was doing and he said, "Because of the LVAD, we have rolled back 4 years of his heart's deterioration." After a while, he was able to go to rehabilitation. Abe was a new person. Physically, he was able to get his body back in shape. Although he was tethered to the machine and batteries, he was able to move around. I can't tell you that it wasn't scary and that we didn't have any questions. |
| **Ed S (born 1956)** **Postoperative recovery** | I had the HeartMate installed on September 20, 2004. It was definitely not a walk in the park. I had never been sicker in my entire life before I had the operation; I was death warmed over! I was knocked down even lower after I had the procedure. My recovery was slow and painful. I needed 4 mg of morphine as needed to overcome the pain for about 2 months after the operation. I had trouble sleeping for a while after getting the pump. I've seen other patients who had the operation recover faster than myself, patients slightly older than myself. I turned 48 years old here in the hospital. I was given a box of Cheerios as a birthday present from the nursing staff! It took quite a while, but after 3 months or so the pain completely subsided. |

**Deborah (mother of Joel L, born 1969)**

**Postoperative situation**

Joel was hooked up to so many monitors and machines. He was intubated, and IVs were running into veins and arteries in his extremities and neck. Various machines were bleeping and blinking. And then there was the LVAD. This bigger-than-a-bread-box black box that had wires going into a wound in Joel's abdomen, whooshing and clicking; each whoosh and click keeping my beautiful son alive. I found myself staring at the machine, watching the digital read-out count beats and whatever else it counted. For the next 2 months, I guarded that machine, making sure no one touched it or tripped over its cord, looking at it as the essence of Joel's life.

Joel was a competitive cyclist before the myocarditis and he was extremely strong. He was able to ride 100 miles on his bike in the daytime and still go to work in the afternoon for a full 8 hours without missing a beat. He could carry in one hand things that took two men to carry. His postop nurse was a tiny Filipina and, although he was unconscious, he grabbed her and threw her across the room. Those first 24 hours, I delighted in his grabbing my hand and squeezing it until it blanched and I struggled to free myself. I would walk from one side of the bed to the other to have him grab at me. Joel was still unconscious and intubated, but I was assured that this was within normal range.

On the second day, I noticed that he was no longer grabbing with his left hand. I checked his reflexes on his left foot and found no reaction. I quickly called the staff, and after a gross examination he was taken for a CT scan, where it was horribly discovered that he had suffered an ischemic stroke. Oh God! My son! Paralyzed, unconscious, unresponsive, being kept alive by an ominous black box. Who was inside that body? Would Joel want to continue being that person? By now, his medical team had expanded to include neurologists and nephrologists. He was still not voiding. His creatinine was dangerously high and he was put on continuous dialysis. He was still unresponsive and unconscious. The neurologists called for another CT scan because they felt that he may have suffered another stroke.

The only sign of responsiveness Joel showed was to grimace in pain. I cried and prayed for him. I asked God to give him the strength to come back from all this, to wake up, to speak, to live, to just be Joel. Alicia and I sat for hours in the waiting room talking to other families and asking everyone to pray for Joel, as we would pray for their family members. I asked strangers on the street to please pray for him.

The CT scan showed that there was no further progression of the stroke, and all that was needed was time for him to regain consciousness. One morning, I walked into the room and saw a crash cart in his room. I turned to his medical student and asked why this was being stored in Joel's room, and he told me that Joel had to be cardioverted during the night. I remember falling into the wall and crying out with the realization that Joel was going to die. No one could assure me that this would not happen. No one knew and Joel was unconscious. In my mind, Joel was unconscious for weeks, but in reviewing his chart at a later date it seems that it was less than 2 weeks. Not for his family it wasn't; for us, it was an eternity.

I remember coming in one morning and finding him awake. He was still intubated and was not focused, but he was awake. We still did not know who was in Joel's body, and he was giving us no indication that he could think or recognize. Multiple times over the course of the next few days, the staff tried to extubate him, but he would bite down on the tube and they could not get his jaw to open. I am not sure when he was finally extubated, but it was a huge milestone. But even then, he would not speak, nor did he appear to know who we were or what was happening.

Finally, on a Sunday, with our dear Reb Terry present, he spoke his first words. I asked him as I did daily, "Do you know who I am?" "You are effing mom," he said. Yes, effing; not fucking because Joel did not swear: effing. That's Joel. He was there inside that poor, weak body, hooked up to all those machines, paralyzed, confused and scared, in pain; but Joel nonetheless.

I was overjoyed. If he never walked again, I would take care of him forever. I had my son back. But I had him tethered to that box, the LVAD. Although Joel was such a strong man, he is not a large man and the LVAD was really too big for his body. It constantly caused him pain. It took up too much space inside him and he was unable to eat more than one bite at a time. Not being able to move his left side made it impossible for him to get out of bed, but I am not sure that he could have anyhow. The device was causing him too much discomfort.

He was losing weight daily. His weight when he arrived at the hospital was somewhere around 155–160 pounds; by the end of March, it was around 103. He would feel hungry and ask that we bring him sandwiches and treats, and Alicia and I would gladly bring them in only to have him take one bite and stop eating. His body was breaking down and his heart was quickly failing.

## General Principles of Postoperative Management After MCSD Implantation

Postoperatively, a standardized multidisciplinary approach represented by an interdisciplinary team composed of cardiothoracic surgeons, anesthesiologists, cardiologists, nurses, physiotherapists, social workers, and other experts is utilized. In the REMATCH study (Rose *et al.*, 2001), the most common adverse events during the trial were bleeding, infection, neurological dysfunction (stroke, TIA, and toxic metabolic encephalopathy), supraventricular arrhythmias, peripheral embolic events, sepsis, local infection, renal failure, and hepatic failure.

## Postoperative Cardiac Management

*Inflammatory Mediator Release.* Within the context of MCSD implantation, a dramatic inflammatory mediator release contributes to the perturbation of cardiovascular and immune homeostasis. While end-stage heart failure patients show immunological alterations compared to controls, patients who are undergoing MCSD implantation exhibit a more pronounced activation of inflammatory markers. This may be due to more advanced heart failure, but the device itself may also contribute to more pronounced inflammation and a temporary suppression of immunocompetent cells (Deng *et al.*, 1999a).

***Cardiovascular Management Goals.***   The main goal during postoperative care management is to optimize end-organ perfusion by ensuring adequate preload, afterload (systemic vascular resistance), contractility, and rhythm, maintaining synchrony between the native ventricle and pulsatile devices to optimize cardiac output. Special considerations should be given to the specific MCSD types in management decisions. The occurrence of cardiac tamponade, as is usual in cardiac periperative situations, may constitute an emergency and require immediate intervention.

## Postoperative Pulmonary Management

Postoperative. pulmonary complications, including pneumonia, bronchospasm, respiratory failure, and prolonged mechanical ventilation, occur commonly and are a significant source of morbidity and mortality. General anesthesia, surgery, and immobility produce changes in the respiratory system and are responsible (along with underlying conditions) for postoperative pulmonary complications. Patients undergoing MCSD implantation often have underlying illnesses, such as intrinsic lung disease (e.g. chronic obstructive pulmonary disease) and pulmonary dysfunction secondary to congestive heart failure, that increase their susceptibility to postoperative respiratory support dependence.

Other risk factors for respiratory failure include upper abdominal or thoracic surgery, chronic respiratory disease, emergency surgery, prolonged anesthetic time, age, renal failure, poor nutritional status, and significant intraoperative blood loss. The inhibition of phrenic nerve output results in postoperative diaphragmatic dysfunction (Weissman, 2004). The implementation of ventilatory support with lower tidal volumes to protect alveoli from pressure damage is related to improved outcomes, and the routine preoperative use of incentive spirometry decreases the rates of postoperative pulmonary complications and hospital lengths of stay in patients undergoing open cardiac surgery.

## Postoperative Renal Management

The risk of perioperative renal dysfunction is extremely high in this group of patients. A wide variety of nephrotoxic insults may also be presented, including antifibrinolytic agents, obstructive jaundice, prostaglandin inhibitors, radiocontrast dyes, and volatile anesthetic agents. Serial decline in creatinine clearance estimation, a measure of the glomerular filtration rate, is the most reliable clinical indicator of progressive renal dysfunction (Sladen, 2000; Byers and Sladen, 2001). Whether the implementation of continuous/intermittent dialysis/ultrafiltration or low-volume continuous hemodiafiltration has excess benefit as an effective strategy to remove fluid excess and inflammatory mediators is controversial.

Most recently, a French prospective multicenter study compared the effect of intermittent hemodialysis and continuous venovenous hemodiafiltration on survival rates in critically ill patients with acute renal failure as part of multiple-organ dysfunction syndrome. Patients in 21 medical or multidisciplinary intensive care units from university or community hospitals in France between October 1, 1999, and March 3, 2003, were included in the study. Guidelines were provided to achieve optimum hemodynamic tolerance and effectiveness of solute removal in both groups. The two groups were treated with the same polymer membrane and bicarbonate-based buffer. A total of 360 patients were randomized, and the primary endpoint was 60-day survival based on an intention-to-treat analysis. The survival rate at 60 days did not differ between the groups [32% in the intermittent hemodialysis group vs. 33% in the continuous renal replacement therapy group (95% CI, $-8.8$ to 11.1)], or at any other time. The authors concluded that, provided strict guidelines to improve tolerance and metabolic control are used, almost all patients with acute renal failure as part of multiple-organ dysfunction syndrome can be treated with intermittent hemodialysis (Vinsonneau *et al.*, 2006).

## Postoperative Hematological/Coagulation Management

Patients undergoing cardiopulmonary bypass (CPB) are at risk for excessive microvascular bleeding, which often leads to the transfusion of allogeneic blood and blood components as well as re-exploration. Excessive

bleeding after cardiac surgery occurs because of alterations in the hemostatic system pertaining to dilutional thrombocytopenia, excessive hemostatic activation, and exposure to long-acting antiplatelet or antithrombotic
agents. Pharmacological interventions to attenuate the alterations in the
hemostatic system and to reduce excessive bleeding during CPB, transfusion, and re-exploration include the prophylactic administration of agents
with antifibrinolytic and anti-inflammatory properties like aprotinin, which
has potent antifibrinolytic and anti-inflammatory effects. Other agents,
including the lysine analogs with isolated antifibrinolytic properties, may
be effective in low-risk patients.

In a recent prospective observational study involving 4374 patients
undergoing revascularization, three agents [aprotinin (1295 patients),
aminocaproic acid (883), and tranexamic acid (822)] were compared with
no agent (1374 patients) with regard to serious outcomes by propensity
and multivariable methods. In propensity-adjusted, multivariable logistic
regression (C-index, 0.72), the use of aprotinin was associated with a dou-
bling in the risk of renal failure requiring dialysis among patients undergoing complex coronary artery surgery (odds ratio, 2.59; 95% CI, 1.36 to
4.95) or primary surgery (odds ratio, 2.34; 95% CI, 1.27 to 4.31), a 55%
increase in the risk of myocardial infarction or heart failure ($P < 0.001$),
and a 181% increase in the risk of stroke or encephalopathy ($P = 0.001$).
Neither aminocaproic acid nor tranexamic acid was associated with an
increased risk of renal, cardiac, or cerebral events. Adjustment according
to propensity score for the use of any one of the three agents as compared
with no agent yielded similar findings. All of the agents reduced blood
loss. The association between aprotinin and serious end-organ damage indicates that continued use may not be prudent. In contrast, the less expensive
generic medications, aminocaproic acid and tranexamic acid, seem to be
safe alternatives (Mangano *et al.*, 2006).

The ability to reduce blood product transfusions and to decrease operative times and re-exploration rates favorably affects patient outcomes, availability of blood products, and overall healthcare costs. The adequacy of
heparin-induced anticoagulation in the perioperative setting is commonly
controlled by the activated clotting time. This method also indicates the
correct reversal of the heparin effect by protamine. The use of thrombelastography has proved to be valuable for the diagnosis of coagulopathy

associated with cardiac surgery. In addition, the use of thrombelastography-based algorithms has been shown to reduce transfusion requirements. In the future, newer interventions such as recombinant activated factor VIIa might prove to be a therapeutic option in patients with otherwise untractable bleeding, but the efficacy of recombinant activated factor VIIa has yet to be defined for this indication.

## Postoperative Immunological/Infection Management

The clinical success of MCSD implantation has nevertheless been accompanied by complications arising from interactions between the implanted biomaterial and the host immune system. The aberrant state of monocyte and T-cell activation resulting from these host/device interactions is accompanied by two parallel processes: the selective loss of Th1 cytokine producing CD4 T cells through activation-induced cell death; and the unopposed activation of Th2 cytokine producing CD4 T cells, resulting in B-cell hyperreactivity and dysregulated immunoglobulin synthesis through Th2 cytokines as well as heightened CD40 ligand–CD40 interactions. The net result of these events is that the LVAD recipient not only develops progressive defects in cellular immunity and has an increased risk of serious infection, but is also more likely to develop allosensitization, thus posing a significant risk to a successful transplant outcome.

Intravenous immunoglobulin therapy is an effective and safe modality for sensitized LVAD recipients awaiting cardiac transplantation, reducing serum antihuman lymphocyte antigen (HLA) alloreactivity and shortening the duration to transplantation. The therapeutic and safety profiles of intravenous immunoglobulin appear to be superior to that of plasmapheresis. Immunosuppression incorporating intravenous cyclophosphamide before and after transplantation is safe and highly effective in sensitized LVAD recipients of cardiac transplantation. When used after transplantation as part of triple immunosuppressive regimens, cyclophosphamide is superior to mycophenolate mofetil in reducing episodes of allograft rejection in these patients (Itescu and John, 2003; Deng *et al.*, 2005b). Because these immune alterations appear to be related to the effects of excessive biomaterial-associated T-cell activation, future efforts will need to be directed at either altering the physical properties of the materials interacting with the host circulation or conducting pharmacological intervention aimed more selectively at inhibiting T-cell activation (Itescu and John, 2003).

Ventricular-assist-device–related infections are typically caused by Gram-positive microorganisms and are usually *Staphylococcus* species, most frequently *epidermidis* (40%), *aureus* (25%–55%), and *enterococcus*. Gram-negative bacilli — including *Pseudomonas aeruginosa*, *Enterobacter* species, and *Klebsiella* species — can also be implicated and might be associated with a worse outcome. Fungal infections might be found in up to 35% of patient recipients of an assist device, most commonly *Candida* spp. Systemic fungal infection holds the highest infection-related mortality rate, and is frequently related to concomitant bacterial infection treated with broad-spectrum antibiotics (Gordon *et al.*, 2001; Gordon *et al.*, 2006).

Pre-emptive antibiotic prophylaxis is a common practice, most frequently directed to the organisms described above. The prophylaxis therapy used in the landmark REMATCH study is provided in Appendix 3 (Rose *et al.*, 2001; Holman *et al.*, 2004). Empirical treatment of suspected MCSD infections may be initiated early, due to the concurrent multiple medical problems that these patients often carry. After repeated blood cultures and once full diagnostic work has been done, the establishment of an effective therapy should not be delayed. In septic patients, broad-spectrum antibiotics directed to the most common pathogens (Gram-positive, Gram-negative, and fungal) may be started and tailored according to institution-specific microbial resistance patterns, the resistance patterns of any organism previously cultured from the patient (i.e. surveillance cultures), and the patient's antibiotic history. Local infections (including those at the driveline exit site) should cover Gram-positive organisms, while systemic Gram-negative coverage may be added for surgical wound and pump pocket infections. Cultures should always be obtained prior to the initiation of antibiotic therapy, which should be accommodated according to the results of the blood cultures.

Definite treatment of serious MCSD-related infections requires removal of the device and is therefore within the context of heart transplantation, which is a limited alternative. Patients with severe device infection are upgraded to prioritize their status as organ recipients. Urgent (Status 1A) cardiac transplantation is effective in stable patients with device-related bloodstream infections (Gordon *et al.*, 2001; Poston *et al.*, 2001; Poston *et al.*, 2003; Morgan *et al.*, 2003). In this high-risk group, the mortality rates at 30 days and 1 year after transplantation in one study were 14% and 26%, respectively (Poston *et al.*, 2003). Our recommendations on infection management for patients undergoing MCSD implantation are summarized in Appendix 3.

Important considerations for the prevention of infections should also be considered in personnel behavior to prevent the cross-infection of patients by healthcare workers with contaminated hands, which are a major source of infections. Despite educational efforts, healthcare workers (including physicians) continue to fail to adhere to standards for hand hygiene, which is universally considered as the single most important method for infection control. The average level of compliance varies among hospitals from 16% to 81%. Barriers to compliance include understaffing and poor design of facilities, confusing and impractical guidelines and policies, failure to fully apply the behavioral change theory, and insufficient commitment and enforcement by infection-control personnel. Remarkably, the use of waterless antiseptic hand rubs — when part of a multifaceted campaign that encourages appropriate hand washing — has been shown to be more practical than standard hand washing alone, and has been shown to improve the adherence of healthcare workers to hand-hygiene guidelines and to prevent the transmission of methicillin-resistant *S. aureus* to patients.

As a general principle of medical therapy, controlling emergent resistant strains and focusing on the most effective antibiotic therapy with the least adverse effects should always be considered. In general, the use of vancomycin should be avoided in patients infected by methicillin-susceptible staphylococci because this treatment is suboptimal, but methicillin-resistant staphylococci should be covered when the microbiological cause has not yet been identified. If the infected implant is retained or if the response to a single antimicrobial agent is inadequate, then the use of combination antibiotic therapy that includes rifampin for staphylococcal infection may be considered. When performing the second stage of implant replacement, provide antibiotic coverage against organisms isolated during the first surgery. Administer long-term antibiotic therapy if a new implant is placed in a grossly infected area. Common principles of surgical therapy include, when possible, the removal of implants infected by virulent organisms such as *Staphylococcus aureus* and *Candida*, although removal may not be required in the case of infection by less pathogenic coagulase-negative staphylococci.

Regardless of the microbiological cause of infection, removal of the infected implant may be necessary if the patient has not had a response to seemingly appropriate antibiotic therapy. When possible, removal of all the components of an infected implant should be considered to prevent a recurrence of infection. The use of a transesophageal echocardiogram might be useful to identify vegetations related to MCSD endocarditis.

***Sepsis and Multiorgan Failure.***    The management of sepsis in patients with MCSDs should be established early to prevent rapid "burn" of the patient that leads multiorgan failure. Sepsis therapy should follow published guidelines (Dellinger *et al.*, 2004), when applicable to MCSD recipients, by following established emergency care during the first 6 hours after diagnosis and critical care of patients in the later stages. The current management status of sepsis has been very well reviewed elsewhere (Russell, 2006). Based on our experience, patients that are recipients of MCSD devices should be managed within similar general guidelines.

Early-goal–directed therapy should be established during the first 6 hours after diagnosing sepsis. During this period, the focus should be to obtain a central catheter to monitor central venous pressure and oxygen saturation, administer crystalloids to maintain a central venous pressure at 8–12 mm Hg, initiate vassopressors when the mean arterial pressure is less than 65 mm Hg, and order blood transfusions to accommodate hematocrit in the 30s and achieve a central $O_2$ saturation of 70%. If the 70% $O_2$ saturation is not fulfilled, dobutamine should be added according to the published protocol (Rivers *et al.*, 2001). This protocol may not necessarily reflect current practice in MCSD patients, but this is to date the best available evidence for the care of patients with sepsis.

The use of vasopressin to support peripheral vascular resistance during postoperative care and during sepsis is a rational approach (Landry and Oliver, 2001). The baroreflex-mediated secretion of arginine vasopressin has been found to be defective in a variety of vasodilatory shock states, such as postcardiotomy shock, and administration of the hormone markedly improves vasomotor tone and blood pressure. Vasopressin at low doses has been shown to be a safe and effective vasopressor in patients with post-cardiotomy vasodilatory shock (Morales *et al.*, 2000), and did not impair blood flow to any of the vascular beds examined in a single-center study of vasopressin in endotoxic shock when it was used in low doses. However, moderately higher doses of vasopressin may induce ischemia in the mesenteric and renal circulations. The range for exogenous vasopressin in septic shock is narrow and is recommended to be used in a fixed low-dose administration, generally 0.04 units/min and in no case exceeding 0.1 units/min (Malay *et al.*, 2004).

Lung-protective ventilation by using low tidal volumes should be considered, as acute lung injury often complicates sepsis. The use of 6 mL/kg of ideal body weight down to 4 mL/kg if the plateau pressure is greater than 30 cm $H_2O$ has been shown to decrease mortality in patients with acute lung injury (Acute Respiratory Distress Syndrome Network, 2000). To avoid prolonged ventilation and nosocomial pneumonia, daily awakenings by interrupting sedation has been found to be effective (Kress *et al.*, 2000). The use of broad-spectrum antibiotics has already been discussed.

To the best of our knowledge, the goal of activated protein C in this specific group of patients has not yet been evaluated. Therapy with activated protein C has been reported to decrease mortality (Bernard *et al.*, 2001) and ameliorate organ dysfunction (Vincent *et al.*, 2003) in patients with severe sepsis. Activated protein C is approved to be administered to patients with an APACHE II score of $\geq 25$ or with a dysfunction of two or more organs (Ely *et al.*, 2003). Similarly, the use of corticosteroids as well as the role and diagnosis of true/relative adrenal insufficiency are still controversial (Annane *et al.*, 2004).

## Postoperative Gastrointestinal Management

The most frequent serious gastrointestinal complications in patients undergoing cardiac surgery include mesenteric ischemia, diverticulitis, pancreatitis, peptic ulcer disease, and cholecystitis. Predictors of death from GI complications include New York Heart Association (NYHA) class III and

IV heart failure, smoking, chronic obstructive pulmonary disease, history of syncope, liver dysfunction, and hemodynamic support requiring intravenous vasoactive drugs. Mesenteric ischemia is frequently fatal. This complication may be a result of atheroembolization, heparin-induced thrombocytopenia, or hypoperfusion (Mangi *et al.*, 2005).

## Postoperative Metabolic Management

The metabolic changes that occur after cardiac surgery result from a complex interaction between the effects of surgery and extracorporeal circulation *per se*, the inflammatory response to surgical trauma and extracorporeal circulation, the perioperative use of hypothermia, the cardiovascular and neuroendocrine responses characteristic of cardiac surgery, and the drugs and blood products used to support circulation during and after the operation. These changes include, among others, increased oxygen consumption and energy expenditure as well as increased secretion of insulin, growth hormone, adrenocorticotropic hormone, cortisol, epinephrine, and norepinephrine. Other changes include decreased total triiodthyronine levels; hyperglycemia; hyperlactatemia; increased glutamate, aspartate, and free fatty acid concentrations; hypokalemia; increased production of inflammatory cytokines; and increased consumption of complement and adhesion molecules.

Tight control of metabolic abnormalities may improve the patients' outcome. Glucose-insulin-potassium (GIK) solutions have been used in cardiac surgery for more than 40 years. Several studies provide evidence for the beneficial effects of insulin and/or GIK in cardiac surgery that go beyond its metabolic benefits, including better recovery of myocardial tissue after ischemia.

## Postoperative Neurological Management

Neurological complications following cardiac surgery result in increased morbidity and mortality. The current understanding of adverse central nervous system events following MCSD implantation involves several identifiable, evidence-based mechanisms that include atherosclerotic emboli, microgaseous and microparticulate emboli, and hypoperfusion. Secondary factors — including patient comorbidities, individual susceptibilities, systemic inflammatory processes, and a suboptimal metabolic milieu — may interact to potentiate the extent of injury. The incidence of stroke is 2% to 7% depending on the MCSD type, and is higher in patients with a prior history of stroke. The success of off-pump techniques in altering this risk is controversial. Postoperative seizures may result from global or focal cerebral ischemia due to hypoperfusion, particulate or air emboli, or metabolic causes.

## Postoperative Psychiatric Management

The specific characteristics of patients referred for MCSDs because of the terminal condition of their underlying heart failure syndrome pose challenges to psychiatric management after MCSD implantation. The risk of cognitive deficits is debatable, but may be due to factors other than the use of bypass and may not differ from similar deficits after noncardiac surgery. Short-term cognitive deficits are usually resolved by 1–3 months. Long-term risks are not clearly established. Different age groups are affected by different forms of the disease; as a result, patients range from newborn infants to those in their 80s. In recent years, attention has begun to focus on the neurocognitive effects of such surgery (Lazar *et al.*, 2004).

## Postoperative Musculoskeletal/Physiotherapeutic Management

The use of long-acting muscle relaxants in cardiac surgical patients is associated with significant residual neuromuscular block in the intensive care unit, including signs and symptoms. A growing body of evidence from randomized trials has identified many anesthetic interventions that can improve the outcome after cardiac surgery. These include new short-acting hypnotic, opioid, and neuromuscular blocking drugs.

An effective fast-track cardiac anesthesia (FTCA) program requires the appropriate selection of suitable patients, a low-dose opioid anesthetic technique, early tracheal extubation, a short stay in the ICU, and coordinated perioperative care. It is also dependent on the avoidance of postoperative complications such as excessive bleeding, myocardial ischemia, low cardiac output state, arrhythmias, sepsis, and renal failure. These complications have a much greater adverse effect on hospital length of stay and healthcare costs. A number of clinical trials have identified interventions that can reduce some of these complications. The adoption of effective treatments in clinical practice should improve the effectiveness of FTCA. Part of this concept is an active physical and respiratory therapy program. Postoperative goals (viewed by organ system) and associated interventions are summarized in Table 5.

**Table 5.** Postoperative goals (viewed by organ system) and associated interventions.

| Organ system | Goal | Intervention |
|---|---|---|
| Cardiovascular system | Optimize cardiac output<br>Optimize inparallel circuit<br>Avoid regurgitant flow | Tailor inotropes and vasodilators;<br>correct device malfunction;<br>correct aortic regurgitation at the<br>time of MCSD implantation |
| Respiratory system | Optimize gas exchange +<br>early extubation | Use low tidal volume ventilation<br>(prevent alveolar damage); avoid<br>dead space (PEEP and alveolar<br>recruitment maneuvers, including<br>the use of incentive spirometer);<br>prevent/reverse pulmonary<br>infections and edema |
| Renal system | Achieve euvolemia +<br>normal renal function<br>(GFR) | Tailor diuretics; minimize<br>nephrotoxic agents and initiate/<br>finalize hemodialysis when indicated |
| Hematology system | Optimize RBC + clotting<br>system | Reoperate; reverse gastrointestinal<br>bleeding, bone marrow<br>depression, anticoagulation;<br>correct heparin-induced<br>thrombocytopenia |
| Immune system | Optimize<br>immunocompetence | Minimize exposure to external<br>surfaces (i.e. CBP); treat infection;<br>ensure accurate nutritional status |
| Gastrointestinal system | Optimize nutrition +<br>bowel movements | Offer tailored nutrition + fiber-rich<br>diet |
| Nervous system | Optimize coordination | Offer physical therapy +<br>rehabilitation exercises |
| Psychology | Maximize patients'<br>understanding + consent to<br>MCSD | Offer information (e.g. this book),<br>counseling, support group |
| Metabolism | Optimize hormonal<br>homeostasis | Fine-tune diabetes management |
| Muscle and skeletal<br>system | Optimize strength +<br>flexbility | Offer physical therapy +<br>rehabilitation exercises |

# LONG-TERM FOLLOW-UP

| | |
|---|---|
| **Jill**<br>**(partner of**<br>**Robert R,**<br>**born 1947)**<br><br>**Postoperative**<br>**recovery** | As his recovery progressed, we learned how to manage the LVAD, me more so as Robert's short-term memory had been much incapacitated. At 56 years of age, being on the cutting edge of technology was daunting to say the least. I'd only just learned how to use a computer, and I had to be hauled out of the primeval swamps and into the 21st century by my children to do that!<br><br>I read that book from cover to cover. I practiced hand pumping, changing the batteries, identifying alarms, even changing the controller if need be — surely the most awkward set of instructions ever. I began to feel confident; I could manage this. Then came the day that they told me to make arrangements for him to go home; he was going to be discharged. I would have done anything to stay in that hospital. |
| **Jill**<br>**(partner of**<br>**Robert R,**<br>**born 1947)**<br><br>**Discharge**<br>**planning** | The sheer contemplation of going home was a nightmare. I have never felt so alone as I did the day he was discharged. That was when learning to live with the LVAD really began. Just getting used to the noise (surely it was never that loud in the hospital) and sleeping with it. The first night, I was so relieved when I woke up the next morning and he was still alive. |
| **Jill**<br>**(partner of**<br>**Robert R,**<br>**born 1947)**<br><br>**Learning the**<br>**battery supply**<br>**logistics** | But I/we learned, sometimes very fast. I had developed a system to make sure that each day when we left for the office 80 miles away, I had adequate batteries and supplies and Robert's batteries had enough juice in them to get him to the office. I was his driver, and at that time he was still having problems remembering the sequence of events when changing his batteries. Heaven knows I didn't want to fight four lanes of I-80 E traffic to the shoulder to change them. It only happened once. |

| | |
|---|---|
| **Jill**<br>**(partner of**<br>**Robert R,**<br>**born 1947)**<br><br>**Emergency at**<br>**home: power**<br>**outage** | We learned to keep a flashlight by the bed the hard way too. One Saturday night, we were awakened from a sound sleep by the loudest alarm I have ever heard. I fell out of bed and groped for the light switch. Nothing. Total darkness. We realized that a power cut had occurred. Trying to remember which end of the power unit the charged batteries were, I managed to change Robert from the power unit to his batteries. We both fled the room before we went insane.<br><br>I returned to shut off the alarm, but nothing I did worked. I called the hospital, who alerted the person on duty, Margaret Flannery. She suggested other things, but nothing would shut the alarm off. So on her advice, I covered it with pillows and blankets and shut the door. I called the electric company, who I may add had already been advised of Robert's situation. They had assured me that they had heard and inwardly digested what I had said. However, when I reminded them, they had no record of it and the lady on the phone didn't understand what I was saying.<br><br>A car wreck just up the road from us had taken out a power line. So we waited. Robert and the dog went to sleep, I chewed on my fingernails, and Margaret kept checking on the situation. Eventually, after several hours and still no word from the electric company, I called them back. No, they had no idea when the power would be back on. I reiterated that I needed to know. "Why?" she said somewhat exasperatedly, "What will happen if it doesn't?" "He could die," I said. There was a long silence before she said, "I think I better call the foreman." "I think you'd better," I said. The power came back on an hour or so later. |
| **Jill**<br>**(partner of**<br>**Robert R,**<br>**born 1947)**<br><br>**Kids' interest** | On a lighter note, it amused us that children were so fascinated by the noise. They'd be near him, trying not to stare at this man who made funny noises. Sometimes we explained and, believe me, Robert would be right up there with the Power Rangers. |

| Jill (partner of Robert R, born 1947) Daily life restrictions | We livened up a couple of restaurants whenever the alarm to change the batteries went off. It was difficult to tell sometimes just how much they were charging, and it seemed as though we were always changing them for new ones. Robert, ever the engineer, questioned from the start the type of batteries used. "Why so big? Why so heavy?" Water loomed large in our lives. Robert never did feel secure about the shower kit. He opted for very thorough washing. The day the garden hose covered him with water gave us a few anxious moments until we were quite sure that the controller hadn't been soaked. He missed fishing from his boat and swimming. The summer of 2002 was very hot. We had a pool, but Robert couldn't go in it. I dressed the driveline exit wound in absolutely sterile conditions and it paid off: we have had no infection problems that I am aware of. |
|---|---|
| Jill (partner of Robert R, born 1947) Love life | Sometimes, Dr Deng, I thought you had an overly healthy interest in our love life. I cannot think why. The LVAD is not conducive to the most romantic of sex lives. As the pace mounts, so does the noise. The first time, I was convinced that he would expire before he ever reached a climax. After a while, we became less anxious. What with drivelines, power lines, and batteries, the whole act could resemble a comedy routine. |
| Jill (partner of Robert R, born 1947) Daily life | Then there was the clothing situation. We never really have solved the problem of not bending the lines back. As for carrying those batteries, I bet we bought every type of fishing vest under the sun, but the holsters made Robert's back ache. |
| Janice (wife of Eric G, born 1950) MCSD training | First came the training for the LVAD. In the beginning, it was scary, especially when things had to be done speedily. There was also the worry that the controller would malfunction. Hopefully, I would not have to be the one to change it if it did fail. That was the most difficult and potentially dangerous part of the training process. |

Once my husband was home, I was more confident because he was quite capable of switching from battery to machine and back again. He is much more technologically savvy than me; his ability helped me get through it. The noise at times was loud and distracting; but for the most part, acceptable. At times, sleeping was quite a struggle because of the buzz of the machine and its projected light. But, as with anything else, we got used to it. He had to make more daily sacrifices than me, even down to the way he could shower. But this was a new life that we all had to accept, so that's what we did.

**Ed S (born 1956)**

**Living with MCSD**

I also wasn't too happy about not being able to swim anymore. But I have a 6-year-old son who is more important to me than being able to swim; and if I hadn't had the pump installed, I'm convinced that I would be doing the dead man's float anyway. Showering was a little difficult at first, but I've learned how to use the shower kit quite well with practice. I needed a lot of help at first, but I can do it by myself now and it doesn't take me as long. My lovely wife helps me with the dressing change. I've been fortunate in the fact that I haven't had an infection near the line that comes out of me for the pump. I'm careful to keep the site as clean as possible.

Slowly but surely, I have regained a lot of my muscle tone and my stamina has increased. My sleeping has returned to normal; after a month or two, I was able to sleep on my side without discomfort. Looking back over the last 7 months since I've had the pump, I can clearly see that it has saved my life. I was coughing so badly before I received the pump that I prayed to Almighty God that I would do anything if He would stop me from constantly choking and hacking. Well, He answered my prayers and sent me to Columbia Presbyterian Hospital!

# Time of Discharge

The time of discharge marks the transition to the long-term, often out-patient, management of the MCSD patient (Holman *et al.*, 2002). At the time of discharge, a stable medical regimen should be in place. Also, the patient should have — with his/her family members — undergone detailed training on (1) lifestyle modification during MCSD support; (2) the medication plan; (3) the handling of the MCSD, including battery and controller changes; and (4) MCSD-associated emergency situations. The outpatient follow-up should be scheduled around predefined appointments, usually in weekly to monthly intervals.

# MCSD Weaning: Rationale and Protocols

***Weaning Protocols.*** In the long-term course after MCSD implantation, it is of major importance to explore the extent to which the heart has recovered. A novel, hemodynamically guided exercise protocol with two different left ventricular assist device settings in long-term recipients has been recommended by the Münster University group in Germany. This protocol allows for quantitation of the contribution of the native left ventricle to total cardiac output. It facilitates an estimation of the risk associated with device dysfunction, the prediction of left ventricular recovery, and the potential for weaning (Deng *et al.*, 1997; Deng *et al.*, 1998).

The group at Advocate Christ Medical Center in Illinois attempted to improve their previous algorithm for the MCSD-weaning evaluation, and tested the hypothesis that LVAD stroke volume reduction produces a steady-state mechanical reloading of left ventricular pressures and volumes (compared with LVAD rate reduction) that results in transient mechanical reloading of the heart due to beat-to-beat variations in LV pressures and volumes, following a similar strategy first suggested by the group at Münster University (Deng *et al.*, 1997).

The relationship of LVAD flow to LVAD stroke volume and systolic interval over a range of LVAD rates (60, 80, 100, 120, and 140 bpm) was validated in a mock circulatory flow loop. In six acute experiments, calves were implanted with a pneumatic paracorporeal LVAD (PVAD, Thoratec,

Pleasanton, CA). The PVAD was operated asynchronously in the auto-volume mode (full decompression) for 30 min to establish a baseline control condition. The calf hearts were then mechanically reloaded by LVAD rate reduction (80, 60, and 40 bpm) or LVAD stroke volume reduction (100, 120, and 140 bpm) protocols, which consisted of 30 min of support at each LVAD beat rate. The order of weaning protocols was randomized with a 30-min recovery period (LVAD volume mode to fully decompress the heart, allowing it to rest) between protocols to enable a return to the baseline control state. Aortic pressure and flow, LV pressure and volume, pulmonary artery flow, and LVAD flow waveforms were recorded for each test condition.

The LVAD stroke volume reduction protocol produced steady-state mechanical reloading compared with LVAD rate reduction, resulting in transient LV mechanical reloading. This distinction was due to differences in their temporal relationships between LVAD and LV filling and emptying cycles. The acute hemodynamic benefit of LVAD stroke volume reduction was a greater reduction in LV end-diastolic pressure and an increase in LV segmental shortening compared to LVAD rate reduction. The long-term effects of steady-state and transient LV mechanical reloading on myocardial structure and function toward achieving sustained myocardial recovery warrant further investigation (Slaughter *et al.*, 2001; Slaughter *et al.*, 2006).

***Preweaning Diagnostic Challenges.***   Depending on the time after MCSD implantation, the preweaning and postweaning periods should be characterized by a thorough re-evaluation of potential complications that the patient may experience during the early period, fine-tuning of every organ system level, recording of baseline variables, and prediction of the potential transplant candidacy or MCSD reimplantation likelihood. Unfortunately, at this time no tests exist to allow a reliable prediction of the likelihood of recurrence of heart failure.

The evaluation may include the search for potential reversible causes; detailed analysis of the patient's history, with specific emphasis on medication and achievement of the goal of recommended medical management of heart failure; nutritional evaluation; normalization of laboratory tests including basic metabolic panel, liver panel, lipid panel, calcium, $PO_4$, total protein, albumin, uric acid, CBC with differential and platelet count, thyroid panel, ANA (if applicable), ESR, and iron binding; serotyping and screening against a panel of donor antigens (PRA) and HLA phenotype to predict the likelihood of future transplantation; 24-h urine for creatinine clearance and total protein; urinalysis; urine culture to rule out potential complications during the early period after explantation; 12-lead electrocardiogram; 24-h Holter monitor; signal-averaged EKG; thallium scan; radionuclide ventriculogram; echocardiogram; serial evaluation of exercise stress test with oxygen uptake measurements ($VO_2$); right and left heart catheterization; endomyocardial biopsy in selected cases where the etiology of heart failure is still in question; update of pulmonary function tests; dental evaluation; psychosocial evaluation and review of the patient's medical insurance and general financial resources; transcranial and peripheral vascular Doppler imaging if not current; and physical therapy and evaluation until mostly during the early postexplantation period.

Other studies may be required according to each individual patient, including updated carotid Doppler in patients older than 55 years, abdominal ultrasound (>55 years), intravenous pyelogram if indicated, upper GI series if indicated, barium enema/gastrointestinal endoscopies, and urological evaluation or other special consults if indicated.

***Weaning Cardiac Surgical Techniques.*** The surgical technique of MCSD explantation varies according to the individual MCSD and the specific patient situation. Since a standardized approach is not yet defined, the surgical principles of "quick, simple, safe" are being applied.

***Postweaning Therapeutic Challenges.*** A major emphasis on patient education by the heart failure/transplant group should be a major focus. Specifically, the patient and family need to understand the uncertainty of sustained recovery of native heart function after weaning. In addition, the potential necessity of defibrillator implantation after MCSD weaning needs to be discussed.

## Living with the MCSD

There are at this time no consensus guidelines for living with an assist device. Therefore, these recommendations are the practice pattern based on personal and institutional experience.

*Infection Control.* It is important that you maintain sterile conditions when changing the driveline dressing. The position of the driveline exit site has an important role in infection prophylaxis.

*Nutrition.* A heart-healthy nutrition is important. However, you do not need to practice the same restrictive precautions with low-salt and low-fluid intake as during your heart failure condition.

*Swimming/Sauna.* With the current generation of assist devices that have a percutaneous driveline exit, you cannot safely go swimming. Care must be taken not to wet the site of the air filter in the HeartMate I.

*Driving a Car.* Although there are no consensus recommendations for driving a car, you are advised to drive with utmost caution and avoid stressful traffic situations.

*Public Transportation.* You can safely use public transportation. For security checks at the airport, you will have to tell security officers that you are wearing the assist device.

*Heavy Equipment Operations.* If you are in a stable, long-term situation on your assist device, you can operate heavy equipment.

*Professions with Elevated Risks.* While wearing the assist device, you should be very careful and refrain from professional activities with elevated responsibilities for others (e.g. pilot, schoolbus driver). In addition, you should be cautious about professions with an elevated risk of trauma and bleeding if you are on blood-thinning medications.

*Sexual Life.* You and your partner should be very creative in continuing your love life while you are wearing the assist device. You can see from the descriptions of patients and their partners in this book that there are no limits (except for the length of the driveline cable and the weight of the batteries and controller ☺).

*Pregnancy.* If you are a female in the appropriate age group, because of risks associated with infection and coagulopathy as well as unscheduled emergency interventions (including heart transplantation), you are not advised to become pregnant during assist device support. If you are a male, there are no restrictions on conceiving children while you are on assist device support.

*Sport.* You can participate in all kinds of sports that do not expose you to risks of driveline fluid exposure or trauma.

*Vacation.* You can go on any vacation while observing the restrictions applying to sports. Also, you should check the availability of emergency services with experience in assist device handling within the vicinity of your vacation place. This will obviously restrict your vacation location choices.

*Work.* You should aim at returning to work once you are back home and feel comfortable handling your MCSD. All of the above continuously need to be observed.

## DIFFERENTIAL MANAGEMENT BY MCSD TYPE

### MCSD-Related Differences

*General Differences.* There are typical differences in the management of different MCSDs, specifically with respect to anticoagulation, infection prophylaxis, afterload and preload management, and integration of native cardiac performance with the MCSD-generated cardiac support.

*Anticoagulation Protocols.* The anticoagulation concept is probably the management aspect that varies the most between different MCSD types. While the HeartMate I MCSD is managed with antiplatelet agents only, all other MCSDs require the additional application of coumadin as per current recommendations (Appendix 4).

***The Vienna Protocol.***    In Vienna, Wieselthaler *et al.* (2000) studied the effect of the DeBakey axial flow VAD on platelets. They identified a triphasic pattern that was initially expressed by an impaired primary hemostasis in the early postoperative period, after which platelet activity reached supernormal levels several days postoperatively. There was no correlation between routine coagulation tests, such as the activated partial thromboplastin time (aPTT) and the prothrombin time, thus suggesting that routine anticoagulation monitoring and special platelet function monitoring are necessary to manage these patients. After the combined anticoagulation and antiaggregation regimes were stabilized in these patients, sensitive markers of platelet activation such as P-selectin were restored to normal.

Because phase II — the phase with substantial hyperaggregability of the platelets — occurs several days postoperatively, the Vienna Group suggested beginning antiplatelet therapy as early as possible. This is a different pattern than the immune and coagulation stimulating pattern that is seen with the HeartMate I volume displacement device, and suggests that the anticoagulation regimen needs to be tailored to the type of device that is being used. This is suggested by the increased thrombin generation and fibrinolysis as well as the upregulation of the immune system with the textured HeartMate device and the platelet activation — probably secondary to high shear rates — that are experienced in the axial flow DeBakey VAD (Wieselthaler *et al.*, 2000).

# CHAPTER 4

# OUTCOMES

## OUTCOME ASSESSMENT/PROGNOSTICATION

### The Challenges of Generating Evidence on the Outcomes of MCSD Therapy

*How to Compare the Performance of Different MCSDs?* In 2001, in the first randomized clinical trial testing the survival benefit of MCSDs in a patient population ineligible for heart transplantation secondary to noncardiac reasons including age and comorbidities, the HeartMate I pulsatile MCSD was shown to improve survival and quality of life (Rose *et al.*, 2001). Within the evolving family of first-, second-, and third-generation MCSDs, comparison has been difficult. The first trials comparing, in patients ineligible for heart transplantation, other MCSDs against the gold standard MCSD HeartMate I are ongoing in the US, testing the pulsatile Novacor MCSD and the DeBakey continuous flow MCSD. The only mechanism of generating scientific evidence in the absence of a randomized comparison would be mandatory participation in an MCSD observational database, which has been inaugurated as a voluntary mechanism by the International Society for Heart and Lung Transplantation during the last 3 years following consensus recommendations of international experts (Deng *et al.*, 2003c; Deng *et al.*, 2004; Deng *et al.*, 2005a).

In the US, the National Institutes of Health are organizing a mandatory MCSD registry for centers participating in lifetime or destination MCSD therapy. This mechanism, hopefully staged as an international registry, will over time provide uniform standards (Wright and Weinstein, 1998) and definitions of morbidity and mortality events, allowing for a comparison of outcomes between different MCSDs.

***Necessity for Translational Outcomes Research.*** The similar profile of complications (such as infections and coagulopathies) in Jarvik 2000 MCSD recipients compared to HeartMate I MCSD recipients warrants a fully developed translational research program that addresses these problems and transitions them from "halfway technology" to mainstream cardiovascular medicine accepted by referring cardiologists, internists, cardiac surgeons, and the general public. Such research funding, as for example with the Specialized Center for Clinically Oriented Research (SCCOR) at Columbia University in New York on the "Biology of Human Long-Term Mechanical Circulatory Support", is essential to foster the translation of this new technology into clinical practice.

***Necessity for MCSD Center Infrastructure Requirements.*** Which centers should be embarking on long-term MCSD therapy? The overall spectrum of centers embarking on this type of therapy should be based on an international and national consensus on the type of expertise that needs to be in the center in order to provide the program with a low morbidity and mortality profile (Smits *et al.*, 2003a). This approach is in line with a consensus recommendation by the International Society for Heart and Lung Transplantation that was endorsed by the American Heart Association, the American College of Cardiology, and the Heart Failure Society of America (Deng *et al.*, 2003c).

***MCSD Outcomes As a Multidisciplinary Task.*** The entire community of advanced heart failure cardiologists and cardiac surgeons, nurses, social workers, psychologists, physiotherapists, and financial experts participating in this mode of therapy has to face the challenge of developing safe and efficacious MCSD therapies. We have the responsibility to counsel our patients regarding their best options, and to allow them to come to an informed decision according to their personal preferences. The type of evidence that has to be generated for this approach includes not only an observational report as detailed in this book, but also a comparison of different MCSDs using a mandatory international registry mechanism as well as (in a complementary manner) a framework of randomized clinical trials (Deng, 2005).

# The Mechanical Circulatory Support Device Database of the ISHLT

*Background.* In 2001, the Scientific Council on Mechanical Circulatory Support Devices of the International Society for Heart and Lung Transplantation (ISHLT) established an international database to provide comparative assessments of efficacy between generic therapies and between individual devices (www.ishlt.org/regist_mcsd_main) (Pae *et al.*, 2001; Stevenson *et al.*, 2001; Deng *et al.*, 2005a). The purposes of the MCSD Database are to capture worldwide data relating to the implantation and outcome of patients receiving mechanical circulatory support devices designed for and capable of use for 30 or more days, to identify the risk factors for complications, to improve patient selection and management before and after device implantation, to generate predictive outcome models for given patient profiles, to generate statistical analyses of the data that can be used for further clinical trials, and to identify trends with the aim of improving current practices.

While some surgical interventions for heart failure — such as MCSD therapy in patients ineligible for cardiac transplantation — have undergone randomized evaluation (Rose *et al.*, 2001) or — as coronary artery bypass grafting in heart failure — are so scheduled (Joyce *et al.*, 2003), others may not reach this stage of clinical testing owing to a lack of consensus about the rationale and clinical equipoise, such as in the case of cardiac transplantation (Deng, 2000; Hunt, 2000; Deng, 2002). Scientific mechanisms of generating evidence beyond randomized clinical trials have to be considered to assess the potential comparative benefit (efficacy) and safety of these interventions according to evidence-based medicine criteria. This alternative mode of analysis is possible by creating databases that represent a longitudinal observational study design.

Here, we summarize the rationale, development, and utility of the Mechanical Circulatory Support Device Database of the ISHLT (www.ishlt. org/regist_mcsd_main), which represents such an evidence-based mechanism in advanced heart failure medicine. The database design requires a high degree of cooperation among participating centers, a high degree of sophistication with respect to validated prognostic tools to assess heart failure severity, and an outcome analysis with sophisticated statistical analysis methods.

***History of the ISHLT MCSD Database.***    The treatment of advanced heart failure (AHF) with MCSDs has evolved rapidly during the last two decades. Since the initiative by the US National Heart, Lung, and Blood Institute in the 1960s to develop long-term artificial heart devices, several types of long-term MCSDs have been developed and implemented in clinical trials and practices. In 1985, the ISHLT and the American Society for Artificial Internal Organs (ASAIO) proposed a combined registry for the clinical use of mechanical ventricular assist devices (VADs) and the total artificial heart (TAH) (Pae and Pierce, 1986). The first report of this voluntary registry was published in 1986, followed by five subsequent reports until 1995. While the initial report included 83 patients, the sixth report analyzed more than 2000 patients. Due to inadequate funding, the project was terminated. An attempt to incorporate the registry into the National Database of the Society of Thoracic Surgeons as a separate module was unsuccessful.

Driven by the evolving MCSD technology and expanding clinical experience, a multidisciplinary conference in June 2000 — jointly sponsored by the American College of Cardiology and a number of major national and international medical and surgical societies — brought together physicians, scientists, the US Food and Drug Administration (FDA), and industry representatives to discuss the future role of mechanical circulatory support and to establish a consensus on the design principles of future MCSD trials (Stevenson *et al.*, 2001). In this conference, a broad consensus was reached that there should be a mandatory registry for all implantable MCSDs to address the following scientific issues:

- Identification of patient populations who would potentially benefit from MCSD implantation
- Characterization of the spectrum, nature, and rates of adverse events associated with MCSD implantation
- Generation of multivariate predictive models for outcomes
- Assessment of the mechanical and biological reliability of current and future MCSDs

With this ambitious agenda in mind, the ISHLT — which had, soon after its inception in 1981, initiated the highly successful Heart and Lung Transplantation Registry — established the Scientific Council on Mechanical Circulatory Support, which was charged to develop an international

MCSD database utilizing the data forms of the European Novacor Registry as a template (Deng *et al.*, 2001a). The ISHLT, a worldwide nonprofit medical subspecialty society with over 2300 members dedicated to the science and management of end-stage heart and lung disease, seemed to be well positioned to take the lead in developing this project.

Upon the solicitation of 30 applications responding to a request for proposals (RFP), the UNOS/Transplantation Informatics Institute (UNOS/TII) in Richmond, VA, was awarded the contract to run this database. Separately, a search for the medical director of this Database was initiated, to follow the founding and interim director, Dr Robert Kormos. Dr Mario Deng was selected to serve as the first appointed medical director of the MCSD Database starting from January 2002.

***Design Considerations of the ISHLT MCSD Database.*** From a scientific point of view, the purposes of the MCSD Database are to capture worldwide data relating to the implantation and outcome of patients receiving cardiac assist devices designed for and capable of use for 30 or more days, to identify the risk factors for complications, to improve patient selection and management before and after device implantation, to generate predictive outcome models for given patient profiles, to generate statistical analyses of the data that can be used as the underlying evidence/justification for government agency–funded studies and clinical trials, and to identify the overall and best practices with the aim of improving current practices.

Several design items have been deemed essential for the new MCSD Database:

- The ISHLT MCSD Database should reflect the overall current practice patterns, not just the practice of selected centers of excellence such as that assembled in the CTRD Database (Jaski *et al.*, 2001), because their results could not be generalized to the average center and the average patient in US and non-US centers. To capture all MCSD implants worldwide, the database should be mandatory and not a voluntary registry such as the ISHLT non-US Transplant Registry (Hosenpud *et al.*, 2001), the early Combined Assist Pump Registry (Pae and Pierce, 1986), the CTRD Database (Jaski *et al.*, 2001), or the European Novacor Registry (Deng *et al.*, 2001a).

- The ISHLT MCSD Database should enable the evaluation of patient safety for all current and future MCSDs that are designed to be capable of supporting the circulation for more than 30 days. This should, for the first time ever, be accomplished by applying uniform consensus definitions of complications to all devices, thus providing a framework for measuring each device along the same set of criteria. This has previously not been accomplished by the ISHLT non-US Transplant Registry (Hosenpud *et al.*, 2001), the early Combined Assist Pump Registry (Pae and Pierce, 1986), the FDA postmarketing surveillance mechanism, or the European Novacor Registry (Deng *et al.*, 2001a).
- The ISHLT MCSD Database should enable the evaluation of MCSD efficacy, as defined by the gain of survival through MCSD intervention in relation to the preimplantation risk of dying from heart failure. This goal should, for the first time ever, be accomplished by integrating validated heart failure risk prediction parameters in the preimplantation assessment form. This has previously not been accomplished by the ISHLT non-US Transplant Registry (Hosenpud *et al.*, 2001), the early Combined Assist Pump Registry (Pae and Pierce, 1986), the FDA postmarketing surveillance mechanism, the CTRD Database (Jaski *et al.*, 2001), or the European Novacor Registry (Deng *et al.*, 2001a).

The database consists of three tiers of data. Tier 1 includes basic data that focus on the specifics of the device type, the surgical implant procedure and indications for implant, and the outcome. Tier 2 includes details regarding the specific patient-related complications and events subsequent to device implantation. Tier 3 consists of device-related events compatible with FDA postmarketing surveillance requirements. These data are expected to be invaluable, as they will be collected at the source by the clinicians using the devices and should reflect an unbiased assessment of what took place. Data such as these are sought out by a number of clinicians and specialties.

All centers worldwide that were known to perform MCSD implantation received an invitation to participate in the MCSD data collection process in December 2001. In February 2002, the ISHLT launched the web-based Tier 1 data entry into the database. More than 150 centers worldwide were invited to participate.

The major logistical challenges for the new MCSD Database included the following:

- Identify all MCSD centers worldwide
- Secure reporting agreements with all centers worldwide
- Solicit compliance from all centers using a three-tiered system
- Establish a web-based system and computer database
- Collect follow-up data at specified time points
- Assure data integrity through periodic auditing
- Ensure patient/institution confidentiality (according to HIPAA requirements in the US)
- Secure third-party financial support

***MCSD Database as a Joint Project of Diverse Professional Interest Groups.*** The challenge for continuous databases such as the ISHLT MCSD Database is a well-defined consensus among the participating societal groups, specifically professional experts, regulatory agencies such as the FDA, patient organizations and third-party payors, and the industry. These groups present complementary, occasionally conflicting interests (Deng *et al.*, 2003c). The combined effort of the various stakeholders is required to address the following issues:

- Goals
- Data format and management
- Funding
- Compliance
- Access

The responsibility to support the Dabatase should be shared between the surgical and medical expert societies representing the physicians involved in using these devices, the industry, the payors, and governmental agencies.

***MCSD Database from an Expert Perspective.*** The counseling of individual patients with advanced heart failure by their physicians about the indication, timing, and choice of MCSD critically depends on the availability of solid MCSD outcome data. Therefore, the goals of the MCSD Database are to capture worldwide data relating to the implantation and outcome of patients receiving cardiac assist devices designed for and capable of use for 30 or more days, to identify the risk factors for complications, to improve patient selection and management before and after device implantation, to generate predictive outcome models for given patient profiles, to generate statistical analyses of the data that can be used as the underlying evidence/justification for government agency–funded studies and clinical trials, and to identify the overall and best practices with the aim of improving current practices.

***MCSD Database from an Industry Perspective.***    The ISHLT has invited the world's leading MCSD companies to participate in this project. By doing so, companies are able to suggest early modifications and improvement of the database (specifically with regard to Tier 2 and Tier 3 data); profile or market their company as a state-of-the-art manufacturer spearheading the implementation of evidence-based high-tech cardiovascular medicine; allow payors/insurers, MCSD centers, and regulatory agencies to recognize their company as a leader in the field; and avoid duplication of reporting. Specific additional benefits for manufacturers include a comprehensive evaluation of their product's strengths and weaknesses in relation to that of their competitors, as assessed by an independent scientific mechanism; and — with improving clinical outcomes as documented by the MCSD Database — a broadening of indications, potentially without having to undergo *de novo* randomized testing.

***MCSD Database from a Payor Perspective.***    The legitimate interest of payors or customers in the MCSD Database includes financing evidence-based medicine, while simultaneously avoiding payment for interventions that have not been demonstrated to be safe or efficacious and are thus not in their best interest. In the case of MCSD therapy, which is rapidly emerging as a potentially life-prolonging and quality-of-life–enhancing intervention, the applicability of the REMATCH results (Rose *et al.*, 2001) to the general advanced heart failure population ineligible for heart transplantation is specifically challenging for two reasons. One reason is the likely postmarketing trend of the selection of AHF patients with a less dismal prognosis than those included in the REMATCH study, and another reason is the likely trend of the start-up of less experienced centers. These opposing trends will reduce the survival benefit of destination MCSD therapy.

As the 2-year survival benefit in the REMATCH study was already marginal, there may no longer be any detectable survival benefit in post-marketing practice, thus implying that destination MCSD therapy may (in the worst-case scenario) result in a mode switch of death. Instead of dying from heart failure, transplant-ineligible AHF patients would just die from infection, coagulopathies, neurological events, or device dysfunction during destination MCSD therapy. Payors clearly would not want to pay for a mode switch of death. Currently, the best and probably only way to ensure the efficacy of chronic MCSD therapy is by utilizing a mechanism such as the ISHLT MCSD Database (Deng *et al.,* 2003c; Deng *et al.*, 2004; Deng *et al.*, 2005a).

***MCSD Database from a Regulatory Perspective.*** Progress in the field requires the establishment and maintenance of a mandatory database that includes all implantable MCSDs, both before and after approval. For example, from a US perspective, MCSD safety and effectiveness are ultimate goals of the FDA in the interest of the public. The FDA is continuously involved as MCSDs move from the design phase through the evolution of lab- and bench-testing to clinical testing.

Potential benefits to the FDA of utilizing this Database include the fact that the MCSD Database is operated by the ISHLT, rendering the foundation and mechanics of the Database least susceptible to criticism of industry bias. Furthermore, the MCSD Database, which the ISHLT has contracted to the UNOS/Transplantation Informatics Institute (TII), is ongoing. This is especially valuable in light of the recently completed REMATCH trial. Also, the database is uniform (as opposed to company-specific postmarketing reporting instruments), thus yielding a gain in the comparability of information.

***MCSD Database from a Patient Perspective.*** To achieve the goal of a mandatory database that incorporates the interests of all participating groups, a continuous dialog based on mutual trust and transparent reliable communication has to be established. With the

MCSD Database in place and the INTERMACS created after the MCSD Database model, it is possible to use parametric methodology to generate patient-specific and clinical profile–specific gain-of-survival predictions.

Only a rigorous analysis of properly selected and accurately collected outcome data for a variety of MCSDs can ultimately provide the individual patient with the best choice of support for long-term quality and duration of life. The care, commitment, and accuracy of the data collected by each participating institution will determine the success or failure of this venture (Kirklin, 2001), which is critically important to advance our knowledge regarding the effectiveness of MCSDs for one of the most difficult and costly medical problems — the malignant syndrome of advanced heart failure.

## US Interagency Registry for Mechanically Assisted Cardiac Support (US INTERMACS)

Based on the MCSD Database organized by the ISHLT between 2001 and 2005 (Deng *et al.*, 2003c; Deng *et al.*, 2004; Deng *et al.*, 2005a), the National Institutes of Health (USA) have funded a new Interagency Registry for Mechanically Assisted Circulatory Support (INTERMACS) to comply with the US national regulatory requirements for long-term (destination) MCSDs to generate critical data in order to advance our knowledge on the effectiveness of MCSD therapy. INTERMACS is the direct successor of the ISHLT MCSD Database. With this successful transition, the international component of INTERMACS has emerged as the seamless successor to the initial ISHLT MCSD Database (Kirklin and Holman, 2006).

## Cardiac Transplant Research Database

The Cardiac Transplant Research Database, in which almost 40 of the most active US cardiac transplant centers participate, has estimated the survival benefit from transplantation in patients with different degrees of heart failure severity as indicated by VAD support vs. inotrope support on the waiting list. The study was designed to compare patients supported by an LVAD before transplant with those treated with intravenous inotropic medical therapy.

Of the 5880 patients transplanted between 1990 and 1997, 502 received support from LVADs and 2514 received intravenous inotropic medical therapy at the time of transplant. Kaplan–Meier analysis showed no significant difference in posttransplant survival between the LVAD and medical therapy groups ($p = 0.09$). The results of a multivariate Cox regression analysis were consistent with that of the Kaplan–Meier analysis and did not identify LVAD as a significant risk factor for mortality. The percentage of patients who received LVADs as a function of total transplants increased from 2% in 1990 to 16% in 1997. Furthermore, although the number of extracorporeal LVADs remained relatively constant, the number of intracorporeal LVADs increased over time. Multivariate parametric analysis found that the risk factors for posttransplant death in the LVAD group were extracorporeal LVAD use ($p = 0.0004$), elevated serum creatinine ($p = 0.05$), older donor age ($p = 0.03$), increased donor ischemic time ($p < 0.0001$), and earlier year of transplant ($p = 0.03$).

It was concluded that, given a limited donor supply, an intracorporeal LVAD helps the sickest patients survive to transplant and provides a posttransplant outcome similar to that of patients supported on inotropic medical therapy. Therefore, patients supported on LVADs before transplant may receive the greatest benefit when compared with other transplant candidates (Jaski *et al.*, 2001).

## BRIDGE-TO-TRANSPLANTATION MECHANICAL CIRCULATORY SUPPORT

| | |
|---|---|
| **Peter P (born 1947)** **Battery charge emergency** | About 2 months after my quadruple bypass and LVAD surgery, I was sent home. I went to work and commuted about half an hour to my office. One day, as I joined the rush hour crowd and entered the ramp to the New Jersey Turnpike, I noticed that it was not moving. The average timeline for my batteries was about 4 hours. I had replaced |

them with my last set of charged batteries, as usual, about 3 hours before the end of the workday. I sat in the car counting the minutes as they went by and worrying about my batteries.

An hour later, I had progressed about halfway home. I got the pump out of the pouch within inches of where it was supposed to be hooked up, and got everything loose and ready for a quick transfer. Luckily, I made it home with a few minutes left on my batteries. After that, I got an extra pair of batteries from the hospital and they have remained in the car.

**Peter P**
**(born 1947)**

**Movie theatre**

One day, my wife and I decided to go to a movie theatre. As the audience settled down and became silent to await the beginning of the movie, the sounds from my LVAD became very noticable. People directly in front of us started to look around in search of the sound. I quickly grabbed my winter leather jacket and suffocated the noise as best as I could. Luckily, the movie started and nobody took further notice.

**Peter P**
**(born 1947)**

**Return to normal life: car racing**

As I have always been an avid car enthusiast and racer, I participated in an autocross (a high-speed course navigated through pylons in a large parking lot). Some of the participants who were aware of my condition moved jokingly to create a special handicapped class for me. I subsequently led the field with first place in my usual class and forgot about any handicaps.

**Peter P**
**(born 1947)**

**LVAD and noise**

While in a crowded elevator, there were a few moments of silence. My LVAD became the only sound heard by the passengers. A young lady at the back became very alarmed and asked, "Oh my, what is that sound? Is there something wrong with the elevator?" I quickly replied in my best southern drawl, "No, honey, it's my heart going pitter-patter over you." My traveling companion, aware of my condition, started laughing out loud.

| | |
|---|---|
| **Peter P (born 1947)** **LVAD and love life** | A few weeks after returning home from all the operations and wearing an LVAD, my wife and I attempted to have sex. I wore the battery packs to give me more flexibility, but that proved to be dangerous as I bruised my wife with them. So, I quickly unplugged them and connected myself to the charger. Now, I was limited to a 5-foot radius from the equipment. |
| **Peter P (born 1947)** **After heart transplantation** | Five months after my heart transplant, my family decided to go on vacation to Club Med at Columbus Isle. Both my wife and I are avid scuba divers. So I checked with Columbia, and they reluctantly agreed to let me go. We went out with a group to a famous reef location where we could see sharks, barracudas, and other sea creatures. The dive was wonderful.<br><br>When I returned to the boat and removed my wetsuit jacket, the dive master noticed the very long scar on my chest. He asked what had happened to me. I promptly answered, "I had a heart transplant a few months ago." His jaw dropped to the floor and he asked with trepidation, "Does your doctor know what you just did?" I asked him if he could keep a secret (in jest). |
| **Eric G (born 1950)** **Daily life with HeartMate I** | Sleeping with an LVAD isn't as challenging as one might suppose. It takes time to position the wires and to comfortably move them, so that you can turn a bit without pulling on anything critical and waking yourself up. As the chest heals, more and more movement becomes possible. Within days, comfortable sleep is possible. After 2 months, I was almost on my stomach, but not quite! That titanium drum is formidable.<br><br>After a short time, it's easy to become comfortable with the unit, much like the comfort one experiences in the presence of a recently tamed wild animal: unfailing trust, but with one eye always open. You can't forget that you have an LVAD, not even for a minute. Are the batteries charged? Am I connected to the base unit? Where is the manual pump and what if I have to use the damn thing? |

A normal daily life is attainable, but there is the constant reminder of the reality. A fair analogy would be Poe's "The Telltale Heart": 80 times a minute, 60 minutes an hour, 24 hours a day, you can hear the pump moving your blood. But unlike the silent pounding in your chest that you're accustomed to, this sound is broadcast to everyone around you. At home, it's a constant reminder to you and to your family of what has transpired and what is to be.

Each day becomes a little better than the last. In the beginning, the idea of leaving the house is absurd. The fear of the device, the awareness of the noise, and not wanting to be noticed are all very much in the forefront of your mind. Then one day, it happens. You go out. Someone looks at you in a strange way and you realize that they are hearing the LVAD, but you aren't. Unabashedly, you say something out loud to answer their silent question: "It's a pump helping my heart." This may end the conversation or it may not. In either case, you are living with this beast in your chest and you're okay with that.

If you're very lucky, you get to the point of full acceptance by both you and your family. That point came for me one night when we were watching TV. My daughter turned to me and said, "I can't hear my show, and you're going to have to either turn that thing off or go in the other room." It's a good thing she loves me; she made sure I could watch what I wanted to in the other room.

It's a challenge, but it's not insurmountable. Once things fall into place, it is workable. Sometimes frustrating, sometimes infuriating; but always workable. Bathing in a tub and swimming are forbidden and for good reason. Movies and quiet restaurants might be difficult. However, with a little planning, most of everything else is possible.

I was able to exercise and regain my strength. I was able to work, play, and drive. I went shopping, and I went to Christmas dinner with my family. Assume that there's a way to do what you want, and then find the way. Ask for help; this is no time to go it alone.

I didn't make the original decision, but in hindsight it was the right decision. There's a balance between staying alive and quality of life. My heart attack was as serious as it gets, but the LVAD gave me the opportunity to recover. I wanted to recover. In the end, my quality of life was not seriously impacted and I am staying strongly alive.

I said that my family made the decision for me. The doctors were concerned about how I would react. My older daughter caught the essence of it. She told them, "He loves all those technical things and he'll think it's totally neat." To think it's "totally neat" might be extreme, but clearly she knows me well. Rarely does a day pass that I don't think, "Unbelievable, it's working."

If you want to keep the LVAD in perfect perspective, consider this very simple question: what's the alternative? To accept the LVAD and all that it entails requires a very simple philosophy: "It is what it is." The device is installed, it's working, and it's helping to make me stronger for the long term. With little exception, the LVAD does not stop me from doing anything that I could do before the implant. It may take creativity, but that's okay. Without it, however, life as I know it would be over and I'm just not ready to go.

**Daughter of Eric G (born 1950)**

**MCSD– transplant transition**

My dad just had a heart transplant 3 weeks ago. Three months on the LVAD made that possible. It is still a struggle. He'll have to constantly be on medication to prevent his body from attacking his new heart, but at least he won't be attached to something every waking (and sleeping, for that matter) moment of his life ... right? Well, maybe.

The thing is, the LVAD was seemingly and comfortingly fail-safe. There were always options: the batteries, the base unit, the independent power generator in case there was a blackout, even the hand pump. It is a machine, and I think my dad trusts technology more than he trusts his own body's capabilities. He knows electronics and programs; he has mastery over them. The body's mechanics, though, will do what they will. With the removal of the

LVAD, my dad's life is back in the hands of the doctors; he has been stripped of his control.

So even though the LVAD is not the most convenient lifestyle accessory, it has its benefits, living being the primary one of course. Having a new, healthy heart was always the goal of placing my father on the LVAD; but now that he has one, he almost misses that titanium metronome and the semi–sense of control it brought with it. Well, almost!

**Deborah (mother of Joel L, born 1969)**

**Pre-heart transplant**

On April 5, 2002, one of the cardiologists told me that if there was no heart over the weekend, there would probably be no Monday for Joel. They were willing to take an old heart, even a not completely healthy heart, just to allow Joel to live. That evening, Alicia and I were sitting in the third-floor waiting room, away from the tumult of the fourth-floor waiting room, when I picked up a newspaper lying on the table. The paper was open to the horoscopes page and I looked at Joel's. "You will have a change of heart," it read. How ironic!

Blessedly, on April 6, 2002, a heart became available. Not just a heart, but a healthy heart, a perfect match. Sadly of course, a family had lost someone, but they had made the decision to donate this person's organs so that others might live and so that the death of a 35-year-old man in NYC would not be in vain.

At Joel's bedside, waiting for the move to the OR with me was Alicia, my nephew and his significant other, my niece, and Alicia's girlfriend from Massachusetts who wanted to be there to give Joel strength. We chatted and joked and cheered Joel on throughout the day, and then some time before 7 PM they came to take Joel to the OR. The medical staff looked at me and asked me to pull the LVAD plug from the wall for the last time. I remember shaking as I went to the wall socket. I pulled the plug, and immediately we were all overwhelmed with the sound of silence. No whooshing, no clicking. The battery pack that controls the device does not make the same sound. Joel was free, and in a few hours his new life would begin.

You know the rest of the story. Joel has had his ups and downs since the transplant. He has regained so much of his strength, but not his balance from the stroke. He walks with a slight limp, and cannot move his hand and fingers as swiftly or deftly as before. His cognitive function is good, but not 100%. However, he works, he lives alone, he drives, he hikes, he plays the piano and guitar, and he knows more about sports then the whole of ESPN. He is being treated for a recurrence of the giant cell, and he will beat this as he has beaten everything else. He feels down, especially when the weather is good and the cyclists are out, but his will to live is so strong.

What you don't know and should know is that he answers questions on Jeopardy that we have no idea from where he would have learned the answers. For this reason, he has invented a biography of his transplanted heart: the brilliant 35-year-old man who worked on Wall Street, enjoyed decorating and cooking, and was educated in the humanities (probably with a Phi Beta Kappa). Joel, being the person that he is, does not want to know any reality of the soul who gave him his second chance at life. This would be too disturbing for him, and I and everyone else respect his wishes.

When you asked us to send you our thoughts on the LVAD, he asked me what you were looking for. I told him to send you his feelings about having had the device in him. I asked him if he was happy to be alive, and he unequivocally said yes. "Then the ends justified the means," I said. And that is the bottom line. Joel is alive. We have him with us to share his life, to hear his laughter, to share his knowledge, to just be with him. For this, we are all grateful.

**Ted L (born 1943)**

**The heart transplant call**

**The Call**

The miracle from God and the gift of life came on June 23, 2005. The transplant team called and said, "We have a donor heart for you, come right away." While I had thought about this moment for over a year, the next few hours were a blur. I was wheeled into the operating room at about midnight, and $5\frac{1}{2}$ hours later Dr Naka told Trina that all had gone well and that I had gotten a good heart. It was as close a match as could have been possible. Within a day, the nurses had me up and walking. By the fifth day, I was doing physical therapy on a stationary bicycle for 20 minutes at a time.

While it took me a number of hours to come around after the operation, my body immediately recognized that it now had a foreign object in it. The brain sent out an all-points message: "Every antibody get to the heart area; we have a foreign object that must be eliminated." My body wanted to reject my new heart and will keep this up as long as I live.

Therefore, the doctors and nurses began an educational program to make me understand the very big responsibility that I had going forward. I would have to take many very powerful medications to suppress my immune system in order to reduce the body's efforts to eliminate my new heart. Since my immune system would be compromised, I would be subject to the slightest cold, flu, or virus. I would have to make sure to avoid sick people and large crowds.

I now take various antibiotics and antiviral medications to fight infections, and will do so for the rest of my life. I also need medications to offset the effects of these strong drugs. There are always trade-offs in life, and a heart transplant patient may possibly get diabetes, coronary artery blockage, or osteoporosis. As time passes from the day of transplantation, many patients can have these medications reduced, but never eliminated.

Twelve days after being admitted to the hospital for the transplant, I was discharged on my wife's birthday. She says it was the best present she has ever received.

**Your Help**

Have any of you ever had someone say to you, "If you could come back to earth a second time and do it all over again, what would you do?" God and I have been having many long chats about what I will do with my new life. I quickly decided that I would not go back to Wall Street. Instead, I would dedicate myself to helping other people by dedicating my life to raising the awareness of the need for and benefits of organ donation. Today, I am continuing my volunteer work at the New York Organ Donor Network and have joined the Board of Trustees of the Transplant Speakers International, an organization that educates the public on the need for organ donation.

According to the latest statistics from the UNOS (the federal agency responsible for organ transplants), there are just over 90 000 people waiting for an organ transplant and not nearly enough donors. One hopeful organ recipient dies every 17 minutes. If we could just get everyone to sign up to donate their organs and to let their wishes be known and accepted by their families, then there would be no waiting lists and everyone would get a transplant.

There is a saying that goes like this:

> Don't take your organs to heaven
> Heaven knows, we need them here on earth!

Would each of you be willing to become an organ donor? Would you be willing to encourage your family, neighbors, and friends? Would you be willing to be ambassadors at your place of work to encourage this?

May God bless each and every one of you, and may you appreciate your good health and that of your family and friends. Not everyone is as lucky as you.

## Observational Non-RCT Studies

*European Bridge-to-Transplant VAD Registry.* In the European Bridge-to-Transplant VAD Registry, clinical factors were analyzed in 258 patients during the period 1986–1993. All variables were analyzed by a univariate and multivariate analysis. The indications for mechanical circulatory support were hemodynamic deterioration before transplantation in 177 (69%)

patients, post–acute myocardial infarction in 40 (15%), postcardiotomy cardiogenic shock in 20 (8%), graft failure in 12 (5%), and cardiac rejection in 9 (3%). The devices implanted were pneumatic VAD in 145 (56%) cases, electromechanical LVAS in 15 (6%), TAH in 78 (30%), and centrifugal pump in 20 (8%). The patients were supported for a period ranging from 2h to 623 days (mean $18.3 \pm 43.2$ days). The types of support were LVAD in 50 (20%) cases, RVAD in 3 (1%), BVAD in 127 (49%), and TAH in 78 (30%). Bleeding occurred in 84 (32.5%) patients, and infections in 83 (32.1%); 21 embolic complications were reported in 16 (6%) patients. Renal failure was noted in 64 (25%) cases, with 33 (13%) requiring dialysis; respiratory failure in 47 (18%); and neurological impairment in 22 (9%).

A total of 160 (62%) patients were transplanted, and 104 were ultimately discharged (40% out of all 258 patients; 65% out of the 160 transplanted patients). Among the postoperative parameters, renal failure, TAH, neurological impairment, and infection showed statistical power. Some preoperative and postoperative variables were identified as independent risk factors for overall mortality: age, indication for graft failure, all indications different from cardiomyopathy, neurological impairment, renal insufficiency, infection, bleeding, and any type of support other than LVAD. The improvement in the success rate in the last 2 years was statistically significant ($P = 0.0282$), considering the percentages of both transplanted patients and discharged patients. The authors concluded that the results are encouraging if mechanical support is performed in patients with deteriorating condition while awaiting transplant, if an LVAD is feasible and effective, and if the ideal timing of transplant during the support period is identified (Quaini *et al.*, 1997).

***The University of Arizona Experience.*** Device selection has historically been supported by minimal comparative data. Since 1994, the group in the University of Arizona has implanted 43 patients with the CardioWest total artificial heart, 23 with the Novacor left ventricular assist system, and 26 with the Thoratec ventricular assist system. This experience has provided a basis for the group's device selection criteria.

The authors retrospectively reviewed the results for survival, stroke, and infection in the three groups. The Thoratec group patients were younger and smaller-sized than the CardioWest group or Novacor group. The CardioWest group had the highest mean central venous pressure and the lowest mean cardiac index. Survival to transplantation was 75% for the CardioWest group, 57% for Novacor, and 38% for Thoratec. Postimplant multiple organ failure caused the most deaths in the CardioWest and Thoratec groups; right heart failure and stroke caused the most Novacor deaths. The linearized stroke rates (event/patient-month) were 0.03 for CardioWest, 0.28 for Novacor, and 0.08 for Thoratec. Serious infections were found in 20% of CardioWest, 30% of Novacor, and 8% of Thoratec patients; but the linearized rates showed little difference and deaths from infection were rare. They concluded that the Novacor device should be used in stable patients with a body surface area greater than $1.7\,m^2$; otherwise, the Thoratec device should be used if they are smaller (Copeland *et al.*, 2001).

***Symbion Total Artificial Heart.*** Several models of total artificial hearts have been used for transient or permanent circulatory support in patients with decompensation. The most successful and widely used device has been the Symbion total artificial heart. From December 12, 1982, to January 1, 1991, a total of 180 Symbion total artificial hearts were implanted in 176 patients in 28 centers. Five patients received a Symbion total artificial heart as a permanent circulatory support device, whereas 171 patients received the device as a bridge to heart transplantation. Of the 175 bridge devices (171 patients), 141 were Symbion J7-70 hearts and 34 were Symbion J7-100 hearts. Four patients received two total artificial hearts, the second one after the failure of a transplanted heart because of either rejection (two patients) or donor heart failure (two patients). Most of the recipients (152) were males. The mean age was $42 \pm 12$ years, and the mean weight was $74 \pm 14\,kg$.

The most common indications for implantation included deterioration while awaiting heart transplant (36%) and acute cardiogenic shock (32%). The cause of heart disease was primarily ischemic (52%) or idiopathic (35%) cardiomyopathy. The duration of implantation ranged from 0 to 603 days (mean, $25 \pm 64$ days). One hundred three (60%) patients had the device for less than 2 weeks, 37 (22%) for 2–4 weeks, and 31 (18%) for more than 4 weeks. Complications during implantation included infection (37%), thromboembolic events (stroke, 7%; transient ischemic attack,

4%), kidney failure requiring dialysis (20%), bleeding requiring intervention (26%), and device malfunction (4%). Of the 171 patients, 118 (69%) underwent orthotopic heart transplantation. The actuarial survival rate for all patients with implants was 62% for 30 days and 42% for 1 year; and for patients with transplants, 72% for 30 days and 57% for 1 year. The main causes of death were sepsis (33%), multiorgan failure (21%), and posttransplant rejection (10%). The results indicated a relative success of this treatment for patients with an otherwise fatal prognosis. The authors also concluded that, as the demand for donor organs far exceeds availability, continued investigation of total artificial hearts seems justified (Johnson *et al.*, 1992).

***The Heart Center Nordrhein-Westfalen (Bad Oeynhausen) Experience.*** Evolving into the world's largest MCSD center since 1986, the group in Bad Oeynhausen has developed specific protocols for patient selection and management for different devices. The principal systems applied in the bridge-to-transplant cohort in this report were the Thoratec ventricular assist device ($n = 144$; mean duration of support, $53 \pm 57$ days), the Novacor left ventricular assist system (LVAS) ($n = 85$; mean duration of support, $154 \pm 15$ days), and the HeartMate LVAS ($n = 54$; mean duration of support, $143 \pm 142$ days). The Thoratec device was used for biventricular assistance or if the duration of support was expected to be less than 6 months; for long-term support, either the Novacor or the HeartMate LVAS was preferred.

Despite careful postoperative patient management, this group of patients were prone to a variety of complications. Bleeding occurred in 22%–35% of patients, right heart failure in 15%–26%, neurological disorders in 7%–28%, infection in 7%–30%, and liver failure in 11%–20%. Complications varied with the device applied and the patient's preoperative condition. The Novacor and the HeartMate systems offered the additional possibility of discharging patients during support if they fulfilled certain criteria. A total of 73 patients were discharged from hospital for a mean period of 184 days; this cumulative experience amounted to 37.5 patient-years. The main reasons for rehospitalization were thromboembolic and infectious complications (El-Banayosy *et al.*, 2001).

# BRIDGE-TO-RECOVERY MECHANICAL CIRCULATORY SUPPORT

## NHLBI Strategy on MCSD-Assisted Cardiac Recovery

Over the past decade, mechanical circulatory support has been beneficial as a bridge to cardiac transplantation, and anecdotal evidence suggests that heart failure patients fitted with mechanical assist devices experience direct cardiac benefits. Moreover, recent trials on limited numbers and subpopulations of patients — notably the Randomized Evaluation of Mechanical Assistance for the Treatment of Congestive Heart Failure (REMATCH) — support earlier observations of improved cardiac function, and point towards the use of assist devices as a destination therapy. To investigate this phenomenon, on August 2–3, 2001, the National Heart, Lung, and Blood Institute (NHLBI) convened the working group "Recovery from Heart Failure with Circulatory Assist" in Bethesda, MD. The team included cardiac surgeons, cardiologists, and experts in experimental research.

The goal was to prioritize recommendations to guide future programs in (1) elucidating the mechanisms leading to reverse remodeling associated with a left ventricular assist device (LVAD); (2) exploring advanced treatments, including novel pharmacologies, tissue engineering, and cell therapies, to optimize recovery with LVAD therapy; and (3) identifying target genes, proteins, and cellular pathways to focus on the production of novel therapies for myocardial recovery and cardiovascular disease. The working group also made the following research and clinical recommendations to eventually translate findings into improved therapeutic strategies and device design: (1) support collaborations among clinical and basic scientists, with an emphasis on clinical/translational research that might eventually lead to clinical trials; (2) identify candidate patients most likely to benefit from LVAD as a destination therapy; (3) explore potential biomarkers indicating when patients can most successfully be weaned from devices; and (4) promote clinical and experimental studies of mechanically assisted organs and the tissues derived from them (Reinlib and Abraham, 2003).

## Observational Non-RCT Studies

*The German Heart Center (Berlin) Experience.*  LVAS support may eventually be used as a bridge to recovery, with explantation of the device without the requirement of cardiac transplantation. The fraction of patients eligible for this mode of therapy is currently under investigation and is being analyzed in an international multicenter observational database (Hetzer *et al.*, 2000; Helman *et al.*, 2000).

Specifically, the group at the German Heart Center in Berlin first reported long-term effects of ventricular unloading on cardiac function, humoral anti–beta1-adrenoceptor autoantibodies, and myocardial fibrosis. Seventeen patients in New York Heart Association functional class IV with nonischemic IDC received MCSS. All had a cardiac index of $<1.6\,L \times min^{-1} \times m^{-2}$ of body surface area, a left ventricular ejection fraction (LVEF) of $<16\%$, and a left ventricular internal diameter in diastole (LVIDd) of $>68\,mm$; and all tested positive for anti–beta1-adrenoceptor autoantibodies. Echocardiographic evaluation, serum tests for anti–beta1-adrenoceptor autoantibodies, and histological assessment of myocardial fibrosis were performed both before and after MCSS implantation. The mean support duration was $230 \pm 201$ days. Six patients died, 4 were transplanted, and 2 are still on MCSS. Five patients with significant cardiac recovery (mean LVIDd, $54 \pm 2.3\,mm$; LVEF, $47\% \pm 3.7\%$) were weaned after 160 to 794 days, and are now device-free. Anti–beta1-adrenoceptor autoantibodies gradually disappeared during MCSS, without any increase after weaning. Cardiac function and volume density of fibrosis remained normal. Nine patients' cardiac function hardly improved during ventricular unloading.

The authors concluded that cardiac function can be normalized in selected patients with end-stage IDC by MCSS. The degree of preoperative myocardial fibrosis may be an indicator of the outcome; anti–beta1-adrenoceptor autoantibodies can be used to monitor myocyte recovery. Weaning from MCSS offers an alternative to cardiac transplantation in certain patients (Müller *et al.*, 1997).

In 1999, they reported their extended clinical experience with the weaning concept. In 19 patients (23–65 years old) with intractable end-stage dilated cardiomyopathy, ventricular assist devices were explanted after support periods of up to 26 months, when repeat off-pump studies had shown either restoration of cardiac function (LVEF >45%) and dimensions (LVIDd <55 mm) or partial recovery (LVEF between 35% and 40%) with serious complications on the device. At the time of device placement, the LVEF was <20%, the LVIDd was >64 mm, and bridge to transplantation had been planned.

Seven patients with persistently restored cardiac function for >8 months and 5 patients for <5 months after weaning were studied. Five patients with recurrent heart failure died within 4–8 months after explantation. Four patients had to be transplanted, and two died for reasons unrelated to cardiac function. Individual optimal LVEFs and LVIDds were reached before pump removal was actually conducted in all patients. These parameters gradually deteriorated until pump removal.

At that time, they concluded that lasting recovery can be reached by ventricular unloading in a subset of patients with intractable end-stage dilated cardiomyopathy. Obviously, there is an individual optimum of recovery that cannot be further improved by prolonged unloading (Hetzer *et al.*, 1999).

As of 2000, a total of 512 cardiac assist devices of various types (Berlin Heart, Berlin, Germany; Novacor, WorldHeart, Ottawa, Ontario, Canada; TCI, ThermoCardio Systems, Inc., Woburn, MA; DeBakey, MicroMed Technology, Inc., Houston, TX) had been implanted in patients with end-stage heart failure in the Berlin Center. Of these, 95 patients belonged to a subgroup of patients with nonischemic, idiopathic, dilated cardiomyopathy who were implanted with a left ventricular support system (Novacor 84, TCI 10, Berlin Heart 1) between 1994 and 2000. All were routinely examined by echocardiography for improvement of cardiac function. The LVIDd and LVEF served as the main parameters to assess changes in cardiac performance. Under the conditions of a running device, an LVIDd below 60 mm and an LVEF above 40% were the criteria to do further echocardiographic studies when the pump was turned off for up to 20 min.

Twenty-eight patients (26 men, 2 women; ages 18 to 64 years; history of heart failure, 1 to 17 years) fulfilled the criteria of improved cardiac performance and were weaned from the device. Since then, 16 patients have continued normal heart function with follow-up times ranging from 1 month to 5.5 years (group B). Three patients died of noncardiac causes (group C). Eight patients were transplanted 1–17 months later, and one died on the waiting list (group A). Statistically significant differences between groups A and B were calculated for the duration of heart failure (9 vs. 2 years, $p = 0.0002$). Differences in LVIDd before removal of the device (57 vs. 51 mm, $p = 0.0420$), LVEF after 2 months of unloading (30% vs. 49%, $p = 0.0300$), and LVEF pre-explantation (43% vs. 52%, $p = 0.0001$) were significant. Overall, 16 (17%) of the cohort of 95 patients were successfully weaned.

The authors concluded at that time that weaning from cardiac assist devices is feasible for selected patients; it saves donor hearts and is preferred to cardiac transplantation. However, as of 2001, no reliable parameter exists to predict the outcome after weaning or to determine the possibility of device removal before implantation in advance (Hetzer *et al.*, 2001).

The extended 9-year experience of the Berlin group in weaning 31 IDCM patients after MCSD, using echocardiographic evaluations during repeated off-pump trials as the cornerstone for the weaning decision, was evaluated to assess the reliability of their weaning criteria in light of the long-term results. They evaluated all of the IDCM patients who were weaned between March 1995 and March 2004 with regard to preservation of cardiac function without LVAD support and survival after weaning, and reviewed their echocardiographic data to assess the predictive value of long-term stability of cardiac function after weaning.

The 32 weaned IDCM patients showed a survival rate of 78.3% $\pm$ 8.1% at 5 years after LVAD explantation. Heart failure recurred during the first 3 years after weaning in 10 (31.3%) patients. Two patients died of heart failure after weaning, while the remaining recurrent patients were successfully transplanted. An off-pump LV end-diastolic diameter of >55 mm and/or an LVEF of <45% before LVAD removal, as well as a history of HF $\geq$5 years before LVAD implantation, appeared to be major risk factors for the early recurrence of HF. Patients without any of these three risk factors showed no HF recurrence during the first 3 years after weaning, but all of those with at least two of these three risk factors developed early recurrence of HF. In patients with HF recurrence during the first 3 postweaning years, a significant LVEF decrease occurred during the first month after weaning; whereas in those with long-term stable cardiac function even at the end of the sixth postweaning month, the LVEF was not different from that before LVAD removal.

The authors showed that for selected patients with IDCM, weaning from LVADs is a clinical option with good results observed for over 9 years and should, therefore, be considered in those with cardiac recovery after LVAD implantation. Their data also suggested that off-pump echocardiography is reliable for the detection of LV recovery and the prediction of long-term cardiac stability after weaning (Dandel *et al.*, 2005).

***The Charite Experience.***   Fulminant myocarditis causes substantial morbidity and mortality, especially in children and young adults. Mechanical circulatory support has become the standard therapy to bridge patients with intractable heart failure to either transplantation or myocardial recovery. Yet, successful weaning from biventricular support with full recovery is extremely rare in the pediatric population.

Hotz *et al.* (2004) described the successful use of the MEDOS HIA ventricular assist device to bridge a 12-year-old girl to myocardial recovery in a biventricular bypass configuration. The left and right ventricles were completely offloaded by the pumps, and the device provided sufficient cardiac output to normalize end-organ function. Anticoagulation was maintained with IV heparin infusion. No neurological complications were detected and the pump system was free of any macroscopic thrombi. After 19 days of support, cardiac function had recovered and the patient was successfully weaned from the device. Following physical rehabilitation, the patient was discharged home (Hotz *et al.*, 2004).

***The Bad Oeynhausen Experience.***   The group at the world's largest MCSD program in the Heart Center Bad Oeynhausen have studied children and adolescents with fulminant myocarditis undergoing prolonged circulatory support with different assist devices. Between 1994 and 2004, seven children and adolescents (aged 7–18 years, mean age 13.5 years) were treated with VADs (5 Thoratec, 1 MEDOS, 1 Novacor) for circulatory support. Three patients underwent left ventricular support; while biventricular support was necessary in four patients. Four patients (three left VADs, one bi-VAD) were successfully bridged to heart transplantation after a mean support time of 163 days (56–258 days). One 7-year-old girl (MEDOS BVAD) died after a support time of 11 days because of irreversible multiorgan failure. One 18-year-old patient was successfully weaned from Thoratec BVAD after 66 days with complete recovery of left ventricular function. As good markers, atrial and brain natriuretic peptides were found to reach normal values after recovery of myocardial function. A 15-year-old girl was still on the device at the time of writing this report.

In children or adolescents with irreversible shock in fulminant myocarditis with an anticipated mortality of 100%, both successful bridging to heart transplantation and successful bridging to recovery are possible. Thus, the authors concluded that young patients with fulminant myocarditis should be rapidly transferred to a clinic with a mechanical circulatory support program so as to offer this life-saving option (Reiss *et al.*, 2006).

***The La Pitie-Salpetriere Experience.***  Fulminant myocarditis (FM) is a rare but life-threatening condition, for which an MCSD can be life-saving. However, the device selection, weaning, and explantation procedures remain poorly defined. At La Pitie-Salpetriere in Paris, four patients were bridged to recovery using the Thoratec biventricular support device. All four were in a state of cardiogenic shock with rapid deterioration of their clinical status, despite increasing doses of inotropes. Three patients required mechanical respiratory support, 3 were anuric, and 1 was dialyzed. Echocardiography showed a mean ejection fraction of $12\% \pm 8\%$. Each Thoratec implantation was performed on cardiopulmonary bypass with a beating heart. Three patients underwent biventricular cannulation; the fourth patient underwent left ventricular and right atrial cannulation.

All patients manifested evidence of moderate-to-severe end-organ dysfunction after device implantation. However, by the time of explantation, end-organ function had recovered in all patients. After a mean duration of $17 \pm 10$ days, all of the patients showed evidence of myocardial recovery. This was confirmed through echocardiography, which showed an opening of the aortic valve and a contraction of both ventricles. The weaning process was performed in 2–5 days by setting the device in a fixed mode and increasing the rate. Device explantation was uneventful in the four patients. During the sixth-month echocardiography follow-up, all patients had normal systolic function.

The authors concluded that in patients with FM, biventricular support allows full circulatory support and unloads both ventricles until recovery occurs. In this set of patients, the weaning and removal procedures were straightforward. Therefore, the authors suggested an aggressive stance toward the implantation of MCSDs in patients with fulminant myocarditis (Leprince *et al.*, 2003).

***The University of Pittsburgh Experience.*** Ventricular assist devices are important bridges to cardiac transplantation. VAD support may also function as a bridge to ventricular recovery (BTR); however, clinical predictors of recovery and long-term outcomes remain uncertain. The Pittsburgh group examined the prevalence, characteristics, and outcomes of BTR subjects in a large single-center series.

The University of Pittsburgh group implanted VADs in 154 adults from 1996 through 2003. Of these implants, 10 were BTR, including 2 (2.5%) out of 80 ischemic patients (who were supported for 42 and 61 days, respectively). Both subjects had surgical revascularization, required perioperative left VAD support, and were alive and transplant-free during the follow-up (232 and 1319 days, respectively). A larger percentage of nonischemic patients underwent BTR [8 (11%) out of 74 patients; age, $30 \pm 14$ years; 7 (88%) female; LVEF, $18\% \pm 6\%$; supported for $112 \pm 76$ days]. Three had myocarditis, 4 had postpartum cardiomyopathy (PPCM), and 1 had idiopathic cardiomyopathy. Five received biventricular support. After explantation, ventricular function declined in two PPCM patients who then required transplantation. Ventricular recovery in the six nonischemic patients who survived transplant-free was maintained (LVEF, $54\% \pm 5\%$; follow-up, $1.5 \pm 0.9$ years). Overall, 8 of the 10 BTR patients were alive and free of transplant (follow-up, $1.6 \pm 1.1$ years).

The authors concluded that BTR is more evident in nonischemic rather than ischemic patients, and that the need for biventricular support does not preclude recovery. For most BTR subjects presenting with acute inflammatory cardiomyopathy, ventricular recovery is maintained in the long term. VAD support as a BTR should be considered in the care of acute myocarditis and PPCM (Simon *et al.*, 2005b).

***The Columbia University Medical Center Experience.*** A retrospective review of patients receiving a mechanical bridge to transplantation at Columbia Presbyterian Hospital after July 21, 1991, was performed to determine the incidence of patients in whom the device was successfully explanted. From August 1, 1996, to February 1, 1998, the team prospectively attempted to identify potential explant candidates by using exercise testing. During this time, they recruited 39 consecutive patients after insertion of the Thermo Cardiosystems vented electric device to participate in the following study. Approximately 3 months after device implantation, a maximal exercise test with hemodynamic monitoring and respiratory gas analysis was performed with the LVAD in the automated mode. The electric device was interfaced with a pneumatic console such that the rate could be decreased to 20 cycles/min. Hemodynamic measurements were recorded as the device rate was decreased. A repeat exercise test was then performed if the patient remained hemodynamically stable.

A retrospective chart review of 111 LVAD recipients at the institution identified only 5 successful explant patients. Eighteen of the 39 patients were studied. Fifteen patients exercised with maximal device support. At peak exercise, $VO_2$ averaged $14.5 \pm 3.6$ mL $\cdot$ kg$^{-1}$ $\cdot$ min$^{-1}$; LVAD flow, $8.0 \pm 1.3$ L/min; Fick cardiac output, $11.4 \pm 3.3$ L/min; and pulmonary capillary wedge pressure, $13 \pm 4$ mm Hg. Seven patients remained normotensive and could exercise at a fixed rate of 20 cycles/min. In these patients, peak $VO_2$ declined from $17.3 \pm 3.9$ mL $\cdot$ kg$^{-1}$ $\cdot$ min$^{-1}$ to $13.0 \pm 6.1$ mL $\cdot$ kg$^{-1}$ $\cdot$ min$^{-1}$. In one of these patients, the device was explanted.

The authors concluded that significant myocardial recovery after LVAD therapy in patients with end-stage congestive heart failure occurs in a small percentage of patients. Most of these patients have dilated cardiomyopathy. Exercise testing may be a useful modality to identify those patients in whom the device can be explanted (Mancini *et al.*, 1998b).

*The Advocate Christ Medical Center Experience.*    At Advocate Christ Medical Center, Oak Lawn, IL, six patients with advanced heart failure and severe mitral regurgitation underwent successful bridge to recovery using a Thoratec left ventricular assist device. Data detailing their myocardial recovery monitoring and their weaning from the left ventricular assist device were prospectively collected. Clinical data collected during the recovery phase included chest roentgenogram, echocardiography, plasma norepinephrine, tumor necrosis factor alpha, bioimpedance, and cardiopulmonary exercise testing (peak oxygen consumption). The normalization of these variables with a 10% increase in the peak oxygen consumption was obtained before weaning. The Thoratec device rate and percent systole were manipulated to allow gradual reloading of the ventricle. The weaning process occurred for more than 5–10 days so as to allow time for observation of the ventricle and its response to the increasing workload.

The authors concluded that select patients with advanced congestive heart failure and severe mitral insufficiency can benefit from mechanical device support. They described their monitoring technique for myocardial recovery using clinical variables. This technique of weaning allows for gradual reloading of the ventricle and a longer period of observation before device removal. Additional research is needed to determine which variables will accurately predict long-term myocardial recovery and the optimal weaning method (Slaughter *et al.*, 2001).

***The Texas Heart Institute Experience.*** The use of dobutamine stress echocardiography (DSE) has also been applied to quantitate myocardial recovery in patients with heart failure supported by LVADs. By recording the hemodynamic response with the use of DSE, the group at Texas Heart Institute evaluated and applied the resulting data in 16 patients who regained functional capacity on full LVAD support and who tolerated decreased mechanical support with no worsening of dyspnea or fatigue. All 16 patients underwent dobutamine stress with increasing doses of dobutamine (5–40 mcg/kg/min). Hemodynamic tests and two-dimensional echocardiography were performed at each dose level. In addition, paired myocardial samples were obtained and histologically analyzed to determine the myocyte size and collagen content.

Dobutamine stress separated the study population into two groups: those who had favorable responses to dobutamine (9 out of 16 patient), and those who had unfavorable responses (i.e. experienced hemodynamic deterioration; 7 out of 16). Favorable dobutamine responses were characterized by improved cardiac index, improved force–frequency relationship in the left ventricle (dP/dt), improved left ventricular ejection fraction, and decreased left ventricular end-diastolic dimension. All nine favorable responders underwent LVAD explantation, and six survived for more than 12 months.

In all of the patients studied, LVAD support resulted in decreased myocyte size ($n = 14, 33.9 \pm 0.9$ microM before support vs. $16.6 \pm 0.8$

microM after support, $p = 0.0001$; normal, 5–15 microM), but resulted in no consistent changes in collagen content. The findings of these authors suggested that DSE with hemodynamic assessment may be a useful tool to assess physiological improvement in the myocardial function of patients with end-stage heart failure who receive LVAD support, and to help predict which patients can tolerate LVAD removal (Khan *et al.*, 2003).

The Texas Heart Institute group have presented their experience with four patients who had acute, severe heart failure without coronary artery disease or biopsy-proven myocarditis. After receiving prolonged ventricular assist system support, all four patients had a significantly improved left ventricular function, returning to New York Heart Association functional class I without inotropic therapy. In each case, dobutamine stress echocardiography and invasive hemodynamic tests were performed to confirm the improvement of cardiac function before device explantation was undertaken. In all four cases, device explantation was followed by early successful maintenance of left ventricular function. These cases reveal a unique clinical syndrome that may be successfully treated with early institution of ventricular assist system support, followed by explantation after myocardial recovery (Frazier *et al.*, 2004a).

***The Guangzhou Experience.***   A multivariate model to predict the likelihood of weaning from ventricular assist devices was recently developed by the group at Jinan University, Guangzhou, China. This group analyzed the factors influencing the cardiac function of patients after weaning from ventricular assist devices, and established a prognostic index by building a Cox proportional hazards model that included the clinical parameters of 28 patients with end-stage heart failure both before implantation of a ventricular assist device and directly before weaning from the device. After weaning from the ventricular assist devices, 14 of the 28 patients showed stable cardiac function, 12 had recurrent heart failure (1 died before either transplantation or implantation of another ventricular assist device), and 2 died of causes unrelated to heart failure.

In addition to left ventricular ejection fraction, the duration of symptomatic heart failure and left ventricular intracavitary dimensions in diastole measured before ventricular assist device weaning were the major factors influencing cardiac function after weaning. In the group of patients with a heart failure duration of <3 years, only 2 out of 13 cases were recurrent; but in the group with a heart failure duration of >3 years, 10 out of 15 cases were recurrent. In 10 patients with 40–50 mm left ventricular intracavitary dimensions in diastole before weaning, only 1 case was recurrent. In 10 patients with 51–55 mm left ventricular intracavitary dimensions in diastole, 3 cases were recurrent. In the group with left ventricular intracavitary dimensions in diastole >56 mm, all 8 cases were recurrent.

A prognostic index was calculated as $-10.10 + 0.208$ (heart failure duration in years) $+0.173$ (pre-explantation left ventricular intracavitary dimensions in diastole in mm). In the group with a prognostic index of <0, only 2 out of 16 cases were recurrent and the rate of stable cardiac function after weaning was 83.6%. In the group with a prognostic index of >0, 10 out of 12 cases were recurrent and the rate of stable function was 0.0%. The authors concluded that in patients with an off-pump left ventricular ejection fraction of >40%, the duration of symptomatic heart failure and the left ventricular intracavitary dimensions in diastole measured before weaning yield a useful index to predict long-term cardiac function after weaning from ventricular assist devices (Liang *et al.*, 2005).

***The STS Cardiac National Database Experience.***    An important retrospective analysis in patients who failed to wean from cardiopulmonary bypass was recently conducted by the group at Duke University by examining the large cardiac national database of the Society of Thoracic Surgeons (STS). A total of 5735 patients underwent MCSD implantation after cardiac surgery during the years 1995–2004, representing 0.3% of the total cardiac surgeries in the database. The overall survival rate to discharge following MCSD placement was 54.1%. Risk-adjusted mortality by periods was 58.1% between January 1995 and June 1997, and 39.1% between July 2002 and December 2004 ($P < 0.0001$).

Perioperative characteristics associated with increased mortality were urgency of procedure, reoperation, renal failure, myocardial infarction, aortic stenosis, female gender, race, peripheral vascular disease, NYHA class IV, cardiogenic shock, left main coronary stenosis, and valve procedure (c-index $= 0.756$). The authors concluded that after adjusting for the clinical characteristics of patients requiring mechanical circulatory support, the survival rates to hospital discharge improved dramatically, and that the insertion of an MCSD for post–cardiac surgery shock is an important thera-peutic intervention that can salvage a majority of these patients (Hernandez *et al.*, in press).

A summary of selected functional recoveries under MCSD support and explantation experience/protocols is provided below (Table 6). A proposed protocol for evaluation and explantation is provided in Appendix 5.

## Mechanisms of Cardiac Recovery During MCSD Support

***Effect of Left Ventricular Unloading on Right Ventricular Recovery.***
Although many reports demonstrate the hemodynamic benefits of left ven-tricular assist devices (LVAD) on right-sided circulation, it is not known whether the right ventricular myocardium goes through reverse remodeling after left ventricular mechanical circulatory support (Rodrigue-Way *et al.*, 2005). Accordingly, the purposes of the studies conducted by the group at Baylor College of Medicine in Houston were (1) to investigate the right ventricular changes that occur in fibrosis, cellular hypertrophy, and intramy-ocardial tumor necrosis factor alpha (TNF-alpha) levels in patients receiv-ing LVAD support; and (2) to determine whether the type of LVAD used influences right ventricular myocardial changes.

The authors measured myocyte size, total collagen content, and TNF-alpha levels using semiquantitative immunohistochemical analysis of myocardial samples from the right and left ventricles of control and failing myocardia, either supported by one of two distinct forms of LVADs or with-out support. They found that, although myocyte size was not increased in the right ventricle of failing myocardia ($p = $ not significant), total collagen content and myocardial TNF-alpha levels were decreased in the right ven-tricle compared with controls ($p < 0.01$ and $p < 0.001$, respectively).

The authors concluded that these data demonstrate that chronic left ven-tricular unloading with either pulsatile or continuous flow devices decreases right ventricular total collagen and myocardial TNF-alpha content. They suggested that the decreased fibrosis and the normalization of the cytokine milieu observed may in part contribute to the recovery of right-sided cardiac function associated with chronic mechanical circulatory support (Kucuker *et al.*, 2004).

**Table 6.** Summary of selected MCSD support explantation protocols.

| Author | Method | Variables | Outcome |
|---|---|---|---|
| Deng et al. (1997) | Exercise protocol Assessment before, during, and after maximum exercise Right heart catheter Echocardiography 2 different MCSD settings: fill rate trigger mode + maximal unloading; fill rate trigger mode + preload and afterload challenge | LVEF Aortic valve flow Hemodynamics Contribution of the native left ventricle to total cardiac output | 2 patients tested 1 patient explanted and transplanted |
| Müller et al. (1997) | Echocardiographic recovery 3-week test in fixed rate/asynchronous mode | Echocardiographic evaluation | Weaning feasible in 29% of patients Device-free for 51–592 days |
| Mancini et al. (1998b) | Exercise testing LVAD (auto mode) pneumatic interface Heart rate decrease to 20 cycles/min Serial hemodynamics Repetition of exercise test if patient remains stable | Maximal exercise test Hemodynamic monitoring Respiratory gas analysis ($VO_2$) LVAD flow Cardiac output PCPW | 39 consecutive patients 18 patients studied 15 patients exercised on maximal device support 7 patients remained normotensive and exercised at 20 cycles/min, but peak $VO_2$ declined 1 patient explanted |
| Hetzer et al. (1999) | Echocardiography: individual optimal LVEF and LVIDd reached before pump removal | LVEF LVIDd | 19 patients studied 7 patients with persistently restored cardiac function 5 patients died of HF 4 patients transplanted 2 patients died of noncardiac causes |
| Hetzer et al. (2001) | Echocardiography on running-device condition: LVIDd <60 mm, LVEF >40% Echocardiography on pump-off condition for up to 20 min | LVEF LVIDd | 95 patients with nonischemic, idiopathic, dilated cardiomyopathy fulfilled the criteria of improved cardiac performance and were weaned from the device 16 patients remained normal (1 month to 5.5 years) 3 patients died |

*(Continued)*

**Table 6.**  (*Continued*)

| Author | Method | Variables | Outcome |
|--------|--------|-----------|---------|
| | | | 8 patients transplanted<br>1 patient died on the waiting list |
| Slaughter et al. (2001) | Postoperative patients failed to wean from surgery<br>Recovery phase: fill mode to empty mode. Monitoring of neurohormonal markers, transthoracic echocardiography, CXR, bioimpedance, cardiopulmonary exercise testing<br>Weaning phase: after assessing the normalization trend of previous parameters. Asynchronous mode, step increase in heart rate during 24–48 h step. Daily transthoracic echocardiography and bioimpedance assessment. Repetition of cardiopulmonary excercise | LV decompression<br>Aortic valve opening<br>Norepinephrine<br>TNF$\alpha$<br>Bioimpedance VO$_2$ | 6 patients studied |
| Khan et al. (2003) | Dobutamine stress echocardiography<br>Patient regained functional capacity on full LVAD support and tolerated reloading with no worsening of dyspnea or fatigue<br>DSE in increasing doses (5–40 mcg/kg/min) | Hemodynamics<br>Cardiac index<br>dP/dt<br>LVEF<br>LVIDd | 16 patients studied<br>9 patients (favorable responders) explanted<br>6 patients survived for more than 12 months |
| Frazier et al. (2004a) | Dobutamine stress echocardiography and invasive hemodynamic tests<br>Significantly improved LVEF<br>NYHA class I (without inotropic therapy) | LVEF<br>NYHA<br>Hemodynamics | 4 patients with nonischemic, nonmyocarditis heart failure |

(*Continued*)

**Table 6.** (*Continued*)

| Author | Method | Variables | Outcome |
|--------|--------|-----------|---------|
| Liang et al. (2005) | Multivariate prediction model, measured before ventricular assist device weaning<br>Calculation of a prognostic index: prognostic index = $-10.10 + 0.208$ (heart failure duration in years) $+ 0.173$ (pre-explantation left ventricular intracavitary dimensions in diastole in mm) | Duration of symptomatic heart failure<br>LVEF<br>LVIDd<br>Index $\geq 0$:<br>index $<0$ = good prognosis;<br>index $>0$ = bad prognosis | 28 patients studied<br>14 patients with stable cardiac function<br>12 patients with recurrent heart failure (1 died before OHT or implantation of another device, 2 deaths unrelated to heart failure)<br>Index $<0$: 2 of 16 patient recurrences; 83.6% stable cardiac function after 51 months<br>Index $>0$: 10 of 12 patient recurrences; 0% stable cardiac function after 57 months |
| Slaughter et al. (2006) | Mechanical reload by LVAD rate reduction (80, 60, and 40 bpm) or LVAD stroke volume reduction (100, 120, and 140 bpm) protocols consisting of 30 min of support at each LVAD beat rate | Aortic pressure/flow<br>LV pressure/volume<br>Pulmonary artery/flow<br>LVAD flow | Experimental protocols in calves<br>LVAD stroke volume reduction protocol produced steady-state mechanical reloading<br>LVAD rate reduction resulted in transient LV mechanical reloading |

***Role of Proinflammatory Cytokines in Reverse Remodeling.*** Proinflammatory cytokine cascades such as tumor necrosis factor and interleukin-6 have been implicated in the progression of heart failure. Individual case reports demonstrate (1) the existence of an intracardiac IL6 and IL6 receptor system; (2) a dynamic regulation of this system in myocarditis-associated low-output syndrome; (3) the temporal association of elevated plasma levels of IL6 with myocardial gene expression and left ventricular dysfunction; and (4) the synchronicity of improvement of left ventricular function with reversal of plasma levels and myocardial IL6 mRNA expression, the cause of which might be LVAD unloading, myocarditis healing, or both. These data support the concept of a pathophysiological role of IL6 in myocarditis and advanced heart failure, potentially based on its intrinsic negative inotropic or hypertrophogenic properties (Plenz *et al.*, 1999).

of the pump. He feels that it keeps him from going to places that are quiet. In his words, "If I'm in the proximity of people in a quiet place or even in the waiting room of doctors' offices, people stare at me because they wonder where the sound (the pump) comes from."

He is frustrated about going on cable at night and not being able to walk into another room of the house. For example, "If I want a drink from the kitchen or if I want to join the family in another room, I can't because I am tied to the PBU." The caregiver has to become accustomed to what I term sedentary behavior. Activity is limited or carefully selected by my husband.

## Randomized Clinical Trial Evidence: The REMATCH Trial

***REMATCH Design.***    The Randomized Evaluation of Mechanical Assistance for the Treatment of Congestive Heart Failure (REMATCH) trial was a prospective randomized trial that evaluated the survival benefit of the HeartMate® left ventricular assist device over medical therapy in patients who are not candidates for cardiac transplantation. The REMATCH trial was a multicenter study supported by the National Heart, Lung, and Blood Institute to compare long-term implantation of left ventricular assist devices (LVADs) with optimal medical management (OMM) for patients with end-stage heart failure who required, but were not qualified to receive, cardiac transplantation (Rose *et al.*, 1999).

***Main Primary Outcomes.***    In REMATCH, 129 patients with end-stage heart failure who were ineligible for cardiac transplantation received an LVAD (68 patients) or OMM (61 patients). All of the patients had symptoms of New York Heart Association class IV heart failure. Kaplan–Meier survival analysis showed a 48% reduction in the risk of death from any cause in the group that received LVADs as compared with the medical therapy group (relative risk, 0.52; 95% CI, 0.34 to 0.78; $P = 0.001$). The survival rate at 1 year was 52% in the device group and 25% in the medical therapy group ($P = 0.002$); and the rates at 2 years were 23% and 8% ($P = 0.09$), respectively. The frequency of serious adverse events in the device group was 2.35 (95% CI, 1.86 to 2.95) times that in the medical therapy group, with a predominance of infection, bleeding, and malfunction of the device. The quality of life was significantly improved at 1 year in the device group.

The authors concluded that the use of an LVAD in patients with advanced heart failure results in a clinically meaningful survival benefit and an improved quality of life, and that an LVAD can be an acceptable alternative therapy in selected patients who are not candidates for cardiac transplantation (Rose *et al.*, 2001).

***Long-Term Survival Outcomes.*** The REMATCH trial (Rose *et al.*, 2001) provided first evidence that lifetime or destination MCSD in patients with advanced heart failure who are not eligible for heart transplantation can prolong and improve the quality of life. The REMATCH trial compared the use of LVADs with OMM for patients with end-stage heart failure. When the trial met its primary endpoint criteria in July 2001, LVAD therapy was shown to significantly improve survival and quality of life. With extended follow-up, two critical questions emerged: (1) did these benefits persist; and (2) did outcomes improve over the course of the trial, given the evolving nature of the technology?

The REMATCH authors analyzed survival in this randomized trial by using the product-limit method of Kaplan and Meier. Changes in the benefits of therapy were analyzed by examining the effect of the enrollment period. The survival rates for patients receiving LVADs ($n = 68$) vs. patients receiving OMM ($n = 61$) were 52% vs. 28% at 1 year and 29% vs. 13% at 2 years, respectively ($P = 0.008$, log-rank test). As of July 2003, eleven patients were alive on LVAD support out of a total of 16 survivors (including three patients receiving OMM who crossed over to LVAD therapy). There was a significant improvement in survival for LVAD-supported patients who enrolled during the second half of the trial compared with those during the first half ($P = 0.03$). The Minnesota Living with Heart Failure scores improved significantly over the course of the trial.

The authors concluded that the extended follow-up confirmed the initial observation that LVAD therapy renders significant survival and quality-of-life benefits compared to OMM for patients with end-stage heart failure. Furthermore, they observed an improvement in the survival of patients receiving LVADs over the course of the trial, suggesting the effect of greater clinical experience (Park *et al.*, 2005).

***Infection Outcomes.***    With respect to infection in lifetime/destination/ permanent MCSD, the analysis of the REMATCH trial focusing on infection is revealing. The REMATCH investigators used the information to suggest ways to decrease the incidence and effects of device-related infection. In REMATCH, patients were prospectively randomized to receive LVADs or OMM for end-stage heart failure. Infection variables included sepsis adjudicated as the cause of death; sepsis reported as a serious adverse event; percutaneous site or pocket infection; and pump housing, inflow tract, or outflow tract infection.

The authors compared the incidence and prevalence of events between the two groups and generated time-related descriptions. Survival with LVAD ($n = 68$ patients) was superior to OMM survival ($n = 61$ patients) with a 47% decrease in the risk of death ($p < 0.001$), but the aggregate adverse event rate was greater for patients with LVADs (risk ratio, 2.29; 95% CI, 1.85–2.84). Freedom from sepsis in patients with LVADs was 58% at 1 year and 48% at 2 years after implantation, with superior survival in nonseptic patients (60% vs. 39% at 1 year and 38% vs. 8% at 2 years in nonseptic vs. septic patients with LVADs, $p < 0.06$). Percutaneous site or pocket infection did not affect survival ($p = 0.86$). The hazard for onset of sepsis peaked within the first 3 weeks after implantation.

The authors concluded that survival is improved with permanent LVAD implantation compared with OMM therapy. However, infection causes substantial morbidity and mortality. The REMATCH investigators concluded that reducing infections increases survival and decreases morbidity in permanent LVAD recipients, and improves the risk-benefit ratio for permanent LVAD therapy (Holman *et al.*, 2004).

## Observational Non-RCT Studies

*INTrEPID.* The INTrEPID trial was a nonrandomized, case-controlled study to evaluate the safety and effectiveness of the Novacor® left ventricular assist system as an alternative to medical therapy in nontransplant eligible patients who are dependent on intravenous inotropic therapy. A retrospective analysis including 255 Novacor assist device recipients showed similar effects as the HeartMate I device (Young *et al.*, 2005).

*ISHLT MCSD Report.* According to the Third Annual ISHLT MCSD Report, the vast majority of patients are triaged to destination MCSD because of advanced age or severe comorbidities, which make them poorly suited for transplantation. The percentage of destination MCSD implantations in this report was around 10%. As expected, most of these patients received pulsatile MCSDs. Among the entire cohort of destination patients, the actuarial survival rate was 65% at 6 months and 34% at 1 year. As shown in the multivariable analysis for the overall group, old age remains a major risk factor for mortality. Among patients less than 65 years of age at the time of destination therapy, the actuarial survival rate at 1 year was 41%, but for those over the age of 65, it was poor (Deng *et al.*, 2005a).

*The German Heart Center Berlin Experience.* Ventricular assist device implantation has become an established therapy in adults and children as a bridge to heart transplantation or to aid myocardial recovery. Recently, the implantation of LVADs as a definitive therapy has been recognized as a better option than pharmacological treatment in patients who are not candidates for heart transplantation. The experience at the German Heart Center Berlin in 27 patients showed that permanent MCSD therapy does have the potential to evolve as a treatment option in selected elderly patients with end-stage HF (Jurmann *et al.*, 2004). In another study presented by the German Heart Center in Berlin, five patients were successfully supported by two different LVADs for over 4 years. This unique experience shows that LVAD support can be extended beyond 4 years with a good quality of life and a low risk, making it a good alternative for nontransplant candidates (Potapov *et al.*, 2006).

# ABIOMED

## Abiomed BVS 5000 Experience

*The Hahnemann University Experience.*   The progress made with the Abiomed Biventricular System (BVS) 5000 (Abiomed, Inc., Danvers, MA) short-term VAD was recently reviewed at Hahnemann University Hospital in Philadelphia, PA. From June 1994 through August 2000, all cardiogenic shock patients who required short-term mechanical assist were supported with the Abiomed BVS 5000. Insertion criteria included any condition that could potentially result in cardiac recovery. A formal algorithm for the timing of insertion was established to standardize the implantation criteria.

A total of 45 patients were supported at Hahnemann University Hospital; of these, 26 were male and 19 were female patients, with a mean age of 57.9 years (range, 33–80 years). Devices were inserted for post-cardiotomy shock in 36 (80%) patients and for precardiotomy shock in 9 (20%) patients. The average duration of support was 8.3 days (range, 1–31 days). Overall, 22 (49%) patients were weaned from support and 14 (31%) were discharged from the hospital. For patients in whom the device was implanted in accordance with an established protocol (group A), the wean and discharge rates were 60% and 43%, respectively. The most common morbidities included bleeding and adverse neurological events.

The authors concluded that the Abiomed BVS 5000 VAD continues to be a valuable form of short-term mechanical assist for acute cardiogenic shock, and that the formation of a uniform VAD insertion algorithm helps to standardize management protocols (Samuels *et al.*, 2001).

## Abiomed AB 5000 Experience

*The Hahnemann University Experience.*   The Abiomed AB 5000 was designed to be an upgrade to the BVS 5000 in terms of patient mobility, blood pump durability, and overall versatility. The Abiomed AB 5000 was implanted in 4 cases, in which 2 AB 5000 systems were placed *de novo* while 2 were transitioned from previously placed BVS 5000 units. Hemolysis was observed in two cases. The AB 5000 VAD flows were generally

4.0 to 4.5 L/min, approximately 0.5 L/min less than that of the BVS 5000. Echocardiography demonstrated high-velocity jets from the inflow cannula in the two hemolysis cases. One patient died of multiorgan system failure while on support, 2 were successfully weaned from support and transferred to long-term care facilities, and 1 was weaned from support and successfully discharged to home.

The authors concluded that the AB 5000 VAD is a versatile paracorporeal pneumatic VAD that can be placed *de novo* or transitioned from a previously placed BVS 5000 unit, without the need for additional surgery. Lower outputs, high-velocity jets, and hemolysis were observed in two of four cases. Modifications in cannula design and placement as well as console reconfiguration may be necessary to optimize performance (Samuels *et al.*, 2005).

# THORATEC

## Thoratec VAD

***Thoratec PVAD.*** As of July 2006, more than 2800 Thoratec paracorporeal VAD (PVAD) MCSD implantations have been performed worldwide in over 170 centers. The Thoratec VAD System is the only system that offers circulatory support for the left side of the heart, the right side of the heart, or both sides of the heart. The Thoratec MCSD has been used to support patients weighing 17–144 kg and as young as 6 years old.

***Thoratec IVAD.*** The implantable VAD (IVAD) is based on the reliable and clinically successful Thoratec® VAD System, which as of July 2006 has been implanted in over 2800 patients worldwide. The result is an implantable VAD with proven technology that can support a wide range of patient sizes. While design attributes integral to the success of the Thoratec VAD System have been kept intact, new features have also been incorporated into the IVAD to allow it to meet the needs and withstand the rigors of an implantable pump, including a smooth external profile and small size, construction from an advanced and durable titanium alloy, a small percutaneous exit site, and an electronic indication of pump empty.

As of September 2003, a total of 30 patients with advanced heart failure have been supported with the Thoratec IVAD for bridge to transplantation or for postcardiotomy ventricular failure in Europe and the US. Sixty-eight percent have been successfully treated through transplantation or ventricular recovery, with many of these patients discharged to their homes through the use of the TLC-II® Portable VAD Driver. The initial IVAD results indicate that the device can successfully treat a wide array of patients with a low incidence of many serious adverse events that are commonly associated with VAD use, such as embolic stroke and systemic infection.

## HEARTMATE

**Peter E (born 1964)**

**Living with an LVAD**

My LVAD experiences, lets see … I was on the golf course that I manage with my then wife Christy chasing the geese (a big problem for sports turfs, parks, and golf courses). I was using a starter-like pistol that shoots whistlers to scare the geese. After we finished, we left the golf course, and we were driving along the road when an off-duty sheriff's officer who had been jogging at the nearby college campus cut me off and pulled me over. He had his gun drawn, thinking that my battery holsters were gun holsters!

The scariest and yet funniest incident, I guess, was at the September 1997 Rolling Stones concert at the Giants Stadium. I had tickets for two nights. The first night's seats were in the third row center. The opening band was fine; but when the Rolling Stones took to the stage, they were just into the beginning of the first song when my LVAD went into the fixed rate of 40 bpm with the alarm going off! Panic city!

I then proceeded to run under the stage with Christy to the first aid tent. I still felt very good. I found a doctor who knew what an LVAD was. He checked me and got me on an ambulance to Columbia Presbyterian. The pump was still alarming on the fixed rate. By the time I reached the George Washington Bridge, the pump had reset itself! I arrived at the emergency room (you know how nice that is!) with Margaret Flannery screaming at me, "Why the hell are you in the emergency room? Go to Milstein!!" I went home after being checked.

Needless to say, I had tickets to the next night's concert that were not quite as close to the stage, so I went. No sooner had the opening band (Foo Fighters) gone on when my pump began alarming and went to the fixed rate again. This time, we called the service and spoke to Dr Oz, asking him what we should do. We decided that although I felt fine, it would be better to go back to the hospital. Dr Oz's comment was, "I will meet you outside for the ticket stubs, okay?" He had me laughing! Another ambulance ride to NY. This time, the pump did not reset itself, and a tech was flown down from Boston to analyze the machine to find the problem. The pump reset itself the next morning. Two weeks later, I received the call from the hospital for the transplant.

Needless to say, I had spent a lot of money on those tickets, so I wrote a letter to the Stones' management to see if I could get my money back. Didn't happen.

## Observational Studies

*The Columbia University Experience.* Between 1990 and 2000, a total of 210 TCI HeartMate LVASs were implanted at Columbia Presbyterian Medical Center (pneumatic, 54; vented electric, 156). Of these, 188 patients survived to transplantation. In 1995, a risk score was derived from 56 patients who had undergone TCI HeartMate LVAS implantation either at the Columbia Presbyterian Medical Center or the Cleveland Clinic, assigning a relative risk-derived weight to oliguria <30 mL (3 points), right heart failure with central venous pressure >16 mm Hg (2 points), ventilator dependence (2 points), hepatic dysfunction with prothrombin time >16 s (2 points), and redo surgery (1 point) (Oz *et al.*, 1995).

This risk score was updated in 130 patients undergoing TCI HeartMate implantation at the Columbia Presbyterian Medical Center between 1996 and 2001. While preoperative renal insufficiency lost its discriminative

power, previous LVAS implantation was identified as an independent predictor of perioperative mortality. It was concluded that improved perioperative management is counterbalanced by an increasingly sick cohort of
patients referred for LVAS implantation (Rao *et al.*, 2003).

***HeartMate I Multicenter Study.***   In a prospective, multicenter clinical
trial conducted at 24 centers in the US, 280 transplant candidates (232
men, 48 women; median age, 55 years; range, 11–72 years) who were
unresponsive to inotropic drugs, intra-aortic balloon counterpulsation, or
both were treated with the HeartMate vented electric left ventricular
assist system (VE LVAS). A cohort of 48 patients (40 men, 8 women;
median age, 50 years; range, 21–67 years) not supported with an LVAS
served as a historical control group. Outcomes were measured in terms
of laboratory data (hemodynamic, hematologic, and biochemical), adverse
events, New York Heart Association functional class, and survival. The
VE LVAS–treated and non-VE LVAS–treated (control) groups were similar in terms of age, sex, and distribution of patients by diagnosis (ischemic
cardiomyopathy, idiopathic cardiomyopathy, and subacute myocardial
infarction).

VE LVAS support lasted an average of 112 days (range, <1–691
days), with 54 patients supported for more than 180 days. The mean VE
LVAS flow (expressed as pump index) throughout support was $2.8 \text{ L} \times \text{min}^{-1} \times \text{m}^{-2}$. The median total bilirubin value decreased from 1.2 mg/dL
at baseline to 0.7 mg/dL ($P = 0.0001$), and the median creatinine value
decreased from 1.5 mg/dL at baseline to 1.1 mg/dL ($P = 0.0001$). VE
LVAS–related adverse events included bleeding in 31 (11%) patients, infection in 113 (40%), neurological dysfunction in 14 (5%), and thromboembolic events in 17 (6%). A total of 160 (58%) patients were enrolled in
a hospital release program. Eight-two (29%) of the 280 VE LVAS–treated
patients died before receiving a transplant, compared with 32 (67%) of the
48 controls ($P < 0.001$). Conversely, 198 (71%) of the 280 VE LVAS–
treated patients survived, 188 (67%) ultimately received a heart transplant,
and 10 (4%) had the device removed electively. The 1-year posttransplant
survival of VE LVAS–treated patients was significantly better than that
of the controls [158 (84%) out of 188 vs. 10 (63%) out of 16; log rank
analysis, $P = 0.0197$].

The authors concluded that the HeartMate VE LVAS provides adequate hemodynamic support, has an acceptably low incidence of adverse effects, and improves survival in heart transplant candidates both inside and outside the hospital (Frazier *et al.*, 2001).

# NOVACOR

## Observational Non-RCT Studies

*European Novacor Multicenter Registry Study.* A large multivariate analysis of 366 unselected consecutive patients who were treated with the Novacor LVAD between 1993 and 1999 in Europe was conducted. The study revealed that respiratory failure associated with septicemia (odds ratio 11.2), right heart failure (odds ratio 3.2), age above 65 years (odds ratio 3.01), acute postcardiotomy (odds ratio 1.8), and acute infarction (odds ratio 1.7) are independent risk factors for survival after LVAS implantation (Deng *et al.*, 2001a).

# DEBAKEY

## BTT Safety and Feasibility Trial

As of December 2004, more than 270 DeBakey MCSD implantations have been performed worldwide. The miniaturization of mechanical support technology has resulted in pumps that can support an expanding pool of patients. Inherent in their design is a limited blood-contacting surface and the lack of valves, air vents, or compliance chambers. The MicroMed DeBakey VAD has been — at the time of this report — the most widely tested of these new miniaturized devices.

Considerations for participation in the trial included the degree of end-organ dysfunction, the condition of the right ventricle, the ability to tolerate chronic anticoagulation, the expected transplantation waiting time, and the patient's desire to participate in the trial, among others. End-organ perfusion was maintained and, despite continuous flow physiology, all the recipients regained some pulsatility owing to the improvement of the left ventricle with unloading. Bleeding requiring reoperation was the most common adverse event observed. Hemolysis rarely occurred and was transient in all three instances.

Remarkably, the incidence of significant device-related infection or malfunction, the two main limitations of pulsatile technology, was almost negligible. The low incidence of infection is likely due to the presence of a low-caliber flexible driveline that readily incorporates to the integument, less torque motion, and the absence of a large preperitoneal pocket. Pump thrombus is a problem more often seen with axial flow technology, and was identified in four patients. In this early experience, pump exchange and high doses of plasminogen activator were used for treatment. None of the patients who developed pump thrombus suffered a stroke or a clinically obvious peripheral embolus.

Not surprisingly, preoperative dependence on intra-aortic balloon support and mechanical ventilation were strong univariate predictors of death before transplantation. Longer CPB time was also a predictor of death and likely reflects previous surgery, technical difficulties, excessive bleeding, and/or right heart dysfunction. Patients were able to ambulate while connected to their portable controller and battery packs, but otherwise were untethered. The nursing staff became readily proficient with axial flow idiosyncrasies, including the lack of an arterial waveform or a palpable pulse and the treatment algorithms for abnormal wave patterns suggestive of ventricular suction.

The trial protocol required that patients remain hospitalized until a suitable donor organ became available. This explains the relatively short mean support time of 42 days observed in the trial. The overall success rate of bridging to transplantation was 67%, and 95% of these patients survived to 30 days after transplantation. Skepticism surrounding the hemodynamics of continuous flow and the ability to maintain end-organ function has abated, as clinical experience with axial flow pumps has grown.

The authors concluded that the results of this first trial of an axial flow pump in the US suggest that the MicroMed DeBakey VAD can provide effective circulatory support in patients with end-stage heart failure. The success rate of bridging to transplantation was similar to that currently achieved with time-tested pulsatile technology. As a result of this initial feasibility trial, the FDA has approved an expanded multicenter evaluation of the MicroMed DeBakey pump as a bridge to transplantation (Goldstein *et al.*, 2005).

# JARVIK 2000

## Feasibility Study

*The Freiburg University Experience.*    The lack of donor hearts has stimulated interest in using blood pumps to treat severe heart failure. The group at Freiburg University tested the hypothesis that a new continuous flow circulatory assist device can be safely employed to relieve symptoms of heart failure, and evaluated its potential to prolong life. An intracardiac axial flow pump was implanted in 17 heart failure patients [idiopathic dilated (12 patients), ischemic (4), or amyloid cardiomyopathy (1)]. All were deemed ineligible for transplantation. Implantation of the device was by left thoracotomy (15 patients) or median sternotomy (2 patients). Power delivery was by a skull-mounted titanium pedestal.

All of the patients survived the surgery. None needed right ventricular support. There were 3 hospital deaths; 2 early from subdural hematoma and aortic thrombosis, and 1 late after switching to transplantation. A total of 14 patients left the hospital with a cumulative support time of 15.9 years (median, 293 days; interquartile range, 286 days; 1–44 months). The actuarial 1-, 2-, and 3-year survival rates were 56%, 47%, and 24%, respectively. There was no pump failure. Quality-of-life scores improved. Two superficial pedestal infections were successfully treated. Four patients had cerebral thromboembolism; 2 early events were attributed to inadequate anticoagulation, and 2 late with near-complete resolution. An improved anticoagulant regime addressed this problem. Late death occurred in five patients from battery disconnection, subdural hematoma, bowel ischemia, respiratory failure, and after cardiac transplantation.

The authors concluded that the continuous flow blood pumps provide symptomatic relief of severe heart failure with a high quality of life. Event-free survival reached 4 years. The analysis of adverse events led to improved management strategies. There is potential for the widespread use of blood pumps in the community, for which a controlled trial is required (Siegenthaler *et al.*, 2005; Deng, 2005).

## OTHER MECHANICAL CIRCULATORY SUPPORT DEVICES

### Cardiowest TAH

***Bridge-to-Transplantation Study.***   The CardioWest total artificial heart orthotopically replaces both native cardiac ventricles and all cardiac valves, thus eliminating problems commonly seen in the bridge-to-transplantation left ventricular and biventricular assist devices, such as right heart failure, valvular regurgitation, cardiac arrhythmias, ventricular clots, intraventricular communications, and low blood flows. The group at the University of Arizona, Tucson, conducted a nonrandomized, prospective study in five centers with the use of historical controls. The purpose was to assess the safety and efficacy of the CardioWest total artificial heart in transplant-eligible patients at risk of imminent death from irreversible biventricular cardiac failure. The primary endpoints included the rates of survival to heart transplantation and of survival after transplantation.

Eighty-one patients received the artificial heart device. The rate of survival to transplantation was 79% (95% CI, 0.68 to 0.87). Of the 35 control patients who met the same entry criteria but did not receive the artificial heart, 16 (46%) survived to transplantation ($P < 0.001$). Overall, the 1-year survival rate among the patients who received the artificial heart was 70%, as compared with 31% among the controls ($P < 0.001$). The 1- and 5-year survival rates after transplantation among the patients who had received a total artificial heart as a bridge to transplantation were 86% and 64%, respectively.

The authors concluded that the implantation of the total artificial heart improves the rates of survival both to and after cardiac transplantation. This device prevents death in critically ill patients who have irreversible biventricular failure and are candidates for cardiac transplantation (Copeland *et al.*, 2004).

# AbioCor TAH

***The University of Kentucky Experience.*** The group at the University of Kentucky in Louisville sought to evaluate the safety and efficacy of the first available totally implantable replacement heart (AbioCor implantable replacement heart system) in the treatment of severe, irreversible biventricular heart failure in human patients. Seven male adult patients with severe, irreversible biventricular failure (>70% 30-day predicted mortality) who were not eligible for transplantation met all the institutional review board study criteria, and had placement of the AbioCor implantable replacement heart. All were in cardiogenic shock despite maximal medical therapy, including inotropes and intra-aortic balloon pumps. The mean age was 66.7 ± 10.4 years (range, 51–79 years). Four of the seven patients had prior operations. Six had ischemic cardiomyopathy, and one had idiopathic cardiomyopathy. All had three-dimensional computer-simulated implantation of the thoracic unit that predicted adequate fit.

At the time of the operation, the internal transcutaneous energy transfer coil, battery, and controller were placed. Biventriculectomy was then performed, and the thoracic unit was placed in an orthotopic position and attached to the atrial cuffs and outflow conduits with quick-connects. The flow was adjusted to 4–8 L/min. The central venous and left atrial pressures were maintained at 5–15 mm Hg. The device is powered through transcutaneous energy transfer. An atrial flow–balancing chamber is used to adjust left/right balance. The balance chamber and transcutaneous energy transfer eliminate the need for percutaneous lines.

There was one intraoperative death caused by coagulopathic bleeding, and one early death caused by an aprotinin reaction. There were multiple morbidities primarily related to pre-existing illness severity: 5 patients had prolonged intubation; 2 had hepatic failure (resolved in 1); 4 had renal failure (resolved in 3); and 1 each had recurrent gastrointestinal bleeding, acute cholecystitis requiring laparotomy, respiratory failure that was resolved after 3 days of extracorporeal membrane oxygenation, and malignant hyperthermia (resolved). There were 3 late deaths: 1 caused by multiple-system organ failure (postoperative day 56), 1 caused by a cerebrovascular accident (postoperative day 142), and 1 caused by retroperitoneal bleeding and resultant multiple-system organ failure (postoperative day 151). This latter patient was not able to tolerate anticoagulation (no anticoagulation or antiplatelet therapy alone for 80% of the first 60 days), and had a transient ischemic attack on postoperative day 61 and a cerebrovascular accident on postoperative day 130. At autopsy, the blood pumps were clean. The two patients who had large cerebrovascular accidents had thrombus on the atrial cage struts, which were removed for future implants.

There were no significant hemolysis or device-related infections or malfunctions. The balance chamber allowed for left/right balance in all patients (left atrial pressure within 5 mm Hg of right atrial pressure). Three patients took multiple (>50) trips out of the hospital, and two were discharged from the hospital. The total days on support with the AbioCor were 759.

The authors concluded that the initial clinical experience suggests that the AbioCor might be an effective therapy for patients with advanced biventricular failure (Dowling *et al.*, 2004).

## DIFFERENTIAL OUTCOMES BY MCSD TYPE

The following Table 7 provides an overview of the published studies comparing the outcomes of different MCSDs. As the Table details, the HeartMate I pulsatile MCSD suggestedly has a lower embolism rate, yet a higher MCSD failure rate than the Novacor MCSD. The second- and third-generation axial flow and centrifugal flow pumps may have a lower infection rate. Hopefully, they will also reduce the surgical implant time and morbidity (because of their smaller size), be more cost-effective, and improve the quality of life.

**Table 7.** Studies addressing differential outcomes by MCSD type.

| Author | Summary |
| --- | --- |
| Hammel *et al.* (1998) | Novacor MCSD is susceptible to driveline fluid exposure |
| Bonkohara *et al.* (1999) | HeartMate I has fatal MCSD dysfunction |
| Schmid *et al.* (1999) | Implantable MCSD allows for patient discharge (OOH) |
| Minami *et al.* (2000) | Implantable MCSD is more durable |
| El-Banayosy *et al.* (2000) | HeartMate has less thromboembolism than Novacor |
| El-Banayosy *et al.* (2003) | Completely implantable MCSD is rare and still too bulky |
| Song *et al.* (2003) | Axial flow MCSD improves morbidity and quality of life, and reduces costs |
| Hetzer *et al.* (2004) | Axial flow LVAD INCOR is durable and reliable |
| Klotz *et al.* (2004) | DeBakey nonpulsatile MCSD unloads as well as pulsatile MCSD |

*(Continued)*

**Table 7.** (*Continued.*)

| Author | Summary |
| --- | --- |
| Bunzel *et al.* (2005) | Partners of patients with pulsatile MCSD have more depression and anxiety |
| Frazier *et al.* (2004b) | AbioCor is bulky and not applicable for small men, women, and children |
| Weitkemper *et al.* (2004) | Implantable MCSD allows for patient discharge (OOH) |
| Chinn *et al.* (2005) | Prevention of device-related infection is crucial for cost-effective use |
| Kalya *et al.* (2005) | Novacor is more durable than HeartMate |
| Schmid *et al.* (2005) | INCOR rotary MCSD reduces infection rate and perioperative bleeding, and improves quality of life. Thromboembolism rates are not lower |
| Klotz *et al.* (2006) | DeBakey and INCOR have similar rates of pretransplant posttransplant mortality, but higher risks of rejection than pulsatile LVAD |
| Miller *et al.* (2006) | Improved management and reduced costs allow for dissemination of new technology |
| Zimpfer *et al.* (2006) | Nonpulsatile MCSD does not mprove neurocognitive function |

# CHAPTER 5
# COMPLICATIONS

## MULTIORGAN FAILURE

Multiorgan failure (MOF) is conceptualized as a rapidly progressive, often irreversible, loss of function of two or more vital organ systems in the context of an initiating critical event. Several clinical studies have demonstrated that after MCSD implantation, MOF is a leading cause of death (Rose *et al.*, 2001; Deng *et al.*, 2005a).

## RIGHT HEART FAILURE

| | |
|---|---|
| **Helen M (born 1969)**<br><br>**Filtered information during BiVAD support** | My husband has told me that I was only the 13th person in the northeast to be on a biventricular assist device (BiVAD). I possess a sarcastic sense of humor, so my first inclination was to wryly say, "Lucky number thirteen." Truth be told, I am lucky. I know from other sources that Number 12 did not make it.<br><br>This is what characterizes my time spent on the BiVAD: information received secondhand, from other sources, filtered, sterilized, in the same way people bathed themselves in disinfectant when they came to visit me. I could not gather my own information, much to my chagrin, due to weakness and immobility. So, I waited for the information to make its way to me, slowly, piece by piece, especially the one piece of information I so fervently craved: that I would be free of the BiVAD because a heart had been found for me. |

**Helen M
(born 1969)**

**Concepts of
disease**

The first information I received on the BiVAD came just after I opened my eyes. My husband leaned over me, as if he had been waiting for me to awaken, I think because he wanted me to know immediately before I realized on my own what had happened. He said, "Helen, they had to put two pumps on you and they couldn't put them on the inside." I was confused, thinking that this would be the way I would have to spend the rest of my life, with these pumps outside my body. How would I dress? I'd have to buy all new clothes. Where do you buy clothes with stretchy waistbands? How would I go to the beach? Would I wear a muumuu to hide my pumps?

I spent a lot of time being confused, wracked with pedestrian thoughts. For example, my kidneys failed while I was on the BiVAD. The doctors came and told me, almost offhandedly, not to worry, for they would give me a heart-kidney transplant. And I wondered, how would you lie in bed with a heart-kidney transplant? You can't lie on your back because of the kidney, and you can't lie on your stomach because of the heart. I resolved not to get a heart-kidney for this reason: I did not want to recuperate standing up.

**Deborah
(mother of
Joel L,
born 1969)**

**Discharge**

Joel was transferred briefly to the seventh floor. During this time, I was asked to learn to care for the LVAD at home. I went through the motions of being shown how to clean the wires and check the machine, but I was saying to myself, "I don't think so." There was no way I was going home with Joel attached to that thing. I slept very little during this time, and I imagined sleeping even less were he able to come home. I imagined sitting there watching the digital read-outs, listening to the sounds and praying that there never be a blackout. To all the patients on an LVAD who went home and to all their families who cared for them during this time, I salute you. You have my utmost admiration. I have no idea how these people could withstand that kind of pressure.

Joel was not to go home. After just a short time on the seventh floor, he was transferred back to the CTICU for heart failure, to either await a heart transplant or die.

## eart Failure Definition

***INTERMACS.*** The INTERMACS database defines right heart failure as the symptoms and signs of persistent right ventricular dysfunction. These include central venous pressure (CVP) of >18 mm Hg with a cardiac index of <2.0 L/min/m$^2$ in the absence of elevated left atrial/pulmonary capillary wedge pressure, tamponade, ventricular arrhythmias, and/or pneumothorax, requiring either right ventricular assist device (RVAD) implantation or inotropic therapy ≥14 days after LVAD implantation.

## Center Experience with Right Heart Failure

***The Columbia University Medical Center Experience.*** Right heart failure (RHF) is a frequent complication of left ventricular assist device (LVAD) implantation, yet few studies have examined the outcomes for LVAD patients who subsequently develop RHF. A recent study at Columbia University has detailed the Center's experience with RHF in chronic congestive heart failure patients. A total of 108 patients with chronic CHF (≥6 months) who underwent HeartMate LVAD implantation were identified between June 1996 and July 2004. Acute heart failure patients requiring LVADs were excluded to eliminate the impact of confounding noncardiac factors. RHF was defined as the need for a subsequent RVAD, ≥14 days of intravenous inotropes/pulmonary vasodilators, or both. Forty-two (38.9%) RHF patients were identified; of these, 14 required RVAD insertion. Outcome parameters included early (≤30-day) mortality, intensive care unit (ICU) length of stay (LOS), incidence of reoperation for bleeding and acute renal failure, stroke, bridge-to-transplantation rate, and posttransplantation survival rate.

More female patients developed RHF than not (73.3% vs. 26.7%, $p = 0.003$). RHF patients had a higher early mortality rate, greater stay in the intensive care unit, higher rates of reoperation for bleeding and renal failure, and a lower bridge-to-transplantation rate than non-RHF patients (19.0% vs. 6.2%, $p = 0.039$; 23.8 ± 23.7 days vs. 9.6 ± 7.1 days, $p < 0.001$; 38.9% vs. 18.3%, $p = 0.026$; 61.0% vs. 22.6%, $p < 0.001$; 65.0% vs. 89.9%, $p = 0.003$; respectively). Fourteen (33.3%) RHF patients required RVAD insertion. Elevated intraoperative central venous pressure was found to be an independent predictor of post-LVAD RHF. The overall bridge-to-transplantation rate for the entire study cohort was 73.1%.

The authors concluded that the development of RHF after LVAD insertion confers significant morbidity and mortality. Judicious application of inotropes and pulmonary vasodilators as well as timely RVAD insertion, if necessary, should be maintained. Further investigations evaluating preoperative and intraoperative risk factors for the development of RHF are warranted (Dang *et al.*, 2006). The Columbia group also reported a technique for the insertion of an RVAD without the need for cardiopulmonary bypass (Rao *et al.*, 2001).

***The Cleveland Clinic Experience.***    Implantable LVAD insertion complicated by early right ventricular (RV) failure has a poor prognosis, and is generally unpredictable. To determine preoperative risk factors for perioperative RV failure after LVAD insertion, patient characteristics and preoperative hemodynamics were analyzed in 100 patients with the HeartMate LVAD (Thermo Cardiosystems, Inc., Woburn, MA) at the Cleveland Clinic.

RV assist device support was required for 11 patients (RVAD group). RVAD use was significantly higher in younger patients, female patients, smaller patients, and myocarditis patients. There was no significant difference in the cardiac index, RV ejection fraction, or right atrial pressure between the two groups preoperatively. The preoperative mean pulmonary arterial pressure (PAP) and RV stroke work index (RV SWI) were significantly lower in the RVAD group ($p = 0.015$ and $p = 0.011$, respectively). The survival rate to transplant was poor (27%) in the RVAD group, but high (83%) in the non-RVAD group. The authors concluded that the need for perioperative RVAD support was only 11%. Preoperative low PAP and low RV SWI are significant risk factors for RVAD use (Fukamachi *et al.*, 1999).

***Other Experiences.***    Milrinone acts as both an inotropic agent and a direct vasodilator, and thus may avoid the need for mechanical support for RV failure due to residual pulmonary hypertension after LVAD implantation (Kihara *et al.*, 2002). The need for right ventricular support as an adjunct to left ventricular assistance is uncommon. When required, the insertion of an RVAD may be complicated by pre-existing hepatic dysfunction, coagulation abnormalities, and renal failure, all of which are exacerbated by cardiopulmonary bypass.

## ARRHYTHMIA

### Ventricular Arrhythmia Definition

***INTERMACS.***    The INTERMACS database defines cardiac arrythmia as any documented arrhythmia resulting in clinical compromise (e.g. diminished VAD flow, oliguria, presyncope, or syncope) that either requires hospitalization or occurs during hospital stay. Cardiac arrhythmias are classified into two types: sustained ventricular arrhythmia requiring defibrillation or cardioversion, and sustained supraventricular arrhythmia requiring drug treatment or cardioversion.

### Center Experience

***The Columbia University Experience.***    Despite the increasing use of LVADs as a bridge to cardiac transplantation, our knowledge regarding its effect on ventricular arrhythmias is currently limited to small series. Little is known about the prevalence, predictors, and clinical consequences of ventricular arrhythmias in LVAD recipients. In a retrospective study, the Columbia University group sought to evaluate the effect of LVAD therapy on ventricular tachyarrhythmias in patients with advanced congestive heart failure.

The Columbia University group reviewed the pre- and post-LVAD courses of the last 100 consecutive adult patients to receive a Heart-Mate LVAD (Thoratec Laboratories Corp., Pleasanton, CA) at their institution. All ventricular arrhythmias sustained for at least 30 s or requiring defibrillation were analyzed. All documented pre- and post-LVAD sustained ventricular arrhythmias were classified either as monomorphic ventricular tachycardia (MVT) or polymorphic ventricular tachycardia (PVT)/ventricular fibrillation (VF). The population had an average age of 51 years, had predominately ischemic cardiomyopathy (63%), and had a mean left ventricular ejection fraction of 20% ± 10%.

New-onset MVT was observed in 18 patients who did not have MVT before the LVAD placement. After LVAD, new-onset MVT was 4.5 times more likely than the elimination of previously present MVT ($p = 0.001$), whereas the effect of LVADs on the incidence of PVT/VF was not significant. In a multivariate Cox proportional hazards regression analysis, serum electrolyte abnormality was an independent predictor of post-LVAD ventricular arrhythmias. Preoperative MVT did not predict postoperative MVT. The authors concluded that after LVAD placement, there is a significant rise in the incidence of *de novo* MVT. In contrast, the incidence of PVT/VF is unaffected by LVAD placement (Ziv *et al.*, 2005).

***Other Experiences.*** Implantable cardioverter defibrillators and MCSDs have been used as a bridge to cardiac transplantation. In selected patients, the combined implantation may be required. A report from the Münster University group was motivated by the case of a 33-year-old female patient with giant cell myocarditis who died of ventricular tachyarrhythmias after having been placed on a VAD, with which she had been treated on an out-of-hospital basis for a prolonged period of time. A subsequent retrospective analysis of their data showed that, of 73 patients who had to be bridged mechanically (54 patients with Novacor, 12 with TCI HeartMate, 4 with Thoratec, 3 with MEDOS) in their institution between 1993 and 1998, ten patients had undergone defibrillator implantation either before ($n = 8$) or after ($n = 2$) VAD implantation. The authors concluded that combination therapy is feasible if the MCSD alone with its combined hemodynamic and antiarrhythmic effect is not sufficient (Deng *et al.*, 1999b).

## INFECTION

| | |
|---|---|
| **Eileen (daughter of Herbert E, born 1930)** **Post-MCSD** | My father has mentioned to me that you would like to receive a copy of my son's essay about his grandfather. It is attached. My son's name is Jacob and he is 9 years old. We're flattered by your interest.<br><br>As you may know, Dr Naka is in the process of attempting to obtain a HeartMate II device for my father. Due to excessive scar tissue from many previous surgeries, the |

opening necessary to accommodate the HeartMate I cannot close and infection has resulted. Dr Naka feels that the HeartMate II is small enough to allow the skin to close, thereby avoiding constant infection.

Without the HeartMate II, it's pretty clear that my father has little or no chance of survival, as the infection will remain and only get worse. We understand that Dr Naka is going to present his case to the IRB in the next day or so. I should note that Dr Naka's efforts on behalf of my father have been extraordinary.

In addition to the medical considerations involved, you are well aware of the emotional and psychological aspects, as evidenced by your interest in my son's essay. Please consider whether you can be of any assistance to Dr Naka in fighting for a HeartMate II for my father.

Thank you very much for your interest, concern, and help.

## Infection Definitions

***INTERMACS Definition of Major Infection.*** The INTERMACS database defines major infection as a clinical infection accompanied by pain, fever, drainage, and/or leukocytosis that is treated by antimicrobial agents (nonprophylactic). A positive culture from the infected site or organ should be present, unless strong clinical evidence indicates the need for treatment despite negative cultures. The general categories of infections are listed below.

***INTERMACS Definition of Sepsis.*** The INTERMACS database defines sepsis as the evidence of systemic involvement by infection, manifested by positive blood cultures and/or hypotension.

***INTERMACS Definition of Localized Nondevice Infection.*** The INTER-MACS database defines localized nondevice infection as an infection localized to any organ system or region (e.g. mediastinitis) without evidence of systemic involvement (see sepsis definition), ascertained by standard clinical methods and either associated with evidence of bacterial, viral, fungal, or protozoal infection and/or requiring empirical treatment.

*INTERMACS Definition of Percutaneous Site and/or Pocket Infection.* The INTERMACS database defines percutaneous site and/or pocket infection as a positive culture from the skin and/or tissue surrounding the external housing of a pump implanted within the body, coupled with the need to treat with antimicrobial therapy, when there is evidence of infection such as pain, fever, drainage, or leukocytosis.

*INTERMACS Definition of Internal Pump Component, Inflow Tract, or Outflow Tract Infection.*   The INTERMACS database defines internal pump component, inflow tract, or outflow tract infection as any infection of LVAD blood-contacting surfaces documented by positive site culture. There should be a separate data file for the paracorporeal pump that describes infection at the percutaneous cannula site (e.g. Thoratec PVAD).

## RCT Studies

*RCT Studies.*   A subanalysis of the REMATCH trial focused on infection, an important source of morbidity and mortality. The REMATCH study participants have used the information to suggest ways to reduce the incidence and effects of device-related infection. Patients were randomized prospectively to receive LVADs or optimal medical management (OMM) for end-stage heart failure. Infection variables included sepsis adjudicated as the cause of death; sepsis reported as a serious adverse event; percutaneous site or pocket infection; and pump housing, inflow tract, or outflow tract infection. They compared the incidence and prevalence of events between the two groups and generated time-related descriptions.

Survival with an LVAD ($n = 68$ patients) was superior to OMM survival ($n = 61$ patients) with a 47% decrease in the risk of death ($p < 0.001$), but the aggregate adverse event rate was greater for patients with LVADs (risk ratio, 2.29; 95% CI, 1.85–2.84). Freedom from sepsis in patients with LVADs was 58% at 1 year and 48% at 2 years after implantation, with superior survival in nonseptic patients (60% vs. 39% at 1 year and 38% vs. 8% at 2 years in nonseptic vs. septic patients with LVADs, $p < 0.06$). Percutaneous site or pocket infection did not affect survival ($p = 0.86$). The hazard for onset of sepsis peaked within the first 3 weeks after implantation.

Survival is improved with permanent LVAD implantation compared with OMM therapy. However, infection causes substantial morbidity and mortality. Reducing infections increases survival and decreases morbidity in permanent LVAD recipients, and improves the risk-benefit ratio for permanent LVAD therapy (Holman *et al.*, 2004).

## Observational Non-RCT Studies

***The Cleveland Clinic Experience.***  The Cleveland Clinic retrospectively reviewed the medical records of all patients with an implantable LVAD with $\geq 72$ h of LVAD support from January 1992 through June 2000 in order to determine the attack rate, incidence, and impact of nosocomial blood stream infection (BSI) in patients with LVADs. A nosocomial BSI was defined using the Centers for Disease Control and Prevention definition. An LVAD-related BSI was defined as one where the same pathogen is cultured from the device and the blood with no other obvious source.

A total of 214 patients were included in the study (17 831 LVAD-days). One hundred forty BSIs were identified in 104 patients for an attack rate of 49% and an incidence of 7.9 BSI per 1000 LVAD-days; of these BSIs, 53 (38%) were LVAD-associated. The most common pathogens causing BSI were coagulase-negative staphylococci ($n = 33$), *Staphylococcus aureus* and *Candida* spp. (19 each), and *Pseudomonas aeruginosa* (16 each). A Cox proportional hazards model found BSI in patients with LVADs to be significantly associated with death (hazard ratio = 4.02, $p < 0.001$). Fungemia had the highest hazard ratio (10.9), followed by Gram-negative bacteremia (5.1) and Gram-positive bacteremia (2.2).

The authors concluded that patients with implantable LVADs have a high incidence of BSI, which is associated with significantly increased mortality. Strategies for the prevention of infection in LVAD recipients should focus on the driveline exit site until technical advances can achieve a totally implantable device (Gordon *et al.*, 2001).

***The Columbia University Experience.*** At Columbia, over a 5-year period, 60 patients underwent the insertion of an LVAD. Detailed medical records were kept prospectively for all patients and a variety of endpoints were analyzed, including the incidence, nature, and sequelae of infections before and after LVAD implantation or after transplantation.

Of the 60 patients who underwent LVAD insertion, 29 (48%) subsequently developed infections. The most frequent sites of infection were blood, LVAD drivelines, and central venous catheters, representing 61% of all infections. At the time of LVAD implantation, 13 (22%) of the 60 patients had culture-proven infections. In spite of an increased incidence of subsequent infection (77% vs. 40%), there were no differences in mortality rates (31% vs. 26%), LVAD endocarditis (23% vs. 11%), and eventual transplantation (62% vs. 57%) between these patients and those without peri-implantation infections. Although the overall mortality rate was not influenced by infections during LVAD support (28% vs. 26%), the development of LVAD endocarditis was associated with a high mortality rate. Finally, although patients with infections during LVAD support had significantly longer median support times than those who remained infection-free (101 vs. 49 days, respectively), there was no difference in the rate of successful transplantation (59% vs. 58%) or in the rate of infection after transplantation (35% vs. 28%).

It was concluded that infections are common in patients undergoing LVAD support, but they do not adversely affect survival, the rate of successful transplantation, or the incidence of posttransplantation infection. Peri-implantation infections may increase the risk of subsequent infections, but they also do not influence survival or transplantability. Patients who develop LVAD endocarditis are at increased risk of morbidity and death, and require early and aggressive therapy, potentially including device explantation (Argenziano *et al.*, 1998).

Fungal infection is a particularly worrisome complication, and LVAD endocarditis does pose a serious threat. Out of the 165 patients who underwent TCI HeartMate LVAD implantation between July 1991 and December 1999 at Columbia University, 37 (22%) developed fungal infections during LVAD support. Five (3%) of them met the institutional criteria for the diagnosis of fungal LVAD endocarditis. Microbial portals of entry were identifiable in all cases. Infections were managed successfully in four (80%) patients.

The authors concluded that the successful management of fungal LVAD endocarditis currently requires early recognition of potentially nonspecific signs and symptoms as well as timely institution of antifungal therapy. In some cases with device-specific manifestations of LVAD endocarditis, device removal and replacement are necessary. In patients with clinical manifestations of sepsis and fungal driveline site or pocket infections without positive blood culture, urgent transplantation may be the appropriate management. In the setting of shortage in donor supply, device removal and replacement are necessary (Nurozler *et al.*, 2001).

***The Temple University Experience.***    Infections acquired during ventricular assist device support may increase the risk of infection and have an impact on transplant survival. At Temple University, 18 patients underwent LVAD implantation followed by heart transplantation. Ten underwent heart transplantation (HT) in the absence of LVAD infection (group 1); and 8, in the presence of LVAD infection (group 2). All patients were treated similarly, except for modification of immunosuppression in group 2 patients. Infectious and noninfectious complications were equivalent between the two groups. There was no difference between group 1 and group 2 with regard to intraoperative deaths (one vs. none, respectively), long-term survival (eight vs. seven), wound complications (three vs. none), and mean length of hospital stay after HT (21 vs. 26 days). The authors concluded that for patients with LVAD infection, transplantation in the face of infection is an effective treatment option (Prendergast *et al.*, 1997).

***The Münster University Experience.***    At Münster University, 25 patients (24 male, 1 female) with end-stage cardiac failure and resulting organ dysfunction were studied. Patients were bridged with the Novacor N100 portable LVAD (median duration of support, 55 days) and were prospectively evaluated by device surface cultures at explantation, molecular typing of isolates, and correlation of infection with survival to transplant. Twelve (48%) of the 25 patients had LVAD infection, as defined by the recovery of multiple isolates of identical genotype from the device surface. Whereas only 5 (42%) of the 12 patients with LVAD infection survived until transplantation, 11 (85%) of the 13 patients without infection were successfully transplanted ($P < 0.05$). The deaths of the seven patients with proven LVAD infection were associated with multiple organ failure or other signs of acute infection. The authors concluded that LVAD infection is associated with a significantly decreased survival probability. It does not preclude successful bridging, but rather may pose an indication for urgent transplantation (Hermann *et al.*, 1997).

***The Rush Medical Center Experience.*** LVAD implantation has become an effective treatment option for patients with severe heart failure awaiting transplantation. Significant infection rates have been reported among LVAD recipients. However, few reports have focused specifically on device infection, its treatment, and the impact of LVAD-related infection on clinical outcome.

Forty-six LVAD-related infections were diagnosed in 38 (50%) of 76 patients who underwent LVAD implantation as a bridge to transplantation. Twenty-nine episodes of LVAD-related bloodstream infection (BSI) (including five that were cases of LVAD endocarditis) and 17 episodes of local LVAD infection were identified. Diabetes mellitus appeared to increase the risk of BSI among patients with LVAD infection. LVAD-related infection delayed transplantation, as reflected by longer device-support times (a mean duration ± SEM of 182.8 ± 31.1 days, compared with 66.3 ± 8.8 days; $P \leq 0.001$). Continuous antimicrobial treatment before, during, and after transplantation was associated with fewer relapses than was a limited course of antibiotics ($P < 0.001$). Longer hospital stays after receipt of a transplant and increased early mortality were observed in the cohort with LVAD-related infection, although long-term survival was similar to that for patients without LVAD-related infection. Posttransplantation invasive vancomycin-resistant *Enterococcus faecium* (VREF) infection was diagnosed in six patients with LVAD-related infection; four of these patients died. No VREF infections were identified in patients without LVAD-related infection.

These observations suggest that LVAD-related infection is common and may require antimicrobial therapy before, during, and after transplantation; but that it does not prevent successful transplantation. However, patients with LVAD-related infection appear to be at increased risk of invasive

VREF infection, which may contribute to early mortality after transplantation (Simon *et al.*, 2005a).

***Other Experiences.*** Between June 1996 and June 1999, eighty-six patients received an LVAD. Fifty patients were transplanted during the same period without prior device support, and were used as controls; they were matched to transplanted LVAD recipients by age, sex, diagnosis, and transplant date. The nature of and actuarial freedom from peritransplant and posttransplant infections were compared at 6 months after transplant; actuarial patient survival was compared at 3 years. Infection was defined as leukocytosis or leukopenia, with a positive culture requiring either medical or surgical intervention.

Forty-four (51%) patients were successfully discharged to home on LVAD support, and 61 (71%) were transplanted. A high incidence of infection during device support did not have an impact on the rates of pretransplant or posttransplant mortality, posttransplant infection, or overall patient survival. Active infections at transplant also did not significantly influence the 6-month mortality rate. In comparison, LVAD recipients had a lower freedom from infection than did controls ($P < 0.05$); however, the 3-year survival rate did not differ (79% and 87% for the LVAD and control groups, respectively).

The authors concluded that although LVADs increase the risk of infection in the early posttransplant period, this appears not to have an impact on transplantability or patient survival and likely reflects effective infection control in both inpatient and outpatient settings (Sinha *et al.*, 2000).

Infectious complications during support with a ventricular assist system (VAS) can cause severe morbidity and mortality, affecting nearly one half of all VAS recipients. Because of the lack of a uniform definition of infection, the incidence of this complication is hard to accurately determine. It is approximately 50% for patients supported by an implantable VAS as a bridge to heart transplantation, and 28% for patients supported by an external short-term VAS. Infections can be classified according to the involvement or noninvolvement of the implanted device and according to the severity of the infection. Severe infections involving the implanted device may preclude heart transplantation for some patients, but numerous patients with milder infections have undergone successful transplantation. A number of factors predispose VAS patients to infection.

Postoperative bleeding necessitating reoperation is an important contributing factor. Endotracheal tubes, intravascular catheters, and other indwelling tubes necessary for the care of postsurgical patients are also common routes of contamination.

Control of infection may be improved with new VAS designs, antibiotic impregnated drivelines, and innovative therapies such as antibiotic beads. The next generation of VASs should be inherently less susceptible to infection because of their smaller size, reduced thrombogenicity, and better flow characteristics. In addition to more effective antibiotics, improved VAS designs that incorporate transcutaneous energy transmission systems may reduce infectious complications and allow safe, long-term VAS support (Myers *et al.*, 2000).

***Wound Complications.***    Wound necrosis and infection pose a tremendous risk for patients with LVADs. The Münster group analyzed their database of patients with LVADs for those who developed wound dehiscence and concomitant infection after LVAD implantation. Of the 66 patients with implantable ventricular assist devices, 3 (4.5%) had severe wound complications with necrosis of the abdominal or thoracic wall uncovering part of the device. The predominant impact on the development of these complications was presumably related to multiple surgical interventions at the same site. Nevertheless, these patients can recover and undergo successful heart transplantation if adequately managed (Tjan *et al.*, 2000).

The device pocket can be the site of infection. One patient developed a wound infection that involved an implanted LVAD. At surgery, the pump was washed with a detergent-containing bacteriocidal solution, and then antibiotic-impregnated polymethylmethacrylate beads were placed around the pump. The wound was revised using rectus muscle to cover the pump. The incisions healed, and the patient was discharged without systemic antibiotics or any evidence of infection 11 months postoperatively (Holman *et al.*, 1999).

## Mechanisms of MCSD-Related Infections

***Overview.***    Heart failure is a leading cause of death in developed nations, despite medical management. Cardiac transplantation is a potentially life-saving intervention for approximately 4000 advanced heart failure patients per year; however, the demand for donor hearts far exceeds the supply. Ventricular assist devices (VADs) provide temporary support for patients with severe heart failure until myocardial recovery occurs or a donor heart becomes available. For those ineligible for transplantation, VADs may be used permanently and have demonstrated reduced mortality and improved quality of life compared with continued medical therapy. Nonetheless, these devices are underused, in part due to the frequency of complications.

Device-related infections are one of the most frequent sequelae of VAD placement, and occur in 18%–59% of patients after VAD implantation. Infections can involve any part of the device and confer substantial morbidity and mortality. Infections are reported to occur in 13%–80% of cases. The true incidence of VAD-related infections is difficult to ascertain for several reasons, including the lack of a universal definition of device-related infection, use of historical data, different interpretations of culture results, and different measures of comparison (prevalence rather than incidence is often reported) (Gordon *et al.*, 2006).

VAD-related infections can involve any aspect of the device: the surgical site, the driveline, the device pocket, or the pump itself. More than half of all VAD-related infections include multiple sites. In general, driveline infection is the most common type of device-related infection. It may remain local and uncomplicated with appropriate antimicrobial treatment and wound care. However, some patients with driveline infection may become systemically ill and the infection may spread to multiple sites, yielding serious complications. These manifestations include bloodstream infection, relapsing bacteremia, sepsis, and VAD-associated endocarditis. Some studies have found locations other than the driveline site to represent the most VAD-related infections. Weyand and colleagues described the predominance of pump chamber infections in infected VAD recipients (41%), of whom 67% died (Hermann *et al.*, 1997).

In another study, more than half of the VAD-infected patients were bacteremic. Bloodstream infection is associated with a poor outcome in this population, including complications such as cerebral emboli and multiorgan failure, and several studies have found sepsis to be the number one cause of death during VAD support. Less common complications of VAD-related infection include mediastinitis, peritonitis, and pseudo-aneurysm. Infections requiring long-term antibiotic use may also predispose patients to *Clostridium difficile* enterocolitis. VAD-related infections are typically caused by Gram-positive organisms and are usually staphylococcal species. Approximately 38% and 24% of bloodstream infections are caused by *Staphylococcus epidermidis* and *Staphylococcus aureus*, respectively. Deng and colleagues demonstrated that staphylococci were cultured in 46% of driveline and device pocket infections and 36% of blood cultures (Deng *et al.*, 2001a). *S. aureus* was responsible for 56% of VAD infection recurrences in one case review. Other commonly implicated Gram-positive organisms are enterococci. In one study, enterococci were responsible for 18% of driveline and device pocket infections, and 20% of bloodstream infections. Enterococci have been associated with a negative outcome (Gordon *et al.*, 2006).

***Immunological T-Cell Defect.*** The development of local and systemic infections is a significant risk factor associated with the implantation of a ventricular assist device. To examine the relation between LVAD-related infection and host immunity, the Columbia group investigated immune responses in LVAD recipients by comparing the rate of candidal infection in 78 patients with New York Heart Association class IV heart failure who received either an LVAD ($n = 40$) or medical management (controls, $n = 38$). Fluorochrome-labeled monoclonal antibodies were used in the analyses of T-cell phenotype. Analysis of T-cell function included intradermal responses to recall antigens and proliferative responses after stimulation by phytohemagglutinin, monoclonal antibodies to CD3, and mixed lymphocyte culture. They measured T-cell apoptosis *in vivo* by annexin V binding, and confirmed the result by assessment of DNA fragmentation. Activation-induced T-cell death was measured after T-cell stimulation with antibodies to CD3. All immunological tests were done at least 1 month after LVAD implantation. Between-group comparisons were by Kaplan–Meier actuarial analysis and Student's $t$ test.

By 3 months after LVAD implantation, the risk of developing candidal infection was 28% in LVAD recipients compared with 3% in controls ($p = 0.003$). LVAD recipients had cutaneous anergy to recall antigens and lower ($< 70\%$) T-cell proliferative responses than the controls after activation via the T-cell receptor complex ($p < 0.001$). T cells from LVAD recipients had a higher surface expression of CD95 (Fas) ($p < 0.001$) and a higher rate of spontaneous apoptosis ($p < 0.001$) than the controls. Moreover, after stimulation with antibodies to CD3, CD4 T-cell death increased by 3.2-fold in LVAD recipients compared with only 1.2-fold in the controls ($p < 0.05$). The authors concluded that LVAD implantation results in an aberrant state of T-cell activation, heightened susceptibility of CD4 T cells to activation-induced cell death, progressive defects in cellular immunity, and increased risk of opportunistic infection (Ankersmit *et al.*, 1999).

The immunological consequence of continuous-flow rotary blood pumps was examined by the Vienna group in six adult male patients (mean age, 47 ± 10.3 years) with end-stage left heart failure who received a DeBakey VAD axial-flow pump for use as a bridge to transplantation (four patients underwent transplantation after a mean of 115 ± 14 days; two patients are still waiting for the allograft). The authors prospectively monitored T-cell populations and apoptosis-specific aberrant T-cell activation via CD95 triggering and annexin V binding to lymphocytes, and identified T cells undergoing early phases of apoptosis within the first 10 weeks. Moreover, the soluble death-inducing receptors soluble CD95 and soluble tumor necrosis factor-R1 were evaluated by enzyme-linked immunosorbent assay.

They found an initial pronounced apoptosis-specific immune alteration by increased annexin V binding to CD3 T cells as well as death-inducing receptors soluble CD95 and soluble tumor necrosis factor-R1 (all $P < 0.001$). All the parameters normalized after 7 weeks to baseline. No blood-borne sepsis was detected (as defined by blood culture) within the first 10 weeks of the cohort study. These results indicate a biphasic immunological response in patients with end-stage heart failure who are treated with nonpulsatile VADs (Ankersmit *et al.*, 2002).

***Immunological B-Cell Hyperreactivity.*** Patients with an LVAD as a bridge to heart transplantation (HT) often have elevated levels of panel-reactive antibodies (PRAs). The clinical significance of antihuman histocompatibility leukocyte antigen (HLA) antibodies detected by flow cytometry in PRA-negative patients remains unclear. At the University of Pennsylvania, 18 patients who underwent LVAD placement as a successful bridge to HT had standard antihuman globulin complement–dependent cytotoxicity and retrospective flow cytometry assays performed to detect class I anti-HLA antibodies. A positive flow result was defined as a fluorescent ratio of 23:1 vs. a negative control. Six patients had anti-HLA antibodies detected by flow cytometry. Univariate analysis demonstrated more moderate-to-severe rejection episodes (ISHLT of $\geq$3A) at 2 months ($0.83 \pm 0.75$ vs. 0; $P = 0.04$) and a trend toward decreased time to first rejection ($61 \pm 17$ days vs. $225 \pm 62$ days; $P = 0.06$) in these patients. No differences were observed in donor–recipient HLA mismatch or 1-year Kaplan–Meier survival between patients with or without anti-HLA antibodies.

The authors concluded that despite a negative PRA, LVAD patients with class I anti-HLA antibodies detected by flow cytometry have a greater incidence of moderate-to-severe rejection in the first 2 months after HT. Flow cytometry may be a useful clinical tool in screening PRA-negative LVAD patients before transplantation. Patients with positive anti-HLA antibody screening by flow cytometry may require more intensive immunosuppression in the early post-HT period (DeNofrio *et al.*, 2000).

In a retrospective analysis of 40 patients with LVADs at the Columbia-Presbyterian Medical Center between 1990 and 1996, age, sex, diagnosis, race, duration of support, transfusions, and infections were studied by univariate and multivariate analyses as predictors for the development of either anti-HLA class I (anti-I) or anti-HLA class II (anti-II) immunoglobulin G (IgG) or M (IgM) antibodies. Eighteen (45%) patients developed anti-I antibodies and 20 (50%) developed anti-II antibodies over the study period. The median time for LVAD support was 142 days (range, 35–439 days).

Only the total number of perioperative platelet transfusions predicted the development of anti-I IgG antibodies ($p = 0.04$). No other associations were found for the development of anti-I IgM or anti-II antibodies of either IgG or IgM specificity. Patients who developed anti-I IgG received a mean of 13.9 (SE $\pm$ 2.6) units of platelets, compared with a mean of 7.7 (SE $\pm$ 2.3) units in those who did not ($p = 0.01$). By Kaplan–Meier analysis, at the median duration of follow-up, 8% of patients receiving <6 units were predicted to have developed anti-I antibodies compared with 63% receiving >6 units ($p = 0.002$). In the last seven patients, leukocyte filters were used to decrease the antigenic load during platelet and red blood cell transfusions; of these patients, only one (14%) developed anti-HLA antibodies compared with 31 (94%) of the 33 patients in whom filters were not used ($p < 0.005$). The authors concluded that platelet transfusion during LVAD implantation is a risk factor associated with the development of HLA class I IgG antibodies. The use of leukocyte filters during platelet transfusion may decrease the risk of developing anti-HLA antibodies (Moazami *et al.*, 1998).

Recipients of LVADs develop prominent B-cell hyperreactivity. The Columbia group investigated the influence of anti-HLA antibodies on the waiting time to cardiac transplantation in LVAD recipients, and compared the effects of two immunomodulatory regimens on anti-HLA serum reactivity. Studies were conducted on 55 previously nonsensitized LVAD recipients of a TCI device that was implanted between 1990 and 1996. Patients with anti-HLA antibodies received monthly courses of either intravenous immunoglobulin (IVIg) or plasmapheresis, in conjunction with cyclophosphamide. The effects of these regimens on anti-HLA alloreactivity and waiting time to transplantation were then determined by Kaplan–Meier log-rank statistics, nonparametric Wilcoxon rank-sum test, and Student's *t* test.

Prolongation in the transplant waiting time was related to serum IgG anti-HLA class I alloreactivity. The infusion of IVIg (2 g/kg) caused a mean reduction of 33% in anti-HLA class I alloreactivity within 1 week. The waiting time to transplantation was significantly reduced by IVIg therapy, and subsequently approximated that in nonsensitized patients. The side-effects of IVIg (2 g/kg) were minimal and primarily related to immune complex disease. Although plasmapheresis caused a similar reduction in alloreactivity to IVIg, this effect was achieved after longer treatment. Moreover, plasmapheresis was associated with an unacceptably high frequency of infectious complications. In patients resistant to low-dose (2 g/kg) IVIg therapy, high-dose (3 g/kg) IVIg was effective in reducing alloreactivity, but was associated with a high incidence of reversible renal insufficiency. The authors concluded that these results indicate that IVIg is an effective and safe modality for sensitized recipients awaiting cardiac transplantation, reducing serum anti-HLA alloreactivity and shortening the duration to transplantation. The therapeutic and safety profiles of IVIg appear to be superior to those of plasmapheresis (John *et al.*, 1999).

The Cleveland group evaluated 60 patients who received the HeartMate LVAD, of whom 53 had PRA results available for analysis. T-lymphocyte PRA levels were examined before LVAD support, at the peak PRA level during LVAD support (PEAK), and just before bridging to transplantation (TX). A PRA level of >10% was considered indicative of sensitization against HLA antigens. The only factor that had a significant effect on PRA levels before LVAD was the patient's sex (1.3% for men vs. 7.4% for women; $p = 0.005$). During LVAD support, peak PRA levels increased significantly and the sex-associated differences were no longer evident (33.3% men, 34.3% women; $p =$ not significant). At the time of TX, PRAs decreased to 10.9% in men and 7.0% in women ($p =$ not significant).

They examined the influence of blood products received before TX on PRA levels. Patients who received less than the median number of total units (<median) had lower peak PRA values (22.3% vs. 49.2%; $p = 0.01$) and TX PRA values (3.5% vs. 22.1%; $p = 0.02$) than those receiving more than the median (>median). When examined by the type of blood product, only the number of platelet transfusions significantly increased the peak PRA (<median, 24% vs. >median, 46.9%; $p = 0.03$). Patients who received leukocyte-depleted blood tended to have lower TX PRA levels (2.9%) compared with those who did not (13.9%, $p = 0.18$). Forty-two patients were successfully bridged to TX, with three early and two late deaths after TX. Whereas 39 patients received transplants without intervention, 3 were treated by plasmapheresis with a 77% reduction in their HLA antibody levels at TX as measured by flow cytometry. They concluded that patients with an implantable LVAD are at significant risk of developing anti-HLA antibodies during support. Although this sensitization is often transient, intervention using plasmapheresis may be useful for some patients (Massad *et al.*, 1997).

*Inflammation.* Elevated levels of cytokines and soluble adhesion molecules were observed in patients with cardiogenic shock, although slightly decreased levels of soluble adhesion molecules were also detectable in patients with chronic heart failure NYHA classes II and III. The signs of systemic inflammation disappeared following successful mechanical circulatory support, but persisted in patients who developed infectious complications. The authors concluded that a systemic hypoxic and inflammatory syndrome is manifested during end-stage heart failure in patients with sepsis or noninfectious insults. During mechanical circulatory support, elevated levels of inflammatory mediators may be indicative of persistent peripheral hypoxia associated with a high risk of infection or sepsis. Therefore, the monitoring of inflammatory mediators should be evaluated as markers of the effectiveness of this therapy (Goldstein *et al.*, 1997; Hasper *et al.*, 1998).

Ventricular assist devices (VADs) are an important form of therapy for end-stage congestive heart failure. However, VAD infection, which is often caused by *Staphylococcus aureus*, poses a major threat to survival. Using a novel *in vitro* binding assay with VAD membranes and a heterologous lactococcal system of expression, the Columbia University Specialized Center for Clinically Oriented Research (SCCOR) group identified three *S. aureus* proteins — clumping factor A (ClfA) and fibronectin-binding proteins A and B (FnBPA and FnBPB) — as the main factors involved in the adherence to VAD polyurethane membranes. Adherence is greatly diminished by long implantation times, reflecting a change in topological features of the VAD membrane, and is primarily mediated by the FnBPA domains in the staphylococcal proteins. The authors also compared the adherence of *S. aureus* mutant strains, and showed that other staphylococcal components appear to be involved in the adherence to VAD membranes and that ClfA, FnBPA, and FnBPB mediate bacterial infection of implanted murine intra-aortic polyurethane patches (Arrecubieta *et al.*, 2006).

***Role of the Endothelial Cell Layer Coating the HeartMate MCSD Membrane.*** The dynamics of infection and related mechanisms can be studied using a murine intravascular infection model. Asai *et al.* (2005) used the textured polyurethane patch material currently used in HeartMate ventricular assist devices as an aortic implant to mimic the interphase between the MCSD membrane and circulation. Mice were infected with *S. aureus* at 1 or 14 days after implantation. Using this model, they found that mice were susceptible to infection in both a dose- and time-dependent fashion. The patch material was significantly more susceptible to infection at day 1 vs. day 14 following surgery.

Immunohistological and morphological studies have demonstrated that the CD31-positive cells deposited on the membrane surface phenotypically appeared to be endothelial cells. *In vitro* adherence studies have found polyurethane membranes coated with endothelial cells to be less susceptible to *S. aureus* binding than membranes coated with fibrinogen. In one study, the authors demonstrated that textured polyurethane membranes were less susceptible to infection as cellular deposition occurred. The timeframe within which these membranes became populated with cellular material was consistent with the time-dependent clinical incidence of infection, thus suggesting that cellular-coated polyurethane may provide a strategy to reduce the risk of infection (Asai *et al.*, in press).

## BLEEDING/HEMOLYSIS

### Bleeding/Hemolysis Definitions

*INTERMACS Definition of Bleeding.* The INTERMACS database defines major bleeding as any episode of internal or external bleeding that results in death; the need for reoperation or hospitalization; or the necessity of red blood cell transfusion of four or more packed units within any 24-hour period during the first 7 days postimplant, or two or more packed units within any 24-hour period after 7 days following implant. In patients over 50 kg, the latter is considered 20 cc/kg or 10 cc/kg, respectively.

*INTERMACS Definition of Hemolysis.* The INTERMACS database defines hemolysis as a plasma-free hemoglobin value of >40 mg/dL, in association with clinical signs associated with hemolysis (e.g. anemia, low hematocrit, hyperbilirubinemia) occurring after the first 72 hours postimplant. Hemolyisis related to documented nondevice-related causes (e.g. transfusion or drug) is excluded from this definition.

### Observational Non-RCT Studies

*The Vienna University Experience.* Ventricular assist device (VAD) implantation is associated with impaired primary hemostasis and thromboembolic complications. Recently, a new generation of implantable continuous-flow axial pumps was introduced into clinical application. To study the potential thrombogenic properties of this type of pump, extensive platelet monitoring was applied. In the authors' institution, 13 patients received the MicroMed DeBakey VAD as a bridge to transplantation. Routine coagulation tests (platelet count, activated partial thromboplastin time, prothrombin time, antithrombin III activity) and platelet function tests (whole blood aggregometry, thrombelastography, flow cytometry) were performed.

No clinically relevant thromboembolic events were detected. No correlation was found between global function tests, platelet aggregation, and thrombelastography. No correlation was detected between platelet activation and hemolysis parameters. Platelet aggregation and coagulation index were significantly suppressed early after operation. A subsequent phase of hyperaggregability, starting at around day 6, suggested the initiation of anti-aggregation therapy. Platelet activation markers were upregulated in the postoperative period, but were returned to preoperative levels after the initiation of aspirin. In contrast to routine coagulation monitoring, platelet function tests reflected in detail the coagulation status of blood pump recipients and the efficiency of antiaggregation therapy. Aspirin and dipyridamole therapy, in addition to oral anticoagulation using phenprocoumon, may contribute to platelet function and clot mechanics restoration, and is therefore recommended for patients after VAD implantation (Bonaros *et al.*, 2004).

***The Baylor University Experience.***   Circulatory support with mechanical devices often leads to bleeding and tamponade. The Baylor University group reported a series of three patients who required mechanical circulatory support for postcardiotomy ventricular dysfunction. Late tamponade occurred in each patient with different clinical presentations. Early postoperative bleeding occurred in two patients. There was no active bleeding in any of the three patients. Transesophageal echocardiography was not helpful in making the diagnosis. They concluded that late tamponade, which may be the result of hematoma with earlier bleeding, can present as dyspnea, hypoxia, or forms of hemodynamic collapse. Exploratory media sternotomy is required to definitively make the diagnosis and to evacuate the hematoma (Smart and Jett, 1998).

***The University of Pittsburgh Experience.***   Ongoing complement activation in patients with a VAD may contribute to observed hemostatic abnormalities and cellular aggregation by mediating leukocyte and platelet activation, the formation of leukocyte–platelet conjugates, and the tissue factor pathway of coagulation. At the University of Pittsburgh, blood from 30 patients was collected before VAD implantation and during the implantation period. Plasma levels of thrombin–antithrombin III complexes, C3a, and SC5b-9 were measured by a commercial enzyme-linked immunosorbent assay. Flow cytometry was used to measure the circulating monocyte tissue factor expression as well as the circulating monocyte–platelet and granulocyte–platelet conjugates.

The thrombin–antithrombin III complex level and monocyte tissue factor expression peaked in the early postoperative period, with maxima occurring on postoperative days 5 and 3, respectively. Levels of C3a and SC5b-9 remained dramatically elevated over normal values for the duration of the study (six and five times upper normal, respectively). Levels of monocyte–platelet conjugates were normal before implantation, decreased during the first four postoperative days, and then increased and remained elevated. Levels of granulocyte–platelet conjugates were elevated over the normal range before implantation, and remained elevated from postoperative days 3 to 21. A positive correlation was found between levels of SC5b-9 and granulocyte–platelet conjugates (Spearman $R = 0.66$; $p < 0.001$), and between levels of C3a and thrombin–antithrombin III complex (Spearman $R = 0.13$; $p = 0.021$). The authors suggested a model in which complement activation mediates the formation of leukocyte–platelet aggregates and may indirectly contribute to thrombin generation through monocyte tissue factor expression (Wilhelm *et al.*, 1998).

*The Henry Mondor Hospital Experience.* The activation of blood coagulation and thromboemboli have been shown to present significant clinical risks in patients supported with a left ventricular assist system (LVAS). The interaction of pseudointima (PI) with blood in the conduits of the device could be involved in these clinical complications. The aim of the group at Henry Mondor was to study the morphology of the PI vs. the duration of circulatory support.

Novacor N100 PC LVASs were explanted from 10 men and 2 women after a mean of 209 days (range, 23–560 days) of circulatory assistance. PI in the inflow and outflow conduits was investigated with immunohistochemical assays. In the inflow conduits, a loosely adherent PI had built up from collagen type I and III fibers growing into and between the fibrin deposits. Disorganized collagenous matrix and longitudinally oriented collagen fibers included alpha-smooth muscle actin–positive cells with random orientation. Macrophages were concentrated in the fibrin and were dispersed throughout the extracellular matrix. In the outflow conduits, a thin adherent PI was composed of regular collagen type I and III layers. Collagen type I fibers had grown into the woven Dacron, and alpha-smooth muscle actin–positive cells were oriented in the axis of the blood flow. Macrophages were concentrated in the Dacron and reached the inner collagen layers.

Venous blood flow in the inflow conduits allows the development of a nonendothelialized irregular collagenous matrix intermingled with fibrin and invaded by macrophages. These persistent structural features progress with the duration of circulatory assistance, and reflect matrix degradation and remodeling. The potential to release thromboembolic fragments from the nonstable, thrombogenic PI may be involved in the thromboembolic or neurologic complications sustained by 5 of the 12 patients who were on circulatory support for as long as 200 days (Houel *et al.*, 2001).

***The University of Alabama Experience.***    The operative technique influences the thromboembolism rate. The University of Alabama in Birmingham group reported on a series of eight Thoratec LVADs for more than 30 days. There were five left atrial (LA) (total, 513 days; range, 33–202 days) and three left ventricular (LV) (total, 484 days; range, 44–247 days) cannulations. The flow provided by LA cannulation was less than that provided by LV cannulation. However, serial measurements of hematologic, renal, and hepatic function were similar for patients with LA and those with LV cannulation throughout support. Plasma-free hemoglobin and lactate dehydrogenase (LDH) levels were similar for LA and LV patients. The five LA patients had one transient ischemic attack, one reversible ischemic neurologic deficit, and one stroke. The LV patients had no neurologic events ($p = 0.20$; LA vs. LV total neurologic events). One LA patient and one LV patient died during support. Three LA patients underwent transplant, and one LA patient recovered native cardiac function. Two LV patients underwent transplant (Holman *et al.*, 1995).

***The Münster University Experience.***    At Münster, 38 Novacor patients (age, $43 \pm 11$ years old) were studied in a nonrandomized manner. Twenty patients were treated with heparin only (control group); whereas in the other 18 patients, aspirin ($3 \times 330$ mg/day) and dipyridamole ($3 \times 75$ mg/day) were added to the treatment protocol (aspirin group). Age, body size, underlying heart diseases, and support interval were comparable among both groups. However, patients in the aspirin group were much sicker with regard to urgency status, postoperative right heart failure, and hematological disorders. Cerebral thromboembolic complications were lower in the aspirin group (33% of patients, $0.4 \pm 0.7$ events) as compared to the control group [55% ($P = 0.18$), $1.4 \pm 2.3$ events ($P = 0.048$)]. Noncerebral thromboembolism of surgical relevance was rare. The incidence of bleeding complications was mildly increased in the aspirin group. It was concluded that the addition of high-dose platelet inhibitors seems to lower the incidence of thromboembolism in Novacor patients (Schmid *et al.*, 2000).

***Use of Transcranial Doppler.***    Since thromboembolism is a major complication, the clinical significance of Doppler microembolic signals (MESs) in patients with LVADs was evaluated at Münster. Six patients with LVADs were monitored for MESs with transcranial Doppler ultrasonography during the first 30 postoperative days. Additionally, repeated (10 per patient per day) and prolonged (3 h per patient) monitorings were performed to assess the adequacy of the 30-min recordings. Three observers evaluated 30 randomly assigned monitorings in a blinded fashion to assess the interobserver variability. The relation between MES counts and clinical, radiological, hemostaseological, and pump flow parameters, as well as the predictive value of MES counts regarding the occurrence of embolic events, was evaluated.

Ten ischemic cerebrovascular accidents and two peripheral thromboembolic events occurred during the observation period of 177 days (total incidence, 6.8%). MESs were found in 143 (84.1%) of 170 monitorings. Their counts were significantly higher on days with clinically manifest embolic events as compared with event-free days [median (95% CI) of 18.5 (0.3–0.74) vs. 4 (0.0–0.52), respectively; $P < 0.001$, Mann–Whitney]. The predictive value of MES counts above 7 per 30 min was high (75%). Significant differences in the incidence and counts of MESs as well as in the

# RENAL DYSFUNCTION

## Renal Dysfunction Definition

*INTERMACS Definiton of Renal Dysfunction.* The INTERMACS database distinguishes between two types of renal dysfunction. Acute renal dysfunction is defined as abnormal kidney function requiring dialysis (including hemofiltration) in patients who did not require this procedure prior to implant, or a rise in serum creatinine of greater than three times the baseline or >5 mg/dL (in children, creatinine greater than three times the upper limit of normal for age) sustained for over 48 hours. Chronic renal dysfunction is defined as an increase in serum creatinine of ≥2 mg/dL above the baseline, or a requirement for hemodialysis sustained for at least 90 days.

## Observational Non-RCT Studies

*The Columbia University Experience.* Postoperative renal failure is a common complication after LVAD implantation. A study was designed to evaluate the predictors and outcomes of acute renal failure after LVAD insertion. A total of 201 patients undergoing LVAD implantation at Columbia from June 1996 through April 2004 were retrospectively analyzed. Patients were categorized into two groups: those who required postoperative continuous veno-venous hemodialysis (CVVHD) (group 1, $n = 65$, 32.3%), and those who did not (group 2, $n = 136$, 67.7%). Independent predictors of postoperative renal failure requiring CVVHD were determined using multivariate logistic regression techniques.

Patients who had postoperative renal failure requiring CVVHD were older ($53.7 \pm 12.9$ years vs. $48.2 \pm 14.2$ years, $p = 0.009$), had a higher incidence of intra-aortic balloon pump use (46.6% vs. 26.2%, $p = 0.006$), and had a higher preoperative mean LVAD score ($5.8 \pm 3.5$ vs. $3.8 \pm 3.3$, $p = 0.001$) than those without renal failure. The LVAD score was the only independent predictor of postoperative renal failure requiring CVVHD (odds ratio = 1.226, $p = 0.006$). The sepsis rate was higher (33.3% vs. 6.9%, $p < 0.001$) and the bridge-to-transplantation rate was lower (52.4% vs. 83.5%, $p < 0.001$) in group 1 than in group 2. The post-LVAD survival rates at 1, 3, 5, and 7 years for group 1 and group 2 were 43.2%, 39.1%, 34.7%, and 34.7% vs. 79.2%, 74.0%, 68.3%, and 66.4%, respectively (log-rank, $p < 0.001$).

Acute renal failure necessitating CVVHD remains a serious complication after LVAD implantation, and confers significant morbidity and mortality. The pre-operative evaluation of patient risk factors and the optimization of perioperative hemodynamics are of the utmost importance to prevent this major complication (Topkara *et al.*, 2006).

***The Papworth/Cambridge University Experience.*** The low-output state associated with end-stage cardiac failure predisposes patients to renal dysfunction and the need for short-term renal support. The use of cardiopulmonary bypass for VAD insertion, VAD, and hemofiltration exposes the blood to mechanical trauma and activated inflammatory cascades that can result in hemolysis. This produces free hemoglobin, a known nephrotoxin; this is a further renal insult.

At Papworth, from July 1999 to December 2000, Thoratec VADs were used in 11 patients. Hemolysis was quantified by plasma-free hemoglobin (PFHb) and hydroxybutyrate dehydrogenase (HBD) levels measured daily, defined as a PFHb level of $>40$ mg/L and a HBD level of $>250$ IU/L. The authors found that Thoratec VADs are associated with a mild degree of hemolysis. This is worsened by the concomitant use of CVVHF. The effect is accentuated if the same CVVHF circuit is used for over 48 hours, but is reversible within 24 hours of stopping the hemofilter (Luckraz *et al.*, 2002).

***The Novacor Experience.*** Among patients who are hospitalized with heart failure (HF), worsening renal function (WRF) is associated with worse outcomes. Whether treatment for HF contributes to WRF is unknown. In one study, the authors sought to assess whether acute treatment for patients who were hospitalized with HF contributes to WRF. Data were collected in a nested case-control study on 382 subjects who were hospitalized with HF [191 patients with WRF, defined as a rise in serum creatinine level of $>26.5 \mu$mol/L (0.3 mg/dL), and 191 control subjects]. The association of medications, fluid intake/output, and weight with WRF was assessed.

Calcium channel blocker (CCB) use and loop diuretic doses were higher in patients the day before WRF (25% vs. 10% for CCB; 199 ± 195 mg vs. 143 ± 119 mg for loop diuretics; both $P < 0.05$). There were no significant differences in the fluid intake/output or weight changes between the two groups. Angiotensin-converting enzyme (ACE) inhibitor use was not associated with WRF. Other predictors of WRF included elevated creatinine level at admission, uncontrolled hypertension, and history of HF or diabetes mellitus. Higher hematocrit levels were associated with a lower risk. Vasodilator use was higher among patients the day before WRF (46% vs. 35%, $P < 0.05$), but was not an independent predictor in the multivariable analysis.

The authors concluded that several medical strategies, including the use of CCBs and a higher dose of loop diuretics (but not ACE inhibitors), are associated with a higher risk of WRF. Although the assessment of in-hospital diuresis was limited, WRF could not be explained by greater fluid loss in these patients. Determining whether these interventions are responsible for WRF or are markers of higher risk requires further investigation (Butler *et al.*, 2004).

## RESPIRATORY DYSFUNCTION

### Respiratory Dysfunction Definition

***INTERMACS Definition of Respiratory Dysfunction.***    The INTERMACS database defines respiratory failure as an impairment of respiratory function requiring reintubation or tracheostomy, or (for patients older than 5 years) the inability to discontinue ventilatory support within 6 days (144 hours) post-VAD implant. This excludes intubation for reoperation, or temporary intubation for diagnostic or therapeutic procedures.

### Observational Non-RCT Studies

***The Cleveland Clinic Experience.***    In critical respiratory dysfunction following MCSD implantation, extracorpreal life support may be indicated. Extracorporeal life support (ECLS) is indicated following an LVAD implant for right heart failure or pulmonary dysfunction. Out of 100 patients on the HeartMate at the Cleveland Clinic, 12 were supported with ECLS post-LVAD implant. Preoperatively, 10 (83%) patients were on an intra-aortic balloon pump, 9 (75%) were intubated, and 8 (67%) required ECLS as a bridge to LVAD implant. Six (50%) patients were men, and the patient age ranged from 28 to 63 years (mean, 46 ± 10 years). The duration of ECLS averaged 3 ± 2 days (range, 1–9 days).

Eight (67%) patients required a right ventricular assist device (RVAD) with an ECLS circuit, 3 (25%) required peripheral veno-venous ECLS, and 1 required peripheral veno-arterial ECLS. Forty-five percent of the patients who were supported with ECLS post-LVAD survived to transplant, compared with the 81% who were supported with LVAD only. Early in this study, three patients had RVAD support only and all three of them died. RVAD support (with or without ECLS) was 11% overall, and declined from 14% in the first 50 patients to 8% in the second 50. The authors concluded that ECLS post-LVAD is relatively uncommon and its use is associated with reduced survival, but it helps salvage these critically ill patients (Wudel *et al.*, 1997).

## GASTROINTESTINAL DYSFUNCTION

### Gastrointestinal Dysfunction Definition

***INTERMACS Definition of Gastrointestinal Dysfunction.*** The INTER-MACS database defines hepatic or gastrointestinal dysfunction as an increase in any two of the three hepatic laboratory values — total bilirubin, aspartate aminotransferase (AST), and alanine aminotransferase (ALT) — to a level greater than three times the upper limit of normal for the hospital beyond 14 days postimplant (or if hepatic dysfunction is the primary cause of death).

### Observational Non-RCT Studies

***The Columbia University Experience.*** MCSD implantation may be complicated by gastrointestinal (GI) events. The Columbia group evaluated GI function in 27 LVAD recipients using interviews, GI contrast studies, endoscopy, and [99m]Tc sulfur colloid studies of esophageal transit and gastric emptying. While on LVAD support (mean duration of 84 days), 19 patients reported early satiety and/or nausea, and 1 was unable to tolerate oral intake. The esophageal transit time (normal, <10 s) was borderline slow at $14 \pm 4$ (mean $\pm$ SEM), and gastric emptying (normal, <90 min) was prolonged (range, 106–506 min; mean, $283 \pm 69$ min).

In a 1–38 month follow-up, the gastric function subjectively improved in all patients. Six patients had intraperitoneal device placement. One patient died of aspiration pneumonia secondary to small-bowel obstruction; and one had a prolonged inability to tolerate oral intake, requiring feeding jejunostomy tube placement. The 21 patients with preperitoneal placement of the device did not require GI operative interventions and had no catastrophic GI events; they had mild-to-no GI complaints. The authors concluded that preperitoneal placement may mitigate early satiety and obviate serious GI complications (El-Amir *et al.*, 1996).

***The Göttingen University Experience.***    The Göttingen group described a patient requiring a HeartMate 1000 IP LVAD due to cardiogenic shock. After prolonged gastrointestinal bleeding, without identifying the source of bleeding, technetium scintigraphy pointed to the right lower abdomen. The patient underwent a laparotomy, and the inflamed ileum was resected. A pathological examination revealed cytomegalovirus ileitis. This was treated with ganciclovir and acyclovir (Aleksic *et al.*, 1998).

***The Osaka University Experience.***    In the condition of pre-existing vital organ failure induced by heart failure, hepatic failure often progresses despite the establishment of adequate hemodynamic support through an LVAD and results in a high mortality rate. At Osaka University, hepatic function and its relation to inflammatory response and hepatic microcirculation were evaluated in 16 consecutive patients who received an LVAD implantation for end-stage cardiomyopathy between 1992 and 2000. The patients were divided into two groups: 5 patients who died from multiple organ failure after severe hepatic failure (group 1), and 11 patients who did not develop severe hepatic failure (group 2). Serum levels of C-reactive protein (CRP), interleukin (IL)-6, IL-8, and hyaluronan (a known indicator of hepatic sinusoidal function) were measured preoperatively and postoperatively in both groups.

Serum ALT and AST levels during LVAD support were similar in the two groups. Serum total bilirubin (T-Bil), CRP, IL-6, and IL-8 levels before and during the first 20 days of LVAD support were significantly higher in group 1 than in group 2 ($p < 0.01$–$0.05$). Serum hyaluronan levels in both groups were significantly correlated with T-Bil levels ($r = 0.60$, $p < 0.05$ in group 1; $r = 0.68$, $p < 0.0001$ in group 2). Histopathological examination by transvenous liver biopsy in a group 1 patient showed hepatic sinusoidal damage as well as cholestasis and fibrosis.

The authors concluded that patients with hyperbilirubinemia and inflammatory reactions before LVAD support show increased hyperbilirubinemia and increased inflammatory cytokine and hyarulonan levels, despite adequate hemodynamics achieved under LVAD support. These results suggest that inflammatory response contributes to the subsequent aggravation of hepatic dysfunction, probably with underlying and continuing derangement in hepatic sinusoidal microcirculation even under systemic circulatory support (Masai *et al.*, 2002).

# MALNUTRITION

## Clinical Experience

Although malnutrition in the context of cachexia secondary to advanced heart failure is one of the risk factors prior to MCSD implantation (Anker *et al.*, 1997), the assist device therapy itself and the associated chronic inflammatory effects can lead to malnutrition. The low-level chronic inflammatory mediator release after MCSD implantation contributes to the clinical syndrome (Deng *et al.*, 1999a). In patients with MSCD support, particularly the elderly, the consequences of poor nutritional status are decreased immune function, higher infection rates, and impaired wound healing. Physical conditioning and rehabilitation efforts might also be compromised, contributing to diminished survival in the acute recovery period (Dang *et al.*, 2005).

***The Columbia University Experience.***  The course and impact of the nutritional status in patients receiving LVAD support were retrospectively reviewed in 99 patients undergoing LVAD implantation from January 1996 through February 2003 at Columbia University. Patients were evaluated according to four preoperative nutritional parameters: serum albumin level, total protein level, absolute lymphocyte count, and body mass index. The mean values of all the nutritional parameters were obtained preoperatively and serially during the postoperative period (at 1, 2, and 3 months).

By 3 months, the mean serum albumin level increased to within normal limits, the mean total protein level increased (although not significantly), and there was a trend toward a decreasing mean absolute leukocyte count and body mass index. During the postoperative period, patients with a low absolute leukocyte count had higher rates of infection and sepsis. There were no differences in infection rates between the subgroups for any of the other parameters. The overall rates of sepsis and of any type of infection were 14.1% and 50.5%, respectively. The mean total hospital length of stay was equivalent among the subgroups, but the mean stay in the intensive care unit was significantly longer in patients with low serum albumin and total protein levels than in those with normal values. The bridge-to-transplantation rate was significantly lower in patients with low serum albumin and total protein levels than in those with normal values; and posttransplantation actuarial survivals at 1, 3, and 5 years were equivalent among all the subgroups.

The authors concluded that malnutrition predisposes LVAD patients to poor clinical outcomes, although protein status improves with LVAD support. Efforts should be made to identify patients at risk and to provide nutritional supplementation throughout the perioperative period (Dang *et al.*, 2005).

## NEUROLOGICAL DYSFUNCTION

### Neurological Dysfunction Definition

*INTERMACS Definition of Neurological Dysfunction.* The INTERMACS database defines neurological dysfunction as any new, temporary, or permanent focal or global neurological deficit ascertained by a standard neurological examination (administered by a neurologist or other qualified physician, and documented with appropriate diagnostic tests and consultation note). The examining physician will distinguish between a transient ischemic attack (TIA), which is fully reversible within 24 h (and without evidence of infarction), and a stroke, which lasts longer than 24 h (or less than 24 h if there is evidence of infarction). The NIH Stroke Scale (for patients over 5 years old) must be readministered at 30 and 60 days following the event to document the presence and severity of neurological deficits.

Each neurological event must be subcategorized as one of the following:

1. Transient ischemic attack (acute event that resolves completely within 24 h with no evidence of infarction); or
2. Ischemic or hemorrhagic cerebrovascular accident (CVA) (event that persists beyond 24 h, or less than 24 h associated with infarction on an imaging study).

In addition to the above, for patients <6 months of age, any of the following should be observed:

3. New abnormality on head ultrasound; or
4. EEG positive for seizure activity, with or without clinical seizure.

## RCT Studies

*The REMATCH Experience.*   The progression of heart failure can lead to cardiac transplantation; but when patients are ineligible, long-term mechanical circulatory support may improve survival. The REMATCH trial showed that LVADs prolong survival in patients with end-stage heart disease, but with a significant number of adverse events. The REMATCH investigators reported on the neurological outcomes in the REMATCH trial. The REMATCH investigators examined new neurological events in 129 patients randomized to either LVAD placement ($n = 68$) or medical management ($n = 61$); and classified them as stroke, transient ischemic attack, toxic-metabolic encephalopathy, or other.

There were 46 neurological events: 42 in 30 LVAD patients, and 4 in 4 patients in the medical arm (chi$^2$, 30 out of 68 patients vs. 4 out of 61 patients, $P < 0.001$). Sixteen percent of the LVAD patients had a stroke at a rate of

0.19 per year (95% CI, 0.10 to 0.33), many occurring in the postoperative period. The stroke rate in the medical arm was 0.052. Kaplan–Meier survival analysis showed a 44% reduction in the risk of stroke or death in the LVAD group vs. the optimal medical group ($P = 0.002$). The mean interval from implantation to stroke was $221.8 \pm 70.4$ days. A history of stroke, age, and sepsis were not stroke risk factors in the LVAD group.

The authors concluded that fewer than half of the patients in the LVAD group had a neurological event, and there were few neurological deaths. Survival analysis combining stroke and death demonstrated a significant benefit for long-term circulatory support with an LVAD over medical therapy. Future trials will need to prospectively address all the neurological outcomes (including neurocognitive function) and the role of long-term neuroprotection (Lazar *et al.*, 2004).

***Observational Studies.***    Observational data for neurological complications in adults (Deng *et al.*, 2005a) and pediatric patients (Cengiz *et al.*, 2005) have recently been published.

## PSYCHIATRIC DYSFUNCTION

### Psychiatric Episode Definition

***INTERMACS Definition of Pyschiatric Episodes.***    The INTERMACS database defines a psychiatric episode as a disturbance in thinking, emotion, or behavior that causes substantial impairment in functioning or subjective distress, requiring intervention. Intervention is the addition of new psychiatric medication, hospitalization, or referral to a mental health professional for treatment. Suicide is included in this definition.

### Observational Center Experience

***The Columbia University Medical Center Experience.***    LVADs driven by external sources and capable of sustaining life for weeks or months as a bridge to heart transplantation have been implanted in over 300 patients in the US. Because of the limited availability of organs for transplantation, the remarkable degree to which LVADs reverse end-organ dysfunction, and patient acceptance, proposals for home LVAD treatment and for the use of the LVAD as a permanent treatment for heart failure are being considered. However, LVAD therapy is associated with characteristic psychiatric and psychosocial problems, which must be addressed to optimize the results.

Among the first 30 LVAD patients treated at the Columbia Center, psychiatric interventions were frequently required for family stress, major depression, organic mental syndromes, and serious adjustment disorders. Psychiatric problems most often occurred in patients with ongoing medical complications following LVAD implantation, and often significantly impaired rehabilitation. Both depression and organic mental syndromes were frequently associated with pre-existing cerebrovascular disease (which was sometimes occult) and with strokes, complicating LVAD therapy. Aggressive treatment of depression played a major role in improving the functional status.

LVADs may decompress heart transplant waiting lists, and may make it possible to optimize patients' physiological and functional status before transplantation. With increased LVAD use, however, neuropsychiatric factors can be expected to play a large role in determining the quality of life and outcome both before and after heart transplantation (Shapiro *et al.*, 1996).

***Other Studies.*** The Hahnemann University group sought to determine the psychosocial and sexual concerns of patients discharged from the hospital with implantable LVADs. Bridge-to-transplant patients with the HeartMate LVAD received a psychosocial and sexual survey at 1 month after discharge from the hospital. The survey consisted of three parts, with five questions in each category. The patients were asked to complete the survey by circling the responses, and to provide more detailed answers when necessary. Eight male patients completed the questionnaire.

Psychologically, all of the patients expressed a positive mood and found support from family or religious sources. The majority described a change in attitude and behavior. Socially, all of the patients described a change in lifestyle as well as a change in the reaction of family and friends. None of the patients went back to work or had the desire to return to work until after transplantation. A minority of patients admitted to smoking or drinking. Sexually, the majority had the desire or participated in sexual activities. The majority of patients either used or were interested in using sexual stimulants. There were no mechanical problems with the LVADs. The authors concluded that psychosocial and sexual conditions are altered in patients with heart failure who are discharged with implantable LVADs (Samuels *et al.*, 2004).

After a 1-month time interval, there was an improvement in mood, an adjustment in lifestyle, and a positive shift in relations with family and friends. There was sexual desire, with an interest in sexual-enhancing medication. The most common concern was related to the pump, such as the durability of the device or damage to the components (Samuels *et al.*, 2004). The implications of MCSD therapy on psychiatric outcomes have been addressed in different studies (Dew *et al.*, 2001a; Grady *et al.*, 2003).

## MECHANICAL CIRCULATORY SUPPORT DEVICE DYSFUNCTION

**Travis B (born 1979)**

**Living with the MCSD**

I do not have many stories for someone who had the LVAD for over 2 years. All LVAD patients need to know how to change their LVAD controller, and the LVAD makers need to do a better job of checking the spare controllers before they give them to people. It was not a problem for me because I was in the hospital. The night I was put on the pneumatic pump, I thought my controller had gone bad. The controller that I was using was my backup because I had to change controllers once during my first year with the LVAD. When I went to change controllers that night in the hospital, the spare controller went right to the red heart when I hooked it up. I was lucky that I never had to change my controller a second time at home, because I would have had to hand pump my LVAD for over 3 hours while driving to the hospital.

During my first year with the LVAD, I felt good enough to play golf until my left hip started to become painful. I stopped playing that fall. The hip limited what I could do on the LVAD during the second year.

Before I was sent to Columbia to have the LVAD implanted, I was at Bassett Hospital. While I was there, one of the residents asked my father and me if we would like to have her Thursday tickets to the 2003 Masters golf tournament. We said that if I was feeling well enough, we would be interested. Shortly after that, I was transferred to Columbia, where I received my LVAD on December 10, 2002.

The following April, we went to the Masters. That Thursday was cold and rainy. The play was canceled that day. On the way out of the golf course, we were interviewed by a reporter from an Atlanta newspaper. It was the first time ever that a day at the Masters had been totally canceled due to rain. During the trip, we also went to Nashville to visit my dad's family. On the way to Nashville, we called the family of the resident to thank them for letting us use her tickets and to tell them that we had made it into the newspaper. They felt so bad because we did not get to see any golf that they said that we could have their tickets for Sunday of the 2004 Masters. We went the next year and the weather was perfect.

We drove to Augusta and Nashville because flying presented too many problems. I did not think flying would be very safe because the PBU could get lost or damaged during the flight. The PBU would probably have been too big to take as a carry-on. I did not want to take the risk of getting to our destination and having the PBU broken in another city. You know how airlines tend to treat your luggage.

## Device Dysfunction Definition

*INTERMACS Definition of Device Dysfunction.* The INTERMACS database defines device malfunction as a failure of one or more of the components of the MCSD system that either directly causes or could potentially induce a state of inadequate circulatory support (low cardiac output state) or death (see also chapter 6). The manufacturer must confirm device failure. A failure that is iatrogenic or recipient-induced is classified as an iatrogenic/recipient-induced failure.

# Center Experience with Device Dysfunction

***The Hahnemann University Experience.***    At Hahnemann University Hospital, Philadelphia, PA, a 57-year-old man with a history of idiopathic dilated cardiomyopathy was admitted with progressive symptoms of heart failure, and was listed for heart transplantation. His condition deteriorated despite the institution of inotropic drug support. An echocardiogram showed global biventricular dysfunction with no aortic stenosis or insufficiency. On June 20, 2000, a TCI VE HeartMate left ventricular assist system (LVAS) (Thoratec Corporation, Pleasanton, CA) was implanted. The patient had an uneventful postoperative course and was discharged to his home on July 23, 2000. He was doing well with LVAS rates between 70 and 80 beats/min and flows ranging between 6 and 8 L/min.

About $2\frac{1}{2}$ months after the implantation, he began to have mild dyspnea with his usual activities. The LVAS rates and flows were inappropriately elevated at rest (rates, 80–100 beats/min; flows, 8–9 L/min). An echocardiogram showed moderate LVAS inflow valve regurgitation and mild native aortic valve insufficiency. On October 3, 2000, orthotopic heart transplantation was performed. The LVAS inflow valve had two small linear perforations in the leaflets and partial dehiscence of two commissures. The LVAS outflow valve was intact. The aortic valve was fused along the anterior aspect of the left noncoronary commissure. The posterior aspect of the commissure was open. A small thrombus was present along the right lunula of the left coronary cusp of the aortic valve. An examination of the ostium of the outflow graft insertion revealed it to be situated above the right coronary cusp, with the angle of the graft directed toward the left coronary cusp. The ostia of the coronary arteries were patent. No mineralization was noted. Microscopic examination of the valve across the area of fusion revealed the fusion tissue to be composed of myxomatous granulation tissue adherent to the inflow aspect of the left and noncoronary cusps. No evidence of remote endocarditis or organizing thrombus at the point of fusion was detected. The remainder of the valve cusps showed no evidence of chronic rheumatic valve disease. The patient recovered well and was discharged home on October 13, 2000, with no shortness of breath (Samuels *et al.*, 2001).

*The Münster University Experience.* The Münster group described an uncommon Novacor N100 PCq LVAS malfunction caused by an internal short circuit of the device due to urine aspiration via the vent line. Device replacement was managed via a subcostal approach without sternotomy. The patient recovery was uneventful, and successful transplantation was performed 1 month after the device exchange (Hammel *et al.*, 1998).

*Native Aortic Valve Regurgitation During MCSD Support.* The management of mild-to-moderate aortic insufficiency in patients with an LVAD remains controversial. The authors at the University of Alabama in Birmingham reported three patients with aortic insufficiency and pulsatile LVADs treated with a central aortic valve coapting suture. Two of the repairs have been durable for more than 1 year, and aspirin appears to be a sufficient anticoagulant (Bryant *et al.*, 2006).

## Monitoring for MCSD Dysfunction and Failure

*Echocardiography.* With the increasing number of LVAD recipients due to the lack of donor availability and the use of LVADs as a destination therapy, a significant proportion of this population will present with device-related complications. The initial evaluation should be with transesophageal echocardiography (TEE) because conduit obstruction would be a significant complication. Echocardiography has been the principal modality used so far to assess the LVAD cannulas. More reliance on Doppler velocities as well as the establishment of a normal range of values and flow profiles of the inflow and outflow cannulas are necessary. Baseline echocardiographic studies could be used for future comparisons. Fluoroscopy and selective angiography have also been reported to be helpful (Park *et al.*, 1998).

Using a transthoracic echocardiography protocol purposely designed to diagnose the common malfunctions of patients on chronic LVAD support, patients were followed up with serial echocardiograms, and the results were validated with clinical observations at the time of catheter evaluation or inspection at the time of cardiac transplant or corrective surgery. Thirty-two patients with 44 LVADs were followed up during a 4-year period using this protocol, which correctly identified 11 patients with inflow valve regurgitation, 2 with intermittent inflow conduit obstruction, 1 with severe kinking of the outflow graft, and 9 with new insufficiency of the native aortic valve. The authors concluded that transthoracic echocardiography provides a practical method to accurately identify the causes of mechanical dysfunction for patients on chronic LVAD support (Horton *et al.*, 2005).

***Hemodynamic Measurements.*** The group at the University of Louisville, KY, have recommended measuring LV hemodynamics as an additional mode of evaluation of this emerging problem, and have suggested the need for additional noninvasive modalities for the diagnosis of ventricular assist device malfunction (Ferns *et al.*, 2001).

# MECHANICAL CIRCULATORY SUPPORT DEVICE FAILURE

## Device Failure Definition

***INTERMACS Definition of Device Failure.*** According to the INTER-MACS database, device failure should be classified according to which components fail as follows:

1. Pump failure (blood-contacting components of the pump, and any other pump-actuating mechanism that is housed with the blood-contacting components). In the special situation of pump thrombosis, thrombus is documented to be present within the device or its conduits, resulting in or potentially inducing circulatory failure.
2. Non-pump failure (e.g. external pneumatic drive unit, electric power supply unit, batteries, controller, interconnect cable, compliance chamber).

## Center Experience with Device Failure

***The ISHLT MCSD Database Experience.*** Device failure, which — in contrast to device dysfunction — may have fatal outcomes if not corrected immediately, has been reported (Deng *et al.*, 2005a).

***Multicenter REMATCH Experience.*** The REMATCH trial was a randomized trial that compared optimal medical management with LVAD implantation for patients with end-stage heart failure. An independent committee adjudicated the patient outcomes. The system failure rate was 0.13 per patient per year, and the confirmed LVAD malfunction rate was 0.90. Freedom from device replacement was 87% at 1 year and 37% at 2 years. The authors concluded that, despite the observed rates of device malfunction and replacement, LVAD implantation confers a clinically significant improvement on survival as compared to medical management (Dembitsky *et al.*, 2004).

## DIFFERENTIAL COMPLICATIONS BY MCSD TYPE

### HeartMate I vs. Novacor

Among the first-generation pulsatile MCSDs, the Novacor was perceived as having a higher rate of neurological complications than the HeartMate I until the REMATCH study — which demonstrated similar rates of neurological complications in the HeartMate I arm — was published (Lazar *et al.*, 2004). The Novacor has higher long-term durability, with less chance of device dysfunction and failure (Deng *et al.*, 2001a).

### Pulsatile vs. Rotary MCSDs

Among the second-generation rotary MCSDs, the DeBakey MCSD was initially perceived to have a fairly high thrombosis rate (Rothenburger *et al.*, 2002). Comparing first-generation pulsatile MCSDs and second-generation rotary MCSDs, the rotary MCSDs are perceived to have a lower infection rate (Deng *et al.*, 2005a).

# CHAPTER 6

# RESEARCH STRATEGIES

## OUTCOMES RESEARCH

### Research Directions in MCSD Outcomes

*Comparative Survival Benefit by Risk-Stratified Analyses.* The definition of patients whose clinical profile is too well for heart support and replacement by either MCSD or cardiac transplantation requires the continuous assessment of survival benefit in different clinical subgroups undergoing MCSD implantation vs. optimal medical treatment and vs. cardiac transplantation (Deng *et al.*, 2005a). The assessment of survival benefit, however, requires adequate methodology in order to be meaningful. Also, the gain in life expectancy is an important measure of the effectiveness of medical interventions, but its interpretation requires that it be placed in context. A gain in life expectancy from a medical intervention can be categorized as large or small by comparing it with the gains from other interventions aimed at the same target population.

Since the REMATCH trial testing the hypothesis that nontransplant candidates derive a survival benefit from chronic MCSD therapy was positive, one of the next hypotheses to be tested may be that MCSD therapy is superior to cardiac transplantation. In this context, to test the hypothesis that there is a survival and quality-of-life benefit associated with cardiac transplantation, a three-stage study has been proposed: (1) to establish a database within the ISHLT/UNOS/EUROTRANSPLANT infrastructure that will provide an estimate of the survival benefit of heart transplantation in different heart failure risk strata; (2) to organize an international consensus conference with the participation of all the expert groups involved in heart failure management that will define, based upon the review of the stage 1 data, the feasibility of a prospective randomized trial; and (3) pending consensus of the conference, to perform a randomized trial, either in a classical design or in an augmented randomized clinical trial design with risk-based allocation of treatment, guaranteeing high-risk patients access to cardiac transplantation and low-risk patients randomization to either conventional treatment or cardiac transplantation (Deng, 2002). There is a medical, ethical, and economic imperative to generate this type of scientific evidence in order to allocate MCSD therapy and cardiac transplantation to those who are in the greatest medical need of it, and in order to prevent the allocation of cardiac transplantation to those who are too well to benefit from it.

## BASIC AND TRANSLATIONAL RESEARCH

### Active Myocardial Recovery Strategies

*Cell Transplantation and Regrowth of Heart Muscle.* The concept of regenerating healthy myocardium in a myopathic heart is in the experimental stage. Several approaches — including transplantation of embryonic cardiomyocytes (Etzion *et al.*, 2001), cryopreserved (Yokomuro *et al.*, 2001) or bioengineered fetal cardiomyocytes (Leor *et al.*, 2000), neonatal cardiac myocytes, skeletal myoblasts (El Oakley *et al.*, 2001), autologous smooth muscle cells (Yoo *et al.*, 2000), and dermal fibroblasts (Hutcheson *et al.*, 2000) — have been proposed. Current problems include chronic rejection in allogeneic cells, lack of intercellular gap junction communication, and differential patterns in excitation–contraction coupling in skeletal and cardiac myocytes.

Alternatively, lineage-negative bone marrow cells (Orlic *et al.*, 2001) or bone marrow–derived endothelial precursor cells with phenotypic and functional characteristics of hemangioblasts have been proposed. The latter can be used to directly induce new blood vessel formation after experimental myocardial infarction, associated with decreased apoptosis of hypertrophied myocytes in the peri-infarct region, long-term salvage and survival of viable myocardium, reduction in collagen deposition, and sustained improvement in cardiac function (Kocher *et al.*, 2001).

*Pharmacological Recovery Strategies.* The Harefield group reported preliminary experience using clenbuterol. This area of research is actively ongoing internationally (Birks *et al.*, 2005). These studies require a coordinated multi-institutional approach, e.g. in the "LVAD recovery study group" (Table 6).

## Xenotransplantation

Xenotransplantation theoretically provides an unlimited supply of cells, tissues, and organs. The immunological challenge is that the favorite source animal of choice — the pig — and the human recipient diverged 90 million years ago during evolution, so biological characteristics such as anatomy, physiology, and immunology have had much time to drift far apart. Thus, rejection remains a large theoretical stumbling block. In addition, the potential individual benefit of a xenograft has to be balanced against the collective risk of transmitting xenozoonoses.

Ethically, all three monotheistic religions and Hinduism support the idea of saving and improving human life with the help of an animal organ (Hammer, 2001). According to a committee of the ISHLT, the existing experimental results do not presently justify the initiation of a clinical trial, but because of the immense potential, research in xenotransplantation should be encouraged (Cooper and Keogh, 2001).

## Collaborative US SCCOR "Biology of Long-Term Human Mechanical Circulatory Support" Grant

*Overview.* Having proven the benefits of LVADs in prolonging the lives of nontransplantable end-stage heart failure patients through the landmark REMATCH trial, its life-saving potential notwithstanding, LVAD implantation remains an invasive and demanding mechanical therapy with significant risks of infection, bleeding, neurological complications, and device failure. In March 2005, a $17-million NIH grant was awarded to the Columbia University College of Physicians and Surgeons to fund multiple basic and clinical studies so as to address these problems, with the goal of transforming LVADs into a safer and more widely accepted therapy (www.columbiasurgery.org/res/sccor/index). This landmark project will — under the direction of Dr Eric Rose (Principal Investigator) as well as Dr Alan Moskowitz and Dr Mario Deng (Coprincipal Investigators) — include patients with advanced heart failure who receive LVADs as a bridge to transplantation, destination therapy, or bridge to recovery.

The Specialized Centers of Clinically Oriented Research (SCCOR) is a program funded by the NHLBI to foster translational research in order to improve the prevention, diagnosis, and treatment of particular diseases. This particular SCCOR program seeks to elucidate and modulate the biology of the interface between implanted long-term MCSDs and patients with end-stage heart failure by a translational research strategy combining animal model and clinical trials. In the initial application, three key problem areas have been prioritized: the feasibility of improving native myocardial function through cellular transplantation to facilitate device removal (Project 1), the evaluation of novel interventions directed at the adverse impact of coagulopathy (Project 2), and the infections resulting from the device–recipient interface (Project 3).

As per July 2006, these research projects are collaboratively pursued among the Columbia University Medical Center (New York), LDS Hospital (Utah), University of Alabama Medical Center (Birmingham), University of Minnesota Medical Center (Minneapolis), Sharp Memorial Hospital (San Diego), University of Iowa (Iowa City), and St. Luke's Medical Center (Milwaukee). Four core units — Data Management and Statistics (Core A), Animal Models (Core B), Clinical Materials (Core C), and Neuroscience (Core D) — are used for central research coordination. Future centers will be joining this collaborative SCCOR program.

*Central Hypotheses.* The central hypotheses underlying the SCCOR grant proposal are as follows:

Project 1: While spontaneous recovery of the myocardium in LVAD recipients is rare, active strategies to regenerate myocardial function allow the potential for device removal. Cell transplantation offers the potential to actively regenerate myocardial function, while the setting of mechanical circulatory assistance offers a circulatory safety net during the process of engraftment.

Project 2: Device surfaces activate the intrinsic coagulation cascade generating a consumptive coagulopathy associated with hemorrhagic complications and fibrin deposition, with its associated thrombotic and embolic complications. Selective blockade of the intrinsic pathway ameliorates this pathophysiology and preserves the function of the extrinsic coagulation cascade, which improves surgical hemostasis at the time of device implantation and prevents late bleeding complications.

Project 3: Staphylococcal infections are among the most common causes of death in device recipients. These pathogens often start as commensals and, due to the presence of selected virulence determinants, are able to initiate infections. Control of this critical initial colonization process may potentially reduce the high incidence of infections in this vulnerable patient population.

***Cell Transplantation and Myocardial Recovery.***   The specific aims are as follows:

1. Perform an exploratory randomized trial evaluating the safety and efficacy of the injection of autologous bone marrow–derived angioblasts in bridge-to-transplant LVAD recipients.
2. Determine the influence of angioblasts on mesenchymal stem cell (MSC) migration, survival, proliferation, and differentiation *in vitro*.
3. Determine if the cotransplantation of mouse or human angioblasts with autologous MSCs enhances engraftment, myogenesis, and cardiac function *in vivo* after myocardial infarction.

***Coagulopathy Aims.***   The specific aims are as follows:

1. Fully characterize the time course of activation of prothrombotic pathways in animals and humans exposed to artificial blood-contacting surfaces acutely using cardiopulmonary bypass (CPB) and chronically after LVAD implantation.
2. Test novel antagonists of the intrinsic pathway of coagulation in CPB and LVAD placement in porcine models.
3. Perform phase II trials in human subjects with advanced heart failure undergoing CPB and LVAD placement with novel small-molecule intrinsic pathway antagonists.

***Infection Aims.***   The specific aims are as follows:

1. Characterize the relationship between cutaneous and nasal surveillance cultures of both coagulase-positive and coagulase-negative

staphylococci and clinical staphylococcal isolates in infected LVAD patients using molecular epidemiological techniques.

2. Conduct two exploratory randomized trials of novel strategies designed to reduce the incidence of *Staphylococcus aureus* infections. Endpoints include the incidence of *S. aureus* infections, the success rate in the eradication of colonization, and risk factor analyses for colonization and infection.

3. Identify the *S. aureus* surface molecules and the LVAD membrane cellular matrix components that mediate adherence to the different device surfaces.

4. Examine the role of specific *S. aureus* adhesins in rodent models of prosthetic intravascular infection (Asai *et al.*, 2005). A brief home-made video of the procedure can be accessed at http://cardiactransplantresearch.cumc.columbia.edu/images/AorticPatchMCSD.rar.

## DIFFERENTIAL DEVELOPMENT BY MCSD TYPE

### Design Development and MCSD Future

The optimization of pulsatile, rotary, and centrifugal MCSD designs remains a challenging research task. From a bioengineering perspective (Chen *et al.*, 2004), the geometry of the surgical integration of the LVAD is an important factor in the flow pattern that develops both in series (aortic valve closed, all flow through LVAD) and in parallel (heart pumping in addition to LVAD).

In one study, computational fluid dynamic models of the aortic outflow conduit (AOC) junctions simulated geometry as cylindrical tubes intersecting at angles ranging from 30° to 90°. Velocity fields were computed over a range of cardiac outputs for both series and parallel flow. The results demonstrated that the flow patterns were significantly affected by the insertion angle of the AOC into the native aorta, both during series and parallel flow conditions. Zones of flow recirculation and high shear stress on the aortic wall were observed at the highest angle, gradually decreasing in size until disappearing at the lowest angle of 30°. The highest velocity and shear stress values were associated with series flow. The results suggest that connecting the LVAD outflow conduit to the proximal aorta at a shallower angle produces fewer secondary flow patterns in the native cardiovascular system (May-Newman *et al.*, 2004).

## FUTURE DIRECTIONS

### MCSD Development

The main focus of MCSD research will be the development of smaller, durable, and completely implantable MCSDs. Combination therapy of active recovery strategies of the left ventricle and a bridge–to-recovery MCSD design, as well as the combination of a partial unloading long-term MCSD design with native left ventricular backup (e.g. by pharmacological or stem cell interventions), will be important. The complications of current MCSD generations, specifically infections and coagulations (including bleeding and embolism), will have to be fundamentally addressed to transition MCSD therapy into fully accepted clinical practice (Table 8).

### Impact of Nonpulsatility on Recipient Biology

At this time, the long-term impact of low-pulsatility (second- and third-generation) MCSDs on recipient biology remains ill understood (Klotz *et al.*, 2004; Thalmann *et al.*, 2005). This area of research will gain increasing importance. Currently, the focus of research is on the effects of blood circulation and exposure to vanes running at high velocity, bearings, and seals. There is also a focus on the effect of blood flow on aortic and arterial walls; cerebral metabolism and cerebral blood flow regulation; neuroendocrine, kidney, splacnic, and pulmonary functions; vasoactive function and baroreceptor reflex; and exercise and oxygen consumption (Thalmann *et al.*, 2005).

### MCSD-Related Clinical Trials

LVAD use is an important step forward as a treatment option for the management of patients with chronic end-stage heart failure, especially those who are not considered candidates for cardiac transplantation because of

**Table 8.** Characteristics of currently available MCSDs within the framework of the "ideal MCSD design".

| Type | Size reduction | Durability | Implantability | Biocompatibility | Cost | Managability |
|---|---|---|---|---|---|---|
| Ideal future MCSD | +++ | +++ | +++ | +++ | +++ | +++ |
| AbioCor | + | | +++ | | + | + |
| Abiomed | | | | | | |
| Berlin Heart INCOR | +++ | +++ | + | | + | ++ |
| CardioWest | + | ++ | + | | + | + |
| CorAide | ++ | | | | | |
| EVAHEART | + | | | | | |
| Jarvik 2000 | ++ | +++ | + | | + | ++ |
| LionHeart | + | | +++ | | + | + |
| MEDOS | | + | | | | |
| MicroMed DeBakey | ++ | | | | | |
| Terumo DuraHeart | ++ | | + | | | |
| Thoratec HeartMate | + | + | + | ++ | + | + |
| Thoratec HeartMate II | ++ | | | | | |
| Thoratec Ventracor | ++ | | + | | + | + |
| WorldHeart Novacor | | +++ | | + | + | + |
| WorldHeart Novacor II | +++ | +++ | +++ | + | + | ++ |

age or comorbidities. As the field of mechanical support progresses, it will be important for physicians involved in the selection of candidates for mechanical support to be familiar with the factors that have been shown to have an adverse impact on the outcome, regardless of the indication. Recent data suggest that well-selected candidates can have a 2-year survival, which may equal or exceed that reported for heart transplantation in an older population.

The development of multiple smaller and more durable devices, which are already in clinical trials, offers hope for even lower morbidity and mortality with this therapy. Future trials with new devices are needed to confirm these findings and to validate the predictive accuracy and benefit of preoperative risk scoring in order to guide patient selection and optimize the results of this therapy (Lietz and Miller, 2005).

# CHAPTER 7
# SOCIETAL PERSPECTIVES

## ROLE OF GOVERNMENTAL AGENCIES

### Industry, Academic Medicine, and Regulatory Agencies

MCSD safety and effectiveness are the ultimate goals of the interaction between academic research and industrial development. In the USA, the FDA becomes increasingly involved as devices move from the design phase through the evolution of lab and bench testing to clinical testing. The FDA's Center for Devices plays a very active role in the premarketing process, marketing approval, and postmarketing surveillance. The Center's mission is clearly defined in the categories of public health, specifically watching for device safety and effectiveness.

### US Food and Drug Administration (FDA)

*Safety and Effectiveness Monitoring.* The FDA conducts a thorough review of drugs, biologics, and medical devices for safety and effectiveness before granting approval for marketing. Before a product is marketed, the sponsor submits an application for approval by the FDA. This application contains a proposed package insert, which may also be referred to as labeling. This insert summarizes what the FDA has determined to be a safe and effective use of the product. The FDA bases its approval decision upon bioresearch data that are generated and reported to the FDA by the sponsor to support the marketing approval of the product. These data are collected by the sponsor during clinical research conducted under an Investigational New Drug (IND) application or an Investigational Device Exemption (IDE).

***Medical Device Definition.*** A medical device is any healthcare product that does not achieve its primary intended purpose by a chemical interaction or by being metabolized. Medical devices include surgical lasers, sutures, pacemakers, and diagnostic aids such as reagents and test kits for *in vitro* diagnoses. An investigational device is a medical device that is undergoing clinical trials to evaluate its safety and effectiveness. The IDE regulations specify how to conduct these clinical trials (21CFR812.2). The regulations require that devices be classified as "significant-risk" or "nonsignificant-risk" devices. The sponsor often first decides on this classification, but the Institutional Review Board (IRB) must agree with the determination.

The risk determination should be based on the proposed use of the device, not on the device alone. A significant-risk device presents a potential for serious risk to the health, safety, or welfare of the subject. More specifically, it is intended to be implanted into a human; is used in supporting or sustaining human life; or is of substantial importance in diagnosing, curing, mitigating, or treating disease, or in preventing the impairment of human health — otherwise, it presents a serious risk to the health, safety, and welfare of the subject [21CFR812.3(5)(m)]. The sponsor must submit an IDE application to the FDA (21CFR812.20). There is no specific form for this purpose, but the regulations list the elements required in the application. The trial cannot begin until the FDA has granted an IDE and the IRB has granted approval for the study. By definition, a study with a significant-risk device poses more than minimal risk to human subjects and requires full IRB review.

***The US Medical Device Laws.*** The Medical Device Amendments of 1976 and the Safe Medical Devices Act of 1990 provide the regulatory framework for medical device development, testing, approval, and marketing. Manufacturers who wish to market a new medical device may need to submit a premarket notification to the FDA. Some medical devices are exempt from the premarket approval process. If the device is not exempt, the FDA determines whether the device is substantially equivalent [21CFR807.81(a)(1)] to similar devices marketed before the 1976 amendment. These devices are often referred to as 510K devices (21CFR807.92). If the new device is not substantially equivalent, the company may need to demonstrate its safety and efficacy in a premarket approval application, which could include clinical trials.

## US Health Insurance Portability and Accountability Act (HIPAA)

The Health Insurance Portability and Accountability Act (HIPAA) was a milestone in federal efforts to facilitate the transfer of healthcare data. The HIPAA, passed by Congress in 1996, mandates regulations protecting the confidentiality of health information and in this way supplements the patchwork of state protections. Issued by the US Department of Health and Human Services (HHS) in 2000 and revised in August 2002, the HIPAA Final Privacy Rule protects oral, written, and electronic protected health information (PHI). PHI is any information that "relates to the past, present, or future physical or mental health or condition of an individual." The regulations went into effect on April 14, 2003, for most organizations.

## US Perspective vs. International Perspective

The creation of a US interagency (NIH/FDA/CMS) national MCSD registry (INTERMACS), which was based on the ISHLT MCSD Database initiative (Deng *et al.*, 2003c; Deng *et al.*, 2004; Deng *et al.*, 2005a), is a good example of a fruitful dialectical/complementary relationship between international/global (ISHLT) and innovative national research and regulatory strategies (NIH).

## QUALITY ASSURANCE CONSIDERATIONS

The best method of ensuring postmarketing quality control is the institution of a mandatory reporting system, as implemented in the USA in 2005 with the INTERMACS registry (Kirklin and Holman, 2006). It can only be hoped for the international heart failure community that the US INTERMACS mechanism, which was blueprinted with the help and resources of the International Society of Heart and Lung Transplantation (ISHLT), will feed back into the international community for international quality control.

# ECONOMIC CONSIDERATIONS

| | |
|---|---|
| **Ed S** **(born 1956)** **Long-term social impact of MCSD** | I've had to go on total disability since I had the pump. The line of work I was doing required some physical prowess. I wasn't fortunate enough to have a profession that I could go back to with the LVAD, so I haven't figured out what to do yet. I'm in the hospital right now waiting for a heart transplant, but I'm one of the healthier patients here on the seventh floor. I'm alive, and that's a miracle of modern science. |

## Current MCSD Costs

***The Columbia University Medical Center Experience.*** We evaluated the hospital costs and reimbursements for patients who were discharged after LVAD implantation and subsequently returned to the hospital for orthotopic heart transplantation (OHT). To control for patient-specific variables, LVAD therapy and OHT therapy were compared in the same patient; that is, only those patients who received an LVAD, were discharged, and returned for OHT were studied. The length of stay (LOS), readmissions and outpatient services were analyzed, including their respective total actual hospital cost (TAHC) and net revenue (NR). The time periods analyzed were the same for LVAD and OHT therapies.

Between December 1996 and June 2000, thirty-six patients out of the LVAD population at Columbia-Presbyterian Medical Center were discharged following HeartMate vented electric (VE) implantation and readmitted for OHT. The mean pre-LVAD implantation LOS was $21.3 \pm 24.1$ days. The post-LVAD LOS was $36.8 \pm 22.2$ days vs. $18.2 \pm 12.2$ days post-OHT ($p < 0.001$). The mean length of LVAD support was $123.4 \pm 77.7$ days. The overall total costs for LVADs exceeded that of OHT, whereas the revenue was relatively lower. The TAHC post-LVAD averaged $197\,957 \pm \$77\,291$, whereas the TAHC post-OHT averaged $151\,646 \pm \$53\,909$ ($p = 0.005$). The NR averaged $144\,756 \pm \$96\,656$ post-LVAD vs. $178\,562 \pm \$68\,571$ post-OHT ($p = 0.09$). LVAD patients had more readmissions compared with OHT patients [1.2 ($\pm 1.7$) out of 123 days vs. 0.3 ($\pm 0.6$) out of 123 days, respectively; $p = 0.005$]. The average

LOS during readmission was similar between the two groups [LVAD, 5.6 ($\pm$10.6) days; OHT, 9.6 ($\pm$8.2) days; $p = 0.18$]. OHT was associated with a significantly greater number of outpatient services compared with LVAD [9.7 ($\pm$6.1) days vs. 3.0 ($\pm$4.7) days; $p < 0.001$]. In contrast to OHT, LVAD revenues did not match the costs of LVAD therapy.

The authors concluded that LVAD implantation is associated with a longer LOS and higher costs for initial hospitalization compared with OHT. LVAD patients have higher readmission rates compared with OHT patients, but similar costs and LOS. OHT is associated with a greater number of outpatient services. Reimbursements for LVAD therapy are relatively low, resulting in significant lost revenue. If LVAD therapy is to become a viable alternative, improvements in both cost-effectiveness and reimbursement will be necessary (Oz *et al.*, 2003; Digiorgi *et al.*, 2005).

***The REMATCH Experience.***    The REMATCH investigators performed a retrospective analysis of 23 consecutive patients who had a HeartMate XVE pump implanted as a destination therapy at two high-volume ventricular assist device implant centers after US FDA approval in October 2003. They evaluated the survival to discharge during implantation hospitalization, the hospital length of stay, and the hospital costs, and compared them with the outcomes reported from the REMATCH (RM) trial. All the patients in this cohort who were implanted post-REMATCH (PRM) had class IV heart failure and were similar in age, gender, and nearly all other preimplantation clinical measures to the RM subjects.

The mean hospital costs for PRM patients was 40% lower than for RM patients when measured from implantation to discharge ($128 084 vs. $210 187, respectively; $p < 0.01$). The PRM patients who survived implantation hospitalization had 48% lower costs than those who did not survive ($114 979 vs. $215 456, $p < 0.01$), a finding similar to the RM experience. The PRM patients in this cohort were more likely to survive to discharge compared with RM patients (87.0% vs. 67.3%, $p = 0.09$). The mean hospital length of stay was 25% lower in the PRM group (44 days vs. 33 days), but did not reach statistical significance ($p = 0.50$). The REMATCH investigators concluded that the outcomes of LVAD use as a destination therapy have improved in the post-REMATCH era, including significantly lower hospital costs as well as strong trends toward better survival to hospital discharge and shorter average length of stay (Miller *et al.*, 2006).

*US National Medicare Coverage Decision.* The intention of the US government agency Centers for Medicare and Medicaid Services (CMS) to issue a national Medicare coverage decision for destination, long-term MCSDs has been estimated to increase the US healthcare budget by as much as 10% over the next few decades.

## ETHICAL CONSIDERATIONS

### General Ethical Problems Arising from MCSD Therapy

The increasingly disseminated implementation of long-term MCSD therapy, specifically destination MCSD therapy, has led to unprecedented ethical questions that the Columbia University team is dealing with under the guidance of the ethics committee (Chairman Dr Kenneth Prager) (Edwards and Prager, 2003).

If a patient supported by a destination MCSD develops multiple organ failure (MOF) and the dying process is interrupted by ongoing MCSD support, is it justified to apply a device-termination protocol? If a patient who has previously agreed to destination MCSD implantation suffers an unacceptable quality of life (QOL), is the patient as the autonomous subject entitled to request device termination? Should a heart transplant allocation policy favor or discourage the transplantation of stable, long-term MCSD patients? In any type of research, but specifically applicable to clinical research with MCSD, the sound conduct of studies according to published ethical guidelines is crucial (www.hhs.gov/ohrp/humansubjects/guidance/belmont.htm#xinform).

### Problem of Emergency Transfer of Patients for MCSD Evaluation

*Scope of Problem.* Currently, there is no protocol in place for the emergency evaluation of patients referred from the ER or from other hospitals who are severely ill with advanced heart failure, and who may need

VAD implantation or OHT. Because of the ethical, medical, personnel, and financial issues involved in undertaking these complex and costly procedures, a more structured approach to the evaluation of these patients is felt necessary. Therefore, the Columbia University Medical Center (CUMC) has set up a Policy Group to develop adequate procedures. This group is tasked to establish a policy and protocol for dealing with advanced heart failure patients referred emergently for possible ventricular assist device implantation or heart transplantation.

***Ethical Issues.*** As is the case with all heart transplant centers, the CUMC/NYPH is entrusted with the societal responsibility of using the extremely scarce medical resource of donated human hearts in a responsible manner. Implied in this trust is the assurance that the heart will be implanted in a recipient who will have an acceptable benefit — in terms of quantity and quality of survival — from the transplant. Implanting the heart in a patient who has a poor expected posttransplant survival and is likely to die may be viewed as a waste of the organ and an abrogation of the hospital's ethical responsibility to use the scarce resource of a donated human organ in the most medically effective way possible. Accordingly, medical and psychosocial criteria have been established to try and select those patients who would benefit the most from the transplant or from the VAD. The adherence to these criteria is carried out in an impartial manner and without consideration of such nonmedical factors as patient gender, race, religion, and occupation.

***Resources.*** Heart transplantation and heart assist devices are very resource-intensive procedures. The NYPH operates under financial constraints, just as every other medical center does. In order to maintain the financial solvency of the heart transplant and VAD services, the hospital finds itself in the sensitive but necessary position of having to consider financial compensation when evaluating patients for these procedures. To do otherwise would place the programs themselves in jeopardy, thereby denying scores of patients the potential of these life-extending procedures.

***Undocumented Non-US Nationals ("Aliens").*** Because of the success of the NYPH heart transplant and VAD programs, patients from other countries frequently arrive at the hospital ER in medically desperate condition. Other patients who are resident aliens lacking both proper papers and insurance also arrive in similar condition. There is every expectation that these dilemmas will continue to occur. Lastly, patients are sometimes transferred from regional hospitals in desperate cardiac straits, and rapid and fateful medical decisions that may involve VAD placement or eventual heart transplantation must be made for them. Traditionally, the hospital has dealt with these situations in an *ad hoc* manner, which has not always been optimal from a medical, ethical, or resource-based point of view.

***Protocol.*** Accordingly, the following protocol was proposed in July 2006 at Columbia University Medical Center in order to deal with these situations in the future in a rational, fair, and efficient manner.

1. The hospital will set up an Emergency Advanced Heart Failure Screening Committee.
2. The Committee will be composed of on-call representatives from the cardiology, cardiac surgery, and social work departments; a pretransplant and VAD coordinator; and the director of the cardiovascular service line. The cardiologist and cardiac surgeon will cochair the Committee.
3. The cardiologist or cardiac surgeon will notify the other Committee members whenever a patient with end-stage heart failure presents with psychosocial issues or financial problems that raise serious questions as to whether steps toward VAD placement or heart transplant should be pursued.
4. The Committee will have access at all times to the medical and psychosocial acceptance criteria for patients presenting for possible VAD or heart transplant procedures.
5. Committee members will rotate at regular intervals; and a schedule of such rotations, member's beepers, etc. will be available to the cardiologist or cardiac surgeon cochairs.
6. The Committee members will be available on a 24/7 basis for the duration of their rotation.
7. The Committee will make decisions concerning the emergency disposition of the patient. The Committee may wish to access the expertise of others in their fields. Ethics consultations will be available as needed. Whenever appropriate, medically acceptable temporizing measures will

be taken to allow a less hurried, in-depth evaluation of the patient by standing committees such as the Heart Transplant Selection Committee.

8. The cardiology department will develop detailed acceptance criteria for potential VAD and heart transplant referrals to this hospital. These criteria, which will include psychosocial as well as medical criteria, will be circulated to referral hospitals. It is assumed that accepting physicians in this hospital will be familiar with these criteria, so that reference to them may be made at the time referrals are requested.

## End-of-Life Challenges and Columbia Protocol

### Guidelines for Treating Terminally Ill Patients with VADs Who Wish to Die at Home

1. It is becoming increasingly common and desirable for physicians to accommodate the wishes of terminally ill patients who express a desire to die at home rather than in the hospital. Similarly, patients with ventricular assist devices who express this desire should be able to do so whenever reasonably possible. Given the advanced cardiac disease of patients in the VAD-as-destination program, such requests may well become common. Because of the unique clinical features of patients with VADs, a policy for dealing with this request is appropriate.

2. Patients being considered for home VAD removal should have clearly expressed a desire to die at home. The family should be in accord with the patient's wish. The medical team should be in agreement that the family will be able to cope emotionally and medically with this event.

3. The patient's family needs to be instructed concerning the likely scenarios that will occur when the patient becomes moribund. In particular, they must be made aware of how the assist device will react and how to deal with such likely occurrences as alarm warnings, etc. Whenever possible, local professional help such as physicians and/or hospice nurses should be contacted, recruited, and instructed so that they will be available to help the family when the end is near.

4. In most cases, it is anticipated that the VAD device will not be disconnected until the patient has been declared dead either by the local physician or by the hospice healthcare provider. It is expected that the patient will be pronounced dead after a suitable period of apnea has

elapsed and the patient has met whatever other clinical guidelines denoting death that the local healthcare provider might use.

5. In some cases, the VAD device may be turned off when the patient is still alive but death is imminent. In such a situation, the decision to discontinue the device will be made by the patient's healthcare proxy in concert with the local physician or other appropriate healthcare provider (such as a hospice nurse). Consultation with the VAD physicians at Columbia may be appropriate as well. Rather than set up strict guidelines for VAD removal in these cases, the VAD Destination Committee feels that the decisions should be made on a case-by-case basis, reflecting the overall policy that the device should be discontinued when it is clearly prolonging the dying process.

6. Finally, every patient receiving a VAD as a destination therapy should have designated a healthcare proxy. Patients with VADs going home to die must also have a do-not-resuscitate (DNR) order form with them (Prager and Oz, 2002).

## PHILOSOPHICAL CONSIDERATIONS

| | |
|---|---|
| **Jill (partner of Robert R, born 1947)** **Philosophical reflection** | The LVAD had a most profound effect on our lives. But we were most grateful to get it, for without it Robert would not be alive today. Despite its problems, awkwardness, and inconvenience, we managed to cope. After a while, our lives took on some semblance of normality. Upon reflection and looking on the positive side, for me it was a very affirming time. I felt that in bringing him through it all, I/we had really achieved something. A small victory over middle age. But to be honest, the one thing that helped to make it bearable was the knowledge that a heart transplant would happen in the future. |
| **Betty (wife of Abraham M, born 1940)** **View of the MCSD concept** | The bottom line is that had the LVAD not existed, my husband would not have been around when a heart became available. The LVAD enabled him to get his body physically ready for when the heart became available. He was physically ready for it. |

We owe a lot to the LVAD. It is a remarkable device. My family and I owe our future to the LVAD for three reasons. The first reason is the simple fact that the LVAD exists; the LVAD gave my family and me hope to endure while we waited for the heart. Secondly, the LVAD acted as a bridge until the doctors were able to find him a heart to replace his heart. Lastly and most important of all, the LVAD made his body strong enough to undergo the transplant operation.

Thank you to Dr Maybaum, Dr Naka, Dr Oz, the committee, the transplant group, and the staff who were there for us during the last few months every step of the way. You cannot imagine how nice and respectful everyone treated my family at Columbia Presbyterian Hospital. Columbia Presbyterian Hospital is a very special place.

**Joel L (born 1969)**

**Living with the MCSD**

Dr Deng, I am here writing you with my thoughts on my LVAD experience from February 12, 2002, to April 6, 2002. I liked it since the device did the job of keeping me alive until a donor heart could be found. But during the time the unit was in me, it was very painful, causing me to need large doses of morphine and sleeping pills to get some rest at night. The size of it also kept me from eating a normal amount of food during mealtimes. I lost 50–60 pounds while I was a patient at Columbia. I would take just a few bites, and not be able to stomach any more. Being a small-framed man with a small body, the size of the unit was big in comparison to the size of the area in my abdomen. Patients with larger body types may not experience this, since they have more room to place the device. The noise of the LVAD was a bit distracting and loud, but I don't think much could be done about that. You can't really expect a chainsaw to be quiet, I suppose. All in all, I'm happy that it was used and that I'm alive to tell you my thoughts on its time in me.

**Ted L
(born 1943)**

**Perspective of
gratefulness**

My name is Ted and on June 24, 2005, I received a heart transplant. It was a miracle from God and a gift of life from a very generous 51-year-old woman and her immediate family, who at a time of profound grief found it in their hearts to donate their loved one's organs. I was told by the hospital that seven lives were saved because of their generous offer.

I want to thank the Columbia Presbyterian Hospital's heart transplant team — the cardiologists, surgeons, nurses, and staff. They are terrific specialists and wonderful, caring people. Over the last 18 months, they have become my family and friends.

**Jacob,
age 9 years
(grandson of
Herbert E,
born 1930)**

**Post-MCSD**

**Trying to Fly**

Grandpa was sitting on a wooden patio chair, loafers on his feet. It was a sunny, breezy, hot day, the sun beating down from the baby blue sky. Beads of sweat danced down my face as I ran barefoot all the way across the lawn, all the way to Grandpa. I rested myself on Grandpa's lap, his face so close his breath tickled my ears. "Want to learn a lesson, Jakey?" Grandpa asked. All enthusiastically, I nodded my head, bouncing up and down, the only way a 4-year-old knows how to. So Grandpa said, "Everyone can fly in their own way ... everyone." Grandpa told me, for the very first time that day. I got all excited and flapped my arms, trying to fly.

Grandpa and I were sitting on a satiny blue couch, flipping through picture albums, the black-and-white torn pictures haphazardly collaged on each page. My 5-year-old hands delicately turned the yellowing pages of the album, knowing how much it meant to Grandpa. A brisk winter storm was whipping outside, but Grandpa and I were safe and warm by the fire. I sat close, resting my head on his clean white polo shirt, it smooth against my cheek. And then, while we were staring at those old pictures, the faces staring back, faces I vaguely knew, in that silence so precious, Grandpa said, "Everyone can fly in their own way ... everyone." Grandpa told me, his voice soothing and calm. At that moment, I started to wonder what Grandpa meant.

As I tiptoed up the polished wooden stairs, my socks slipping and sliding, I saw Grandpa sleeping peacefully, curled up like a ball, wearing red plaid boxers and a thin white undershirt. I crawled into the blue-and-white patterned covers, thumping down, waking him from his doze. When he first woke up, he looked startled. He smiled widely at me, his silver hair messy and knotted, and gave me a tight good morning hug. Grandpa took one look at my 6-year-old head and exclaimed, "The wolf has arrived!" gleaming at his own joke. Though I didn't say it, his hair was worse than mine. Gingerly, Grandpa patted down my hair, I ruffled his, and thus the hair war began. At the end, we always had a contest on whose hair was messier. Grandpa usually won, but I'm not too unhappy about that, for it is a contest for the worst looks. When we were lying in bed, hushed for a moment, Grandpa said, "Everyone can fly in their own way ... everyone." Grandpa told me. "What do you mean, Grandpa?" I asked. Grandpa told me that the meaning would come when the time was right.

Grandpa sat on the cushioned strawberry silk chair, a newspaper covering his face, the headlines screaming. The autumn leaves were thick and many on the backyard lawn, brilliant yellows, rich crimsons, and dazzling oranges. I was playing with an antique perfume bottle, and even though it was empty, the smell of lavender perfume wafted off my hands. Grandpa said, "Hey! Watcha doing with my perfume?!" We both laughed, his laugh louder and richer than anybody else's; mine just a 7-year-old laugh, nothing special. I secretly admired Grandpa's laugh. I went to sit by him, me on the arm of the chair, Grandpa in the middle. He looked down and smiled a sweet Grandpa smile. "Everyone can fly in their own way ... everyone." Grandpa told me, his voice blanketed with love and emotion. The time was not yet right. Little did I know the time would come soon.

Grandpa sat on the green booth, a blue shirt on, bright against the dreary day outside. My mouth tingled from the warmth of the hot chocolate. We chatted about what we wanted, the news, ourselves, our feelings … anything. The only Saturday morning I had ever imagined, chatting, sipping, nibbling, and being with Grandpa. Perfect. Grandpa called me over, ran his soft hands through my hair, and said, "Everyone can fly in their own way … everyone." Grandpa told me. At the tip of my tongue, the answer was there, but I couldn't grab hold of it. The questions kept coming, but were left unanswered.

Grandpa was lying on the hospital bed, starched white sheets gauntly laid over him. Tubes and wires snaked out of him and down to the floor. A worn look washed across his face, a sorrow-sweet smile. I stood up, went over to Grandpa, and sat by his side. Tightly, Grandpa gave me a hug, his arms cradled around me. At that moment, I never wanted to let go, feeling safe in Grandpa's arms. But I did let go, and when I did Grandpa said, "Everyone can fly in their own way … everyone." Grandpa told me, his voice a whisper. And at that very moment, it all made sense. Everything. All those years of wondering, and now it had finally come to me. "The right time is here, Jacob," Grandpa said to me. And on that day, I flew. I flew to the top of the world with Grandpa.

## Complementary Perspectives in Medicine

*High-Technology Modern Medicine and Humanism.*    The revolutionary concept of heart replacement, initially by biological heart transplantation and now by long-term MCSD implantation, is based on a mechanistic concept of human biology, similar to the concept of a motor exchange in a car. The scientific concept is based on the mechanistic scientific concepts of Newtonian/Descartian paradigms. They need to be reconceptualized within a framework of systems theory and humanistic medicine.

*Irreducibility of Complementary Perspectives.*    What is most important in the concept of differing perspectives of patients, relatives, and healthcare professionals — as outlined in this book — is that all these perspectives are complementary. They fit together, each one sharing in telling the story of every patient's experience. They are, in this complementarity, irreducible in their view and number: no one perspective can replace any other, nor can it be reduced to the perspective of any other. A physician report does not capture the patient's perception of the situation, for instance. The patient's account report does not — and of course should not attempt to — capture the details of the physician report (Moose, 2005).

***Consequences for Modern Medicine.*** This "shared perspectives" insight has important consequences for contemporary, modern, high-tech medicine. Healthcare professionals are basically aware of the complementary perceptions of all the people involved in healthcare situations, as captured so remarkably in our patients' and their relatives' vignettes. To this end, medical school and professional teaching and training must seek to implement strategies for healthcare professionals continuously developing this insight; achieving this teaching goal is essential to the claim of humanistic practice of modern medicine. It is a vision with stunning ramifications for the healing process. If this vision were to become routine in the daily care of our patients in all the societies of the world, several beneficial consequences could result:

1. An increased awareness would yield a strengthened perception of the differing roles of patients, relatives, and healthcare professionals in the recovery process — the role of healthcare professionals being that of "consultants", based on their expertise. The professionals would counsel patients and relatives about the different aspects of appropriate diagnostic and therapeutic options. The patient's role would explicitly be that of a person in charge of his/her own destiny, making the decisions for or against the specific options presented. Honoring the patient's preferences would implicitly assist in the healing process.
2. Based on this many-options aspect of high-tech modern medicine, the greater weight being placed on the patient's preferences might not necessarily coincide with the standard teachings of modern medicine textbooks. This respect for preferences would influence not only the patient's perspective of life, but also healthcare resource consumption itself: "more is not always better."

3. The complementary perceptions of human experience in general — and of illness in particular — confirm that a patient's suffering is not eliminated merely by the physician's perspective of scientific developments. Among all healthcare professionals, therefore, an even greater responsibility lies in being available for moments of listening, encouraging, and connecting with the patient as two individuals sharing their concerns. Maintaining eye contact and holding hands are not outdated in the world of contemporary high-tech modern medicine. They are a healing aspect that is more welcome and more powerful than ever before.

# SUMMARY

Heart failure is now acknowledged as the most common malignant disease in industrialized countries, with advanced heart failure having a worse prognosis than most forms of cancer (McMurray and Stewart, 2000). Transplantation provides the most effective therapy for this condition (Deng, 2002), but the shortage of donor organs results in less than 10% of potential recipients actually receiving a transplant. The ISHLT Registry reports that the 1-year posttransplant survival rate has remained below 80% over the past 5 years, with a 5-year survival rate of about 60% and thereafter a steady attrition rate of 4% per year (Hosenpud *et al.*, 2001). Furthermore, recent research suggests that the benefit from heart transplantation may be even lower than expected (Deng *et al.*, 2000).

Over the last two decades, MCSDs have been developed at a rapid pace with the goal of supporting patients with advanced heart failure as a bridge to cardiac transplantation (BTT), a bridge to recovery (BTR), or an alternative to transplantation (ATT). The current generation of devices provides a differentiated spectrum of circulatory support, ranging from short-term to intermediate and long-term duration. Also, partial left ventricular support, more complete left ventricular support, right ventricular support, and biventricular support options can be tailored to the hemodynamic needs of the patient. On a technical level, the device positions range from paracorporeal pumps and intracorporeal pumps with transcutaneous drivelines to completely implantable systems. The major current limitations are infection, coagulopathies, and device dysfunction. In this book, we present a state-of-the-art overview of the currently available MCSD options designed and capable of supporting blood circulation for 30 days or longer as well as future trends.

Since transplantation is able to meet less than 10% of the need for cardiac replacement therapy and xenografting is also unlikely to provide a clinical solution within the next 10 years, at present MCSD therapy provides the only practical alternative to heart transplantation. As a current landmark in generating scientific evidence for the benefit of MCSD therapy, the Randomized Evaluation of Mechanical Assistance for the Treatment of Congestive Heart Failure (REMATCH) trial has set standards. The REMATCH trial was a multicenter study supported by the National Heart, Lung, and Blood Institute to compare the long-term implantation of LVADs with OMM for patients with end-stage heart failure who require, but do not qualify to receive, cardiac transplantation. In the REMATCH trial, 129 patients with end-stage heart failure who were ineligible for cardiac transplantation received either an LVAD (68 patients) or OMM (61 patients). All of the patients had symptoms of New York Heart Association class IV heart failure. Kaplan–Meier survival analysis showed a 48% reduction in the risk of death from any cause in the group that received LVADs as compared with the medical therapy group. The authors concluded that the use of LVADs in patients with advanced heart failure results in a clinically meaningful survival benefit and an improved quality of life, and that LVADs could be an acceptable alternative therapy for selected patients who are not candidates for cardiac transplantation (Rose *et al.*, 2001). The REMATCH trial has created an enormous motivational uptrend for the other devices described above.

Challenges for the future development of MCSD technology result from the impact of MCSDs on the biology of the recipient (Frazier and Delgado, 2003). Advanced heart failure is associated with a systemic inflammatory response (Ankersmit *et al.*, 1999) that is interactive with MCSD therapy, compounding the already considerable challenges of recipient management. The preponderance of early complications (e.g. right heart failure, renal failure, stroke, respiratory infections) suggests the strong influence of patient selection and reflects preimplant morbidity. Major morbidity has been declining as centers have gained wider experience in recipient management, despite the enrollment of sicker patients (Deng *et al.*, 2001b). Infection rates, in particular driveline infection rates, are diminishing as a result of better prophylaxis and management of the exit site. The replacement of valved conduits for endocarditis has been straightforward, due to the modular design of the system. Design changes can have a major impact, as demonstrated by changing the inflow conduit to an uncrimped, integrally supported, and gelatin-coated graft, resulting in a 50% reduction in embolic complications (Portner *et al.*, 2001).

It has recently been demonstrated that MCSD patients can achieve a near-normal exercise response equivalent to that of patients with mild heart failure (Mancini *et al.*, 1998a). While the majority of MCSD applications have been as a bridge to transplant, a growing number of patients are now implanted with a view to the recovery of native left ventricular function. A recent single-center publication has demonstrated that as many as 24% of supported patients may recover sufficient ventricular function to allow weaning from the MCSD (Müller *et al.*, 1997). The process of reverse remodeling of the unloaded left ventricle is currently being studied in international multicenter trials.

In conclusion, patients, industry, and regulatory agencies have to reliably cooperate in order to generate sufficient evidence allowing continued societal resource allocation to this mode of modern medicine. The mechanisms of generating continued evidence may be different from the classical approaches used in drug-based interventions (Stevenson *et al.*, 2001; Deng, 2005).

# REFERENCES

Aaronson KD, Mancini DM. Mortality remains high for outpatient transplant candidates with prolonged (>6 months) waiting list time. *J Am Coll Cardiol* 1999;**33**:1189–95.

Aaronson KD, Patel H, Pagani FD. Patient selection for left ventricular assist device therapy. *Ann Thorac Surg* 2003;**75**(6 Suppl):S29–35.

Aaronson KD, Schwartz JS, Chen TM, *et al.* Development and prospective validation of a clinical index to predict survival in ambulatory patients referred for cardiac transplant evaluation. *Circulation* 1997;**95**:2660–7.

Acute Respiratory Distress Syndrome Network. Ventilation with lower tidal volumes as compared with traditional tidal volumes for acute lung injury and the acute respiratory distress syndrome. The Acute Respiratory Distress Syndrome Network. *N Engl J Med* 2000;**342**:1301–8.

Aleksic I, Baryalei MM, Schorn B, *et al.* Resection for CMV ileitis in a patient supported by a left-ventricular assist device. *Thorac Cardiovasc Surg* 1998;**46**:105–6.

Andrus S, Dubois J, Jansen C, *et al.* Teaching documentation tool: building a successful discharge. *Crit Care Nurse* 2003;**23**:39–48.

Angermann CE, Costard-Jaeckle A, Deng MC, for the EFICAT Investigators. Efficacy and safety of carvedilol in severe heart failure patients accepted for heart transplantation (abstr). *J Am Coll Cardiol* 2001;**37**(Suppl A):179A.

Anker SD, Ponikowski P, Varney S, *et al.* Wasting as independent risk factor for mortality in chronic heart failure. *Lancet* 1997;**349**:1050–3.

Ankersmit HJ, Tugulea S, Spanier T, *et al.* Activation-induced T-cell death and immune dysfunction after implantation of left-ventricular assist device. *Lancet* 1999;**354**:550–5.

Ankersmit HJ, Wieselthaler G, Moser B, *et al.* Transitory immunologic response after implantation of the DeBakey VAD continuous-axial-flow pump. *J Thorac Cardiovasc Surg* 2002;**123**:557–61.

Annane D, Bellissant E, Bollaert PE, *et al.* Corticosteroids for severe sepsis and septic shock: a systematic review and meta-analysis. *BMJ* 2004;**329**:480.

Aretz HT, Billingham ME, Edwards WD, *et al.* Myocarditis. A histopathologic definition and classification. *Am J Cardiovasc Pathol* 1987;**1**:3–14.

Argenziano M, Chen JM, Choudhri AF, *et al*. Management of vasodilatory shock after cardiac surgery: identification of predisposing factors and use of a novel pressor agent. *J Thorac Cardiovasc Surg* 1998;**116**:973–80.

Aronson S, Blumenthal R. Perioperative renal dysfunction and cardiovascular anesthesia: concerns and controversies. *J Cardiothorac Vasc Anesth* 1998;**12**:567–86.

Arrecubieta C, Asai T, Bayern M, *et al*. The role of Staphylococcus aureus adhesins in the pathogenesis of ventricular assist device-related infections. *J Infect Dis* 2006;**193**(8):1109–19.

Asai T, Baron HM, von Bayern MP, *et al*. A mouse aortic patch model for mechanical circulatory support. *J Heart Lung Transplant* 2005;**24**:1129–32.

Asai T, Lee M, Arrecubieta C, *et al*. Cellular coating of the left ventricular assist device textured polyurethane membrane reduces adherence of Staphylococcus aureus. *Thorac Cardiovasc Surg* (in press).

Athanasuleas CL, Buckberg GD, Stanley AW, *et al*.; RESTORE group. Surgical ventricular restoration in the treatment of congestive heart failure due to post-infarction ventricular dilation. *J Am Coll Cardiol* 2004;**44**:1439–45.

Athanasuleas CL, Stanley AW Jr, Buckberg GD, *et al*. Surgical anterior ventricular endocardial restoration (SAVER) in the dilated remodeled ventricle after anterior myocardial infarction. *J Am Coll Cardiol* 2001;**37**:1199–209.

AVID Investigators. A comparison of antiarrhythmic-drug therapy with implantable defibrillators in patients resuscitated from near-fatal ventricular arrhythmias. The Antiarrhythmics versus Implantable Defibrillators (AVID) Investigators. *N Engl J Med* 1997;**337**:1576–83.

Barbone A, Pini D, Grossi P, *et al*. Aspergillus left ventricular assist device endocarditis. *Ital Heart J* 2004;**5**:876–80.

Barbone A, Rao V, Oz MC, Naka Y. LVAD support in patients with bioprosthetic valves. *Ann Thorac Surg* 2002;**74**:232–4.

Bardy GH, Lee KL, Mark DB, *et al*.; Sudden Cardiac Death in Heart Failure Trial (SCD-HeFT) Investigators. Amiodarone or an implantable cardioverter-defibrillator for congestive heart failure. *N Engl J Med* 2005;**352**:225–37.

Basso K, Margolin A, Stolovitzky G, *et al*. Reverse engineering of regulatory networks in human B cells. *Nat Genet* 2005;**37**(4):382–90.

Baudouin SV, Evans TW. Nutritional support in critical care. *Clin Chest Med* 2003;**24**(4):633–44.

Bennett M, Horton S, *et al*. Pump-induced haemolysis: a comparison of short-term ventricular assist devices. *Perfusion* 2004;**19**(2):107–11.

Bernard GR, Vincent JL, Laterre PF, *et al*.; Recombinant Human Protein C Worldwide Evaluation in Severe Sepsis (PROWESS) Study Group. Efficacy and safety of recombinant human activated protein C for severe sepsis. *N Engl J Med* 2001;**344**:699–709.

Bigger JT Jr. Prophylactic use of implanted cardiac defibrillators in patients at high risk for ventricular arrhythmias after coronary-artery bypass graft surgery. Coronary Artery Bypass Graft (CABG) Patch Trial Investigators. *N Engl J Med* 1997;**337**:1569–75.

Birks EJ, Hall JL, Barton PJ, *et al.* Gene profiling changes in cytoskeletal proteins during clinical recovery after left ventricular-assist device support. *Circulation* 2005;**112**(9 Suppl):I57–64.

Bolling SF, Pagani FD, Deeb GM, Bach DS. Intermediate-term outcome of mitral reconstruction in cardiomyopathy. *Thorac Cardiovasc Surg* 1998;**115**:381–6.

Bonaros N, Mueller MR, Salat A, *et al.* Extensive coagulation monitoring in patients after implantation of the MicroMed DeBakey continuous flow axial pump. *ASAIO J* 2004;**50**:424–31.

Bonkohara Y, Minami K, Arusoglu L, *et al.* A fatal mechanical disorder of the TCI HeartMate left ventricular assist system. *J Thorac Cardiovasc Surg* 1999;**118**:769–70.

Bramstedt KA, Nash PJ. When death is the outcome of informed refusal: dilemma of rejecting ventricular assist device therapy. *J Heart Lung Transplant* 2005;**24**:229–30.

Brandt M, Koch MT, Steinhoff G, *et al.* Do long-term results justify bridging to heart transplantation in patients with multi-organ dysfunction? *Thorac Cardiovasc Surg* 1996;**44**:277–81.

Braunwald E (ed.). *Heart Disease. A Textbook of Cardiovascular Medicine* (4th ed.). Saunders, Philadelphia, 1992.

Bristow MR, Feldman AM, Saxon LA. Heart failure management using implantable devices for ventricular resynchronization: Comparison of Medical Therapy, Pacing, and Defibrillation in Chronic Heart Failure (COMPANION) trial. COMPANION Steering Committee and COMPANION Clinical Investigators. *J Card Fail* 2000;**6**:276–85.

Bristow MR, Saxon LA, Boehmer J, *et al.* Comparison of Medical Therapy, Pacing, and Defibrillation in Heart Failure (COMPANION) Investigators. Cardiac-resynchronization therapy with or without an implantable defibrillator in advanced chronic heart failure. *N Engl J Med* 2004;**350**:2140–50.

Bryant AS, Holman WL, Nanda NC, *et al.* Native aortic valve insufficiency in patients with left ventricular assist devices. *Ann Thorac Surg* 2006;**81**:e6–8.

Bunzel B, Laederach-Hofmann K, Wieselthaler GM, *et al.* Posttraumatic stress disorder after implantation of a mechanical assist device followed by heart transplantation: evaluation of patients and partners. *Transplant Proc* 2005;**37**:1365–8.

Butler J, Forman DE, Abraham WT, *et al.* Relationship between heart failure treatment and development of worsening renal function among hospitalized patients. *Am Heart J* 2004;**147**(2):331–8.

Butler J, Howser R, Portner PM, Pierson RN III. Body mass index and outcomes after left ventricular assist device placement. *Ann Thorac Surg* 2005; **79**(1): 66–73.

Buxton AE, Lee KL, Fisher JD, *et al.* A randomized study of the prevention of sudden death in patients with coronary artery disease. Multicenter Unsustained Tachycardia Trial Investigators. *N Engl J Med* 1999;**341**:1882–90.

Byers J, Sladen RN. Renal function and dysfunction. *Curr Opin Anaesthesiol* 2001;**14**:699–706.

Cadeiras M, Von Bayern MP, Pal A, *et al.* Destination therapy: an alternative for end-stage heart failure patients not eligible for heart transplantation. *Curr Opin Organ Transplant* 2005;**10**:369–75.

Califf RM, Adams KF, Mckenna WJ, *et al.* A randomized controlled trial of epoprostenol therapy for severe congestive heart failure: the Flolan International Randomized Survival Trial (FIRST). *Am Heart J* 1997;**134**:44–54.

Cappuccio FP. Commentary: epidemiological transition, migration, and cardiovascular disease. *Int J Epidemiol* 2004;**33**:387–8.

Cazeau S, Leclercq C, Lavergne T, *et al.*; Multisite Stimulation in Cardiomyopathies (MUSTIC) Study Investigators. Effects of multisite biventricular pacing in patients with heart failure and intraventricular conduction delay. *N Engl J Med* 2001;**344**:873–80.

Cengiz P, Seidel K, Rycus PT, *et al.* Central nervous system complications during pediatric extracorporeal life support: incidence and risk factors. *Crit Care Med* 2005;**33**:2817–24.

Cesario DA, Dec GW. Implantable cardioverter-defibrillator therapy in clinical practice. *J Am Coll Cardiol* 2006;**47**:1507–17.

Chen L, McCulloch AD, May-Newman K. Nonhomogeneous deformation in the anterior leaflet of the mitral valve. *Ann Biomed Eng* 2004;**32**:1599–606.

Chinn R, Dembitsky W, Eaton L, *et al.*; Multicenter experience: prevention and management of left ventricular assist device infections. *ASAIO J* 2005;**51**: 461–70.

Christensen E. Prognostic models including the Child–Pugh, MELD and Mayo risk scores — where are we and where should we go? *J Hepatol* 2004;**41**: 344–50.

CIBIS-II Study Group. The Cardiac Insufficiency Bisoprolol Study II (CIBIS-II): a randomised trial. *Lancet* 1999;**353**:9–13.

Cleland JG, Coletta AP, Lammiman M, *et al.* Clinical trials update from the European Society of Cardiology meeting 2005: CARE-HF extension study, ESSENTIAL, CIBIS-III, S-ICD, ISSUE-2, STRIDE-2, SOFA, IMAGINE, PREAMI, SIRIUS-II and ACTIVE. *Eur J Heart Fail* 2005;**7**:1070–5.

Cleland JG, Freemantle N, Coletta AP, Clark AL. Clinical trials update from the American Heart Association: REPAIR-AMI, ASTAMI, JELIS, MEGA, REVIVE-II, SURVIVE, and PROACTIVE. *Eur J Heart Fail* 2006;**8**:105–10.

Cohn JN, Goldstein SO, Greenberg BH, *et al.* A dose-dependent increase in mortality with vesnarinone among patients with severe heart failure. Vesnarinone Trial Investigators. *N Engl J Med* 1998;**339**:1810–6.

Cohn JN, Tognoni G, for the Valsartan Heart Failure Trial Investigators. A randomized trial of the angiotensin receptor blocker valsartan in chronic heart failure. *New Engl J Med* 2001;**345**:1667–75.

Consales G, De Gaudio AR. Sepsis associated encephalopathy. *Minerva Anestesiol* 2005;**71**:39–52.

Cooper DK, Keogh AM. The potential role of xenotransplantation in treating endstage cardiac disease: a summary of the report of the Xenotransplantation Advisory Committee of the International Society for Heart and Lung Transplantation. *Curr Opin Cardiol* 2001;**16**:105–9.

Cooper LT Jr. Giant cell myocarditis: diagnosis and treatment. *Herz* 2000;**25**: 291–8.

Cooper LT Jr., Berry GJ, Shabetai R. Idiopathic giant-cell myocarditis — natural history and treatment. Multicenter Giant Cell Myocarditis Study Group Investigators. *N Engl J Med* 1997;**336**:1860–6.

Copeland JG, Smith RG, Arabia FA, *et al.*; CardioWest Total Artificial Heart Investigators. Cardiac replacement with a total artificial heart as a bridge to transplantation. *N Engl J Med* 2004;**351**:859–67.

Copeland JG 3rd, Smith RG, Arabia FA, *et al.* Comparison of the CardioWest total artificial heart, the Novacor left ventricular assist system and the Thoratec ventricular assist system in bridge to transplantation. *Ann Thorac Surg* 2001;**71**(3 Suppl):S92–7.

Cowie MR, Wood DA, Coats AJ, *et al.* Survival of patients with a new diagnosis of heart failure: a population based study. *Heart* 2000;**83**:505–10.

Crespo Leiro MG, Paniagua Martin MJ. Management of advanced or refractory heart failure. *Rev Esp Cardiol* 2004;**57**:869–83.

Cuffe MS, Califf RM, Adams KF Jr., *et al.*; Outcomes of a Prospective Trial of Intravenous Milrinone for Exacerbations of Chronic Heart Failure (OPTIME-CHF) Investigators. Short-term intravenous milrinone for acute exacerbation of chronic heart failure: a randomized controlled trial. *JAMA* 2002;**287**: 1541–7.

D'Aiuto F, Casas JP, Shah T, *et al.* C-reactive protein (+1444C > T) polymorphism influences CRP response following a moderate inflammatory stimulus. *Atherosclerosis* 2005;**179**:413–7.

Dandel M, Weng Y, Siniawski H, *et al.* Long-term results in patients with idiopathic dilated cardiomyopathy after weaning from left ventricular assist devices. *Circulation* 2005;**112**(Suppl 9):I37–45.

Dang NC, Topkara VK, Kim BT, *et al.* Nutritional status in patients on left ventricular assist device support. *J Thorac Cardiovasc Surg* 2005; **130**:e3–4.

Dang NC, Topkara VK, Mercando M, *et al.* Right heart failure after left ventricular assist device implantation in patients with chronic congestive heart failure. *J Heart Lung Transplant* 2006;**25**:1–6.

DeBakey ME. Development of mechanical heart devices. *Ann Thorac Surg* 2005;**79**:S2228–31.

Dellinger RP, Carlet JM, Masur H, *et al.*; Surviving Sepsis Campaign Management Guidelines Committee. Surviving Sepsis Campaign guidelines for management of severe sepsis and septic shock. *Crit Care Med* 2004;**32**: 858–73.

Dembitsky WP, Tector AJ, Park S, *et al.* Left ventricular assist device performance with long-term circulatory support: lessons from the REMATCH trial. *Ann Thorac Surg* 2004;**78**:2123–9.

Deng MC. Cardiac transplantation. *Heart* 2002;**87**:177–84.

Deng MC. The challenges of generating evidence to guide mechanical circulatory support-based management of advanced heart failure (editorial). *Eur Heart J* 2005;**26**:953–5.

Deng MC, De Meester JMJ, Smits JMA, on behalf of COCPIT Study Group. The effect of receiving a heart transplant: analysis of a national cohort entered onto a waiting list, stratified by heart failure severity. *Br Med J* 2000;**321**:540–5.

Deng MC, Edwards LB, Hertz MI, *et al.* Mechanical Circulatory Support Device Database of the International Society for Heart and Lung Transplantation: second annual report — 2004. *J Heart Lung Transplant* 2004;**23**: 1027–34.

Deng MC, Edwards LB, Taylor DO, *et al.* Mechanical Circulatory Support Device Database of the International Society for Heart and Lung Transplantation: third annual report — 2005. *J Heart Lung Transplant* 2005a;**24**:1182–7.

Deng MC, Erren M, Tamminga N, *et al.* Left ventricular assist system support is associated with persistent inflammation and temporary immunosuppression. *Thorac Cardiovasc Surg* 1999a;**47**(Suppl):326–31.

Deng MC, Loebe M, El-Banayosi A, *et al.* Mechanical circulatory support for advanced heart failure: effect of patient selection on outcome. *Circulation* 2001a;**103**:231–7.

Deng MC, Mehra MC, Eisen HJ, *et al.* Cardiac allograft monitoring using a novel clinical algorithm based on peripheral leukocyte gene expression profiling (abstr). *Circulation* 2003a;**108**:IV–398.

Deng MC, Naka Y. Circulatory support in advanced heart failure. *Cardiol Rev* 2002;**19**:28–35.

Deng MC, Ranjit J, Baron H, *et al.* Transplantation immunology. In: Compston J, Shane E (eds.). *Bone Disease of Organ Transplantation.* Elsevier Academic Press, San Diego, 2005b, pp. 3–29.

Deng MC, Smits JMA, De Meester J, *et al.* Heart transplantation is indicated only in the most severely ill patient: perspectives from the German heart transplant experience. *Curr Opin Cardiol* 2001b;**16**:97–104.

Deng MC, Smits JMA, Packer M. Selecting patients for heart transplantation: which patients are too well for transplant? *Curr Opin Cardiol* 2002;**17**: 137–44.

Deng MC, Smits JMA, Young JB. Proposition: the benefit of cardiac transplantation in stable outpatients with heart failure should be tested in a randomized trial. *J Heart Lung Transplant* 2003b;**22**:113–7.

Deng MC, Tjan TD, Asfour B, *et al.* Combining nonpharmacologic therapies for advanced heart failure: the Münster experience with the assist device-defibrillator combination. *Am J Cardiol* 1999b;**83**:158D–60D.

Deng MC, Wilhelm M, Weyand M, *et al.* Long-term left ventricular assist device support: a novel pump rate challenge exercise protocol to monitor native left ventricular function. *J Heart Lung Transplant* 1997;**16**:629–35.

Deng MC, Wilhelm MJ, Scheld HH. Effects of exercise during long-term support with a left ventricular assist device (letter). *Circulation* 1998;**97**: 1212–3.

Deng MC, Young JB, Stevenson LW, *et al.*; Board of Directors of the International Society for Heart and Lung Transplantation. Destination mechanical circulatory support: proposal for clinical standards. *J Heart Lung Transplant* 2003c;**22**:365–9.

DeNofrio D, Rho R, Morales FJ, *et al.* Detection of anti-HLA antibody by flow cytometry in patients with a left ventricular assist device is associated with early rejection following heart transplantation. *Transplantation* 2000;**69**: 814–8.

Dew MA, Kormos RL, DiMartini AF. Prevalence and risk of depression and anxiety-related disorders during the first three years after heart transplantation. *Psychosomatics* 2001a;**42**:300–13.

Dew MA, Kormos RL, Winowich S, *et al.* Quality of life outcomes in left ventricular assist system inpatients and outpatients. *ASAIO J* 1999;**45**: 218–25.

Dew MA, Kormos RL, Winowich S, *et al.* Quality of life outcomes after heart transplantation in individuals bridged to transplant with ventricular assist devices. *J Heart Lung Transplant* 2001b;**20**:1199–212.

Di Carli MF, Asgarzadie F, Schelbert HR, *et al.* Quantitative relation between myocardial viability and improvement in heart failure symptoms after revascularization in patients with ischemic cardiomyopathy. *Circulation* 1995;**92**: 3436–44.

Digiorgi PL, Reel MS, Thornton B, *et al.* Heart transplant and left ventricular assist device costs. *J Heart Lung Transplant* 2005;**24**:200–4.

DiNardo MM, Korytkowski MT, Siminerio LS. The importance of normoglycemia in critically ill patients. *Crit Care Nurs Q* 2004;**27**:126–34.

Doval HC, Nul DR, Grancelli HO, *et al.* Randomised trial of low-dose amiodarone in severe congestive heart failure. *Lancet* 1994;**344**:493–8.

Dowling RD, Gray LA Jr, Etoch SW, *et al.* Initial experience with the Abio-Cor implantable replacement heart system. *J Thorac Cardiovasc Surg* 2004; **127**:131–41.

Dreyfus G, Duboc D, Blasco A, *et al.* Coronary surgery can be an alternative to heart transplantation in selected patients with end-stage ischemic heart disease. *Eur J Cardiothorac Surg* 1993;**7**:482–8.

Edwards NM, Prager KM. Nothing is fair or good alone. *J Thorac Cardiovasc Surg* 2003;**125**:23–4.

El Oakley RM, Ooi OC, Bongso A, Yacoub MH. Myocyte transplantation for myocardial repair: a few good cells can mend a broken heart. *Ann Thorac Surg* 2001;**71**:1724–33.

El-Amir NG, Gardocki M, Levin HR, *et al.* Gastrointestinal consequences of left ventricular assist device placement. *ASAIO J* 1996;**42**:150–3.

El-Banayosy A, Arusoglu L, Kizner L, *et al.* Novacor left ventricular assist system versus HeartMate vented electric left ventricular assist system as a long-term mechanical circulatory support device in bridging patients: a prospective study. *J Thorac Cardiovasc Surg* 2000;**119**:581–7.

El-Banayosy A, Arusoglu L, Kizner L, *et al.* Preliminary experience with the LionHeart left ventricular assist device in patients with end-stage heart failure. *Ann Thorac Surg* 2003;**75**:1469–75.

El-Banayosy A, Fey O, Sarnowski P, *et al.* Midterm follow-up of patients discharged from hospital under left ventricular assistance. *J Heart Lung Transplant* 2001;**20**:53–8.

Elefteriades JA, Tolis G, Levi E, *et al.* Coronary artery bypass grafting in severe left ventricular dysfunction: excellent survival and improved EF and functional state. *J Am Coll Cardiol* 1993;**22**:1411–7.

Ely EW, Laterre PF, Angus DC, *et al.*; PROWESS Investigators. Drotrecogin alfa (activated) administration across clinically important subgroups of patients with severe sepsis. *Crit Care Med* 2003;**31**:12–9.

Etzion S, Battler A, Barbash IM, *et al.* Influence of embryonic cardiomyocyte transplantation on the progression of heart failure in a rat model of extensive myocardial infarction. *J Mol Cell Cardiol* 2001;**33**:1321–30.

Federal Register. April 2, 1998;**63**:16296.

Feldman AM, Bristow MR, Parmley WW, *et al.* Effects of vesnarinone on morbidity and mortality in patients with heart failure. Vesnarinone Study Group. *N Engl J Med* 1993;**329**:149–55.

Felker GM, Rogers JG. Same bridge, new destinations: rethinking paradigms for mechanical cardiac support in heart failure. *J Am Coll Cardiol* 2006;**47**:930–2.

Ferns J, Dowling R, Bhat G. Evaluation of a patient with left ventricular assist device dysfunction. *ASAIO J* 2001;**47**:696–8.

Fonarow GC, Stevenson LW, Walden JA, *et al.* Impact of a comprehensive heart failure management program on hospital readmission and functional status of patients with advanced heart failure. *J Am Coll Cardiol* 1997;**30**:725–32.

Frazier OH. Mechanical circulatory support: new advances, new pumps, new ideas. *Semin Thorac Cardiovasc Surg* 2002;**14**:178–86.

Frazier OH, Delgado RM. Mechanical circulatory support for advanced heart failure: where does it stand in 2003? *Circulation* 2003;**108**:3064–8.

Frazier OH, Delgado RM 3rd, Scroggins N, *et al.* Mechanical bridging to improvement in severe acute "nonischemic, nonmyocarditis" heart failure. *Congest Heart Fail* 2004a;**10**:109–13.

Frazier OH, Dowling RD, Gray LA Jr, *et al.* The total artificial heart: where we stand. *Cardiology* 2004b;**101**:117–21.

Frazier OH, Kirklin JK (eds.). *Mechanical Circulatory Support* (ISHLT Monograph Series, Vol. 1). Elsevier, Philadelphia, 2006.

Frazier OH, Rose EA, Oz MC, *et al.*; HeartMate LVAS Investigators. Multicenter clinical evaluation of the HeartMate vented electric left ventricular assist system in patients awaiting heart transplantation. *J Thorac Cardiovasc Surg* 2001;**122**:1186–95.

Frigerio M, Gronda EG, Mangiavacchi M, *et al.* Restrictive criteria for heart transplantation candidacy maximize survival of patients with advanced heart failure. *J Heart Lung Transplant* 1997;**16**:160–8.

Fukamachi K, McCarthy PM, Smedira NG, *et al.* Preoperative risk factors for right ventricular failure after implantable left ventricular assist device insertion. *Ann Thorac Surg* 1999;**68**:2181–4.

Gelijns AC, Richards AF, Williams DL, *et al.* Evolving costs of long-term left ventricular assist device implantation. *Ann Thorac Surg* 1997;**64**:1312–9.

Gibbons RD, Meltzer D, Duan N, and other members of the Institute of Medicine Committee on Organ Procurement and Transplantation. Waiting for organ transplantation. *Science* 2000;**287**:237–8.

Golding LAR, El-Banayosy A, Kormos RL, *et al.* Emerging left ventricular assist devices. In: Frazier OH, Kirklin JK (eds.). *Mechanical Circulatory Support* (ISHLT Monograph Series, Vol. 1). Elsevier, Philadelphia, 2006, pp. 205–18.

Goldstein D, Oz MC (eds.). *Cardiac Assist Devices.* Futura Publishing, New York, 2000.

Goldstein DJ, Moazami N, Seldomridge JA, *et al.* Circulatory resuscitation with left ventricular assist device support reduces interleukins 6 and 8 levels. *Ann Thorac Surg* 1997;**63**:971–4.

Goldstein DJ, Zucker M, Arroyo L, *et al.* Safety and feasibility trial of the MicroMed DeBakey ventricular assist device as a bridge to transplantation. *J Am Coll Cardiol* 2005;**45**:962–3.

Gordon D, Shore E. University of Pennsylvania VAD/Heart Transplantation Psychosocial Evaluation Tool. 2000.

Gordon RJ, Quagliarello B, Lowy FD. Ventricular assist device-related infections. *Lancet Infect Dis* 2006;**6**:426–37.

Gordon SM, Schmitt SK, Jacobs M, *et al.* Nosocomial bloodstream infections in patients with implantable left ventricular assist devices. *Ann Thorac Surg* 2001;**72**:725–30.

Grady KL, Jalowiec A, White-Williams C. Improvement in quality of life in patients with heart failure who undergo transplantation. *J Heart Lung Transplant* 1996;**15**:749–57.

Grady KL, Jalowiec A, White-Williams C. Quality of life 6 months after heart transplantation compared with indicators of illness severity before transplantation. *Am J Crit Care* 1998;**7**:106–16.

Grady KL, Meyer P, Mattea A, *et al.* Predictors of quality of life at 1 month after implantation of a left ventricular assist device. *Am J Crit Care* 2002;**11**: 345–52.

Grady KL, Meyer PM, Dressler D, *et al.* Longitudinal change in quality of life and impact on survival after left ventricular assist device implantation. *Ann Thorac Surg* 2004;**77**:1321–7.

Grady KL, Meyer PM, Mattea A, *et al.* Change in quality of life from before to after discharge following left ventricular assist device implantation. *J Heart Lung Transplant* 2003;**22**:322–33.

Granfeldt H, Koul B, Wiklund L, *et al.* Risk factor analysis of Swedish left ventricular assist device (LVAD) patients. *Ann Thorac Surg* 2003;**76**: 1993–8.

Gwechenberger M, Hülsmann M, Berger R, *et al.* Interleukin-6 and B-type natriuretic peptide are independent predictors for worsening of heart failure in patients with progressive congestive heart failure. *J Heart Lung Transplant* 2004;**23**:839–44.

Hammel D, Tjan DT, Scheld HH, *et al.* Successful treatment of a Novacor LVAD malfunction without repeat sternotomy. *Thorac Cardiovasc Surg* 1998;**46**: 154–6.

Hammer C. Xenotransplantation: perspectives and limits. *Blood Purif* 2001;**19**: 322–8.

Hampton JR, van Veldhuisen DJ, Kleber FX, *et al.* Randomised study of effect of ibopamine on survival in patients with advanced severe heart failure. Second Prospective Randomised Study of Ibopamine on Mortality and Efficacy (PRIME II) Investigators. *Lancet* 1997;**349**:971–7.

Hasper D, Hummel M, Kleber FX, *et al.* Systemic inflammation in patients with heart failure. *Eur Heart J* 1998;**19**:761–5.

Hauptman PJ, Havranek EP. Integrating palliative care into heart failure care. *Arch Intern Med* 2005;**165**:374–8.

Hausmann H, Topp H, Siniawski H, *et al.* Decision-making in end-stage coronary artery disease: revascularization or heart transplantation? *Ann Thor Surg* 1997;**64**:1296–302.

Helman DN, Maybaum SW, Morales DL, *et al.* Recurrent remodeling after ventricular assistance: is long-term myocardial recovery attainable? *Ann Thorac Surg* 2000;**70**:1255–8.

Henger A, Kretzler M, Doran P. Gene expression fingerprints in human tubulo-interstitial inflammation and fibrosis as prognostic markers of disease progression. *Kidney Int* 2004;**65**:904–17.

Hermann M, Weyand M, Greshake B, *et al.* Left ventricular assist device infection is associated with increased mortality but is not a contraindication to transplantation. *Circulation* 1997;**95**:814–7.

Hernandez AF, Grab J, Gammie JS, *et al.* A decade of acute outcomes in post cardiac surgery ventricular assist device implantation: data from the Society of Thoracic Surgeons' National Cardiac Database. *Circulation* (in press).

Hetzer R, Muller J, Weng Y, *et al.* Cardiac recovery in dilated cardiomyopathy by unloading with a left ventricular assist device. *Ann Thorac Surg* 1999;**68**: 742–9.

Hetzer R, Muller JH, Weng Y, *et al.* Bridging-to-recovery. *Ann Thorac Surg* 2001;**71**(3 Suppl):S109–13.

Hetzer R, Muller JH, Weng YG, *et al.* Midterm follow-up of patients who underwent removal of a left ventricular assist device after cardiac recovery from end-stage dilated cardiomyopathy. *J Thorac Cardiovasc Surg* 2000;**120**: 843–55.

Hetzer R, Weng Y, Potapov EV, *et al.* First experiences with a novel magnetically suspended axial flow left ventricular assist device. *Eur J Cardiothorac Surg* 2004;**25**:964–70.

Hogness JR, VanAntwerp M (eds.). The artificial heart program. In: *The Artificial Heart: Prototypes, Policies, and Patients*. National Academy Press, Washington, 1991, pp. 14–25.

Hohnloser SH, Kuck KH, Dorian P, *et al.* Prophylactic use of an implantable cardioverter-defibrillator after acute myocardial infarction. *N Engl J Med* 2004;**351**:2481–8.

Holman WL, Bourge RC, Fan P, *et al.* Influence of longer term left ventricular assist device support on valvular regurgitation. *ASAIO J* 1994;**40**:M454–9.

Holman WL, Bourge RC, Murrah CP, *et al.* Left atrial or ventricular cannulation beyond 30 days for a Thoratec ventricular assist device. *ASAIO J* 1995;**41**:M517–22.

Holman WL, Davies JE, Rayburn BK, *et al.* Treatment of end-stage heart disease with outpatient ventricular assist devices. *Ann Thorac Surg* 2002;**73**:1489–93.

Holman WL, Fix RJ, Foley BA, *et al.* Management of wound and left ventricular assist device pocket infection. *Ann Thorac Surg* 1999;**68**:1080–2.

Holman WL, Park SJ, Long JW, *et al.*; REMATCH Investigators. Infection in permanent circulatory support: experience from the REMATCH trial. *J Heart Lung Transplant* 2004;**23**:1359–65.

Horton SC, Khodaverdian R, Chatelain P, *et al.* Left ventricular assist device malfunction: an approach to diagnosis by echocardiography. *J Am Coll Cardiol* 2005;**45**:1435–40.

Hosenpud JD, Bennett LE, Keck BM, *et al.* The Registry of the International Society for Heart and Lung Transplantation: sixteenth official report — 1999. *J Heart Lung Transplant* 1999;**18**:611–26.

Hosenpud JD, Bennett LE, Keck BM, *et al.* The Registry of the International Society for Heart and Lung Transplantation: eighteenth official report — 2001. *J Heart Lung Transplant* 2001;**20**:805–15.

Hotz H, Linneweber J, Dohmen PM, *et al.* Bridge-to-recovery from acute myocarditis in a 12-year-old child. *Artif Organs* 2004;**28**:587–9.

Houel R, Mazoyer E, Boval B, *et al.* Platelet activation and aggregation profile in prolonged external ventricular support. *J Thorac Cardiovasc Surg* 2004;**128**:197–202.

Houel R, Moczar M, Ginat M, Loisance D. Pseudointima in inflow and outflow conduits of a left ventricular assist system: possible role in clinical outcome. *ASAIO J* 2001;**47**:275–81.

Hunt SA. A fair way of donating hearts for transplantation. *BMJ* 2000; **321**:526.

Hunt SA, Abraham WT, Chin MH, *et al.* American College of Cardiology; American Heart Association Task Force on Practice Guidelines; American College of Chest Physicians; International Society for Heart and Lung Transplantation; Heart Rhythm Society. ACC/AHA 2005 guideline update for the diagnosis and management of chronic heart failure in the adult. *Circulation* 2005;**112**: e154–235.

Hunt SA, Baker DW, Chin MH, *et al.*; American College of Cardiology/American Heart Association. ACC/AHA guidelines for the evaluation and management of chronic heart failure in the adult: executive summary. A report of the American College of Cardiology/American Heart Association Task Force on Practice Guidelines (Committee to Revise the 1995 Guidelines for the Evaluation and Management of Heart Failure). *J Am Coll Cardiol* 2001;**38**: 2101–13.

Hunt SA, Rider AK, Stinson EB, *et al.* Does cardiac transplantation prolong life and improve its quality? An updated report. *Circulation* 1976;**54**(Suppl III):56–60.

Hutcheson KA, Atkins BZ, Hueman MT, *et al.* Comparison of benefits on myocardial performance of cellular cardiomyoplasty with skeletal myoblasts and fibroblasts. *Cell Transplant* 2000;**9**:359–68.

Itescu S, John R. Interactions between the recipient immune system and the left ventricular assist device surface: immunological and clinical implications. *Ann Thorac Surg* 2003;**75**:S58–65.

Jaski BE, Kim JC, Naftel DC, *et al.*; Cardiac Transplant Research Database Research Group. Cardiac transplant outcome of patients supported on left ventricular assist device vs. intravenous inotropic therapy. *J Heart Lung Transplant* 2001;**20**:449–56.

John R, Lietz K, Burke E, *et al.* Intravenous immunoglobulin reduces anti-HLA alloreactivity and shortens waiting time to cardiac transplantation in highly sensitized left ventricular assist device recipients. *Circulation* 1999;**100**(19 Suppl):II229–35.

Johnson KE, Prieto M, Joyce LD, *et al.* Summary of the clinical use of the Symbion total artificial heart: a registry report. *J Heart Lung Transplant* 1992;**11** (1 Pt 1):103–16.

Joyce D, Loebe M, Noon GP, *et al.* Revascularization and ventricular restoration in patients with ischemic heart failure: the STICH trial. *Curr Opin Cardiol* 2003;**18**:454–7.

Jurmann MJ, Weng Y, Drews T, *et al.* Permanent mechanical circulatory support in patients of advanced age. *Eur J Cardiothorac Surg* 2004;**25**:610–8.

Kalya AV, Tector AJ, Crouch JD, *et al.* Comparison of Novacor and HeartMate vented electric left ventricular assist devices in a single institution. *J Heart Lung Transplant* 2005;**24**:1973–5.

Kao W, McGee D, Liao Y, *et al.* Does heart transplantation confer additional benefit over medical therapy to patients who have waited >6 months for heart transplantation? *J Am Coll Cardiol* 1994;**24**:1547–51.

Katsumata T, Westaby S. Implantable axial flow impeller pumps. *J Circ Support* 1998;**1**:13–9.

Khan T, Delgado RM, Radovancevic B, *et al.* Dobutamine stress echocardiography predicts myocardial improvement in patients supported by left ventricular assist devices (LVADs): hemodynamic and histologic evidence of improvement before LVAD explantation. *J Heart Lung Transplant* 2003;**22**:137–46.

Kihara S, Kawai A, Fukuda T, *et al.* Effects of milrinone for right ventricular failure after left ventricular assist device implantation. *Heart Vessels* 2002;**16**:69–71.

Kirklin JK. The importance of the Mechanical Circulatory Support Database. A plea for commitment. *J Heart Lung Transplant* 2001;**20**:803–4.

Kirklin JK. Developmental history of mechanical circulatory support. In: Frazier OH, Kirklin JK (eds.). *Mechanical Circulatory Support* (ISHLT Monograph Series, Vol. 1). Elsevier, Philadelphia, 2006, pp. 1–8.

Kirklin JK, Holman WL. Mechanical circulatory support therapy as a bridge to transplant or recovery (new advances). *Curr Opin Cardiol* 2006;**21**:120–6.

Kirklin JW, Barratt-Boyes BG. *Cardiac Surgery* (2nd ed.). Churchill-Livingstone, New York, 1992.

Klotz S, Deng MC, Stypmann J, *et al.* Left ventricular pressure and volume unloading during pulsatile versus nonpulsatile left ventricular assist device support. *Ann Thorac Surg* 2004;**77**:143–9; discussion 149–50.

Klotz S, Stypmann J, Welp H, *et al.* Does continuous flow left ventricular assist device technology have a positive impact on outcome pretransplant and post-transplant? *Ann Thorac Surg* 2006;**82**:1774–8.

Kocher AA, Schuster MD, Szabolcs MJ, *et al.* Neovascularization of ischemic myocardium by human bone-marrow–derived angioblasts prevents cardiomyocyte apoptosis, reduces remodeling and improves cardiac function. *Nat Med* 2001;**7**:430–6.

Koelling TM, Joseph S, Aaronson KD. Heart failure survival score continues to predict clinical outcomes in patients with heart failure receiving beta-blockers. *J Heart Lung Transplant* 2004;**23**:1414–22.

Koster A, Loebe M, Hansen R, *et al.* Alterations in coagulation after implantation of a pulsatile Novacor LVAD and the axial flow MicroMed DeBakey LVAD. *Ann Thorac Surg* 2000;**70**:533–7.

Kress JP, Pohlman AS, O'Connor MF, Hall JB. Daily interruption of sedative infusions in critically ill patients undergoing mechanical ventilation. *N Engl J Med* 2000;**342**:1471–7.

Kron IL, Flanagan TL, Blackbourne LH, *et al.* Coronary revascularization rather than cardiac transplantation for chronic ischemic cardiomyopathy. *Ann Surg* 1989;**210**:348–54.

Kucuker SA, Stetson SJ, Becker KA, *et al.* Evidence of improved right ventricular structure after LVAD support in patients with end-stage cardiomyopathy. *J Heart Lung Transplant* 2004;**23**(1):28–35.

Landry DW, Oliver JA. The pathogenesis of vasodilatory shock. *N Engl J Med* 2001;**345**:588–95.

Lansman SL, Cohen M, Galla JD, *et al.* Coronary bypass with ejection fraction of 0.20 or less using centigrade cardioplegia: long-term follow-up. *Ann Thorac Surg* 1993;**56**:480–6.

Lazar RM, Shapiro PA, Jaski BE, *et al.* Neurological events during long-term mechanical circulatory support for heart failure: the Randomized Evaluation of Mechanical Assistance for the Treatment of Congestive Heart Failure (REMATCH) experience. *Circulation* 2004;**109**:2423–7.

Leor J, Aboulafia-Etzion S, Dar A, *et al.* Bioengineered cardiac grafts: a new approach to repair the infarcted myocardium? *Circulation* 2000;**102**(19 Suppl 3):III56–61.

Leprince P, Combes A, Bonnet N, *et al.* Circulatory support for fulminant myocarditis: consideration for implantation, weaning and explantation. *Eur J Cardiothorac Surg* 2003;**24**:399–403.

Levine TB, Levine AB, Goldberg AD, *et al.* Clinical status of patients removed from a transplant waiting list rivals that of transplant recipients at significant cost savings. *Am Heart J* 1996;**132**:1189–94.

Levy D, Kenchaiah S, Larson MG, *et al.* Long-term trends in the incidence of and survival with heart failure. *N Engl J Med* 2002;**347**:1397–402.

Liang H, Lin H, Weng Y, *et al.* Prediction of cardiac function after weaning from ventricular assist devices. *J Thorac Cardiovasc Surg* 2005;**130**:1555–60.

Liaw PC, Esmon CT, Kahnamoui K, *et al.* Patients with severe sepsis vary markedly in their ability to generate activated protein C. *Blood* 2004;**104**:3958–64.

Lietz K, Miller LW. Will left-ventricular assist device therapy replace heart transplantation in the foreseeable future? *Curr Opin Cardiol* 2005;**20**:132–7.

Lowes BD, Shakar SF, Metra M, *et al.* Rationale and design of the enoximone clinical trials program. *J Card Fail* 2005;**11**:659–69.

Lucas C, Johnson W, Hamilton MA, *et al.* Freedom from congestion predicts good survival despite previous class IV symptoms of heart failure. *Am Heart J* 2000;**140**:824–6.

Luckraz H, Woods M, Large SR; Papworth VAD Group. And hemolysis goes on: ventricular assist device in combination with veno-venous hemofiltration. *Ann Thorac Surg* 2002;**73**:546–8.

MacDonald PS, Keogh A, Mundy J. Adjunctive use of inhaled nitric oxide during implantation of left ventricular assist device. *J Heart Lung Transplant* 1998;**17**:312–6.

Malay MB, Ashton JL, Dahl K, *et al.* Heterogeneity of the vasoconstrictor effect of vasopressin in septic shock. *Crit Care Med* 2004;**32**:1327–31.

Mancini D, Goldsmith R, Levin H, *et al.* Comparison of exercise performance in patients with chronic severe heart failure versus left ventricular assist devices. *Circulation* 1998a;**98**:1178–83.

Mancini DM, Beniaminovitz A, Levin H, *et al.* Low incidence of myocardial recovery after left ventricular assist device implantation in patients with chronic heart failure. *Circulation* 1998b;**98**:2383–9.

Mancini DM, Eisen H, Kussmaul W, *et al.* Value of peak exercise oxygen consumption for optimal timing of cardiac transplantation in ambulatory patients with heart failure. *Circulation* 1991;**83**:778–86.

Mangano DT, Tudor IC, Dietzel C; Multicenter Study of Perioperative Ischemia Research Group; Ischemia Research and Education Foundation. The risk associated with aprotinin in cardiac surgery. *N Engl J Med* 2006;**354**:353–65.

Mangi AA, Christison-Lagay ER, Torchiana DF, *et al.* Gastrointestinal complications in patients undergoing heart operation: an analysis of 8709 consecutive cardiac surgical patients. *Ann Surg* 2005;**241**:895–901.

Marzo KP, Wilson JR, Mancini DM. Effects of cardiac transplantation on ventilatory response to exercise. *Am J Cardiol* 1992;**69**:547–553.

O'Neill AJ, Doyle BT, Molloy E, *et al.* Gene expression profile of inflammatory neutrophils: alterations in the inhibitors of apoptosis proteins during spontaneous and delayed apoptosis. *Shock* 2004;**21**:51–8.

Ochiai Y, McCarthy PM, Smedira NG, *et al.* Predictors of severe right ventricular failure after implantable left ventricular assist device insertion: analysis of 245 patients. *Circulation* 2002;**106**(12 Suppl 1):I198–202.

Olman MA, White KE, Ware LB, *et al.* Pulmonary edema fluid from patients with early lung injury stimulates fibroblast proliferation through IL-1 beta-induced IL-6 expression. *J Immunol* 2004;**172**:2668–77.

Olson PS, Kassis E, Niebuhr-Jorgensen U. Coronary artery bypass surgery in patients with severe left ventricular dysfunction. *Thorac Cardiovasc Surg* 1993;**41**:118–20.

Orlic D, Kajstura J, Chimenti S, *et al.* Bone marrow cells regenerate infarcted myocardium. *Nature* 2001;**410**:701–5.

Ostermann ME, Chang RW; Riyadh ICU Program Users Group. Prognosis of acute renal failure: an evaluation of proposed consensus criteria. *Intensive Care Med* 2005;**31**:250–6.

Oz MC, Gelijns AC, Miller L, *et al.* Left ventricular assist devices as permanent heart failure therapy: the price of progress. *Ann Surg* 2003;**238**:577–83.

Oz MC, Goldstein DJ, Pepino P, *et al.* Screening scale predicts patients successfully receiving long-term implantable left ventricular assist devices. *Circulation* 1995;**92**(9 Suppl):II169–73.

Oz MC, Rose EA, Slater J, *et al.* Malignant ventricular arrhythmias are well tolerated in patients receiving long-term left ventricular assist devices. *J Am Coll Cardiol* 1994;**24**:1688–91.

Pachot A, Monneret G, Brion A, *et al.* Messenger RNA expression of major histocompatibility complex class II genes in whole blood from septic shock patients. *Int Care Med* 2005;**33**:31–8.

Packer M, Abraham W, for the MIRACLE Trial. Effect of cardiac resynchronization on a composite clinical status endpoint in patients with chronic heart failure: results of the MIRACLE trial (abstr). *J Card Fail* 2001;**17**(Suppl 2):53.

Packer M, Carver JR, Rodeheffer RJ, *et al.* Effect of oral milrinone on mortality in severe chronic heart failure. The PROMISE Study Research Group. *N Engl J Med* 1991;**325**:1468–75.

Packer M, Coats AJ, Fowler MB, *et al.*; Carvedilol Prospective Randomized Cumulative Survival Study Group. Effect of carvedilol on survival in severe chronic heart failure. *N Engl J Med* 2001;**344**:1651–8.

Pae WE, Pierce WS. Combined registry for the clinical use of mechanical ventricular assist pumps and the total artificial heart. *J Heart Transplant* 1986;**5**:6–7.

Pae WE Jr, Kormos RL, Greene PS, Sapirstein W. Database: relevant or not. *Ann Thorac Surg* 2001;**71**:S204–9.

Park MH, Goudreau E, Tolman DE, *et al.* Fluoroscopy and selective angiography of left ventricular assist system inflow cannula as a method of detecting cannula entrapment. *Cathet Cardiovasc Diagn* 1998;**44**:47–51.

Park SJ, Liao KK, Segurola R, *et al.* Management of aortic insufficiency in patients with left ventricular assist devices: a simple coaptation stitch method (Park's stitch). *J Thorac Cardiovasc Surg* 2004;**127**:264–6.

Park SJ, Tector A, Piccioni W, *et al.* Left ventricular assist devices as destination therapy: a new look at survival. *J Thorac Cardiovasc Surg* 2005;**129**:9–17.

Parker RA, Himmelfarb J, Tolkoff-Rubin N, *et al.* Prognosis of patients with acute renal failure requiring dialysis: results of a multicenter study. *Am J Kidney Dis* 1998;**32**:432–43.

Philbin EF. Comprehensive multidisciplinary programs for the management of patients with congestive heart failure. *J Gen Intern Med* 1999;**14**:130–5.

Pitt B, Zannad F, Remme WJ, *et al.* The effect of spironolactone on morbidity and mortality in patients with severe heart failure. Randomized Aldactone Evaluation Study Investigators. *N Engl J Med* 1999;**341**:709–17.

Plenz G, Baba HA, Erren M, *et al.* Reversal of myocardial interleukin-6-mRNA expression following long-term left ventricular assist device support for myocarditis-associated low output syndrome (letter). *J Heart Lung Transplant* 1999;**18**:923–4.

Poirier V. Worldwide experience with the TCI HeartMate system: issues and future perspective. *Thorac Cardiovasc Surg* 1999;**47**(Suppl 2):316–20.

Poole-Wilson PA, Swedberg K, Cleland JG, *et al.*; Carvedilol or Metoprolol European Trial Investigators. Comparison of carvedilol and metoprolol on clinical outcomes in patients with chronic heart failure in the Carvedilol or Metoprolol European Trial (COMET): randomised controlled trial. *Lancet* 2003;**362**:7–13.

Portner PM, Jansen PG, Oyer PE, *et al.* Improved outcomes with an implantable left ventricular assist system: a multicenter study. *Ann Thorac Surg* 2001;**71**:205–9.

Portner PM, Oyer PE, Pennington DG, *et al.* Implantable electrical left ventricular assist system: bridge to transplantation and the future. *Ann Thorac Surg* 1989;**47**:142–50.

Poston RS, Husain S, Sorce D, *et al.* LVAD bloodstream infections: therapeutic rationale for transplantation after LVAD infection. *J Heart Lung Transplant* 2003;**22**:914–21.

Poston RS, Sorce DN, Husain S, *et al.* LVAD blood stream infection: therapeutic rationale for transplantation. *J Heart Lung Transplant* 2001;**20**:241–2.

Potapov EV, Jurmann MJ, Drews T, *et al.* Patients supported for over 4 years with left ventricular assist devices. *Eur J Heart Fail* 2006;**8**:756–9.

Prager KM, Oz M. Proposed policy for VAD removal. *Ann Thorac Surg* 2002;**73**:1688.

Prendergast TW, Todd BA, Beyer AJ 3rd, *et al.* Management of left ventricular assist device infection with heart transplantation. *Ann Thorac Surg* 1997;**64**:142–7.

Quaini E, Pavie A, Chieco S, Mambrito B. The Concerted Action 'Heart' European registry on clinical application of mechanical circulatory support systems: bridge to transplant. The Registry Scientific Committee. *Eur J Cardiothorac Surg* 1997;**11**:182–8.

Rao V, Oz MC, Edwards NM, Naka Y. A new off-pump technique for Thoratec right ventricular assist device insertion. *Ann Thorac Surg* 2001;**71**:1719–20.

Rao V, Oz MC, Flannery MA, *et al.* Revised screening scale to predict survival after insertion of a left ventricular assist device. *J Thorac Cardiovasc Surg* 2003;**125**:855–62.

Redfield MM. Heart failure — an epidemic of uncertain proportions. *N Engl J Med* 2002;**347**:1442–4.

Reinhartz O, Farrar DJ, Hershon JH, *et al.* Importance of preoperative liver function as a predictor of survival in patients supported with Thoratec ventricular assist devices as a bridge to transplantation. *J Thorac Cardiovasc Surg* 1998;**116**:633–40.

Reinlib L, Abraham W. Recovery from heart failure with circulatory assist: a working group of the National Heart, Lung, and Blood Institute. *J Card Fail* 2003;**9**:459–63.

Reiss N, El-Banayosy A, Arusoglu L, *et al.* Acute fulminant myocarditis in children and adolescents: the role of mechanical circulatory assist. *ASAIO J* 2006;**52**:211–4.

Rich MW, Beckham V, Wittenberg C, *et al.* A multidisciplinary intervention to prevent the readmission of elderly patients with congestive heart failure. *N Engl J Med* 1995;**333**:1190–5.

Richardson P, McKenna W, Bristow M, *et al.* Report of the 1995 World Health Organization/International Society and Federation of Cardiology Task Force on the Definition and Classification of Cardiomyopathies. *Circulation* 1996;**93**:841–2.

Richenbacher WE, Seemuth SC. Hospital discharge for the ventricular assist device patient: historical perspective and description of a successful program. *ASAIO J* 2001;**47**:590–5.

Rivers E, Nguyen B, Havstad S, *et al.*; Early Goal-Directed Therapy Collaborative Group. Early goal-directed therapy in the treatment of severe sepsis and septic shock. *N Engl J Med* 2001;**345**:1368–77.

Robbins RC, Oyer PE. Bridge to transplant with the Novacor left ventricular assist system. *Ann Thorac Surg* 1999;**68**:695–7.

Rodrigue-Way A, Burkhoff D, Geesaman BJ, *et al.* Sarcomeric genes involved in reverse remodeling of the heart during left ventricular assist device support. *J Heart Lung Transplant* 2005;**24**:73–80.

Rose EA, Gelijns AC, Moskowitz AJ, for the Randomized Evaluation of Mechanical Assistance for the Treatment of Congestive Heart Failure (REMATCH) Study Group. Long-term use of a left ventricular assist device for end-stage heart failure. *N Engl J Med* 2001;**345**:1435–43.

Rose EA, Moskowitz AJ, Packer M, *et al.* The REMATCH trial: rationale, design, and end points. Randomized Evaluation of Mechanical Assistance for the Treatment of Congestive Heart Failure. *Ann Thorac Surg* 1999;**67**: 723–30.

Rose EA, Stevenson LW (eds.). *Management of End-Stage Heart Disease.* Lippincott-Raven Publishers, Philadelphia, 1998.

Rothenburger M, Wilhelm MJ, Hammel D, *et al.* Treatment of thrombus formation associated with the MicroMed DeBakey VAD using recombinant tissue plasminogen activator. *Circulation* 2002;**106**(12 Suppl 1):I189–92.

Ruf AE, Kremers WK, Chavez LL, *et al.* Addition of serum sodium into the MELD score predicts waiting list mortality better than MELD alone. *Liver Transpl* 2005;**11**:336–43.

Russell JA. Management of sepsis. *N Engl J Med* 2006;**355**:1699–713.

Ryden L, for the Xamoterol in Severe Heart Failure Study Group. Xamoterol in severe heart failure. *Lancet* 1990;**336**:1–6.

Sabol VK. Nutrition assessment of the critically ill adult. *AACN Clin Issues* 2004;**15**:595–606.

Samuels LE, Holmes EC, Garwood P, Ferdinand F. Initial experience with the Abiomed AB5000 ventricular assist device system. *Ann Thorac Surg* 2005;**80**:309–12.

Samuels LE, Holmes EC, Petrucci R. Psychosocial and sexual concerns of patients with implantable left ventricular assist devices: a pilot study. *J Thorac Cardiovasc Surg* 2004;**127**:1432–5.

Samuels LE, Thomas MP, Holmes EC, *et al.* Insufficiency of the native aortic valve and left ventricular assist system inflow valve after support with an implantable left ventricular assist system: signs, symptoms, and concerns. *J Thorac Cardiovasc Surg* 2001;**122**:380–1.

Savage L. Quality of life among patients with a left ventricular assist device: what is new? *AACN Clin Issues* 2003;**14**:64–72.

Schmid C, Hammel D, Deng MC, *et al.* Ambulatory care of patients with left ventricular assist devices. *Circulation* 1999;100(Suppl II):II224–8.

Schmid C, Tjan TD, Etz C, *et al.* First clinical experience with the Incor left ventricular assist device. *J Heart Lung Transplant* 2005;**24**:1188–94.

Schmid C, Wilhelm M, Rothenburger M, *et al.* Effect of high dose platelet inhibitor treatment on thromboembolism in Novacor patients. *Eur J Cardiothorac Surg* 2000;**17**:331–5.

Schmidt LE, Dalhoff K. Alpha-fetoprotein is a predictor of outcome in acetaminophen-induced liver injury. *Hepatology* 2005;**41**:26–31.

Schonhofer B, Guo JJ, Suchi S, *et al.* The use of APACHE II prognostic system in difficult-to-wean patients after long-term mechanical ventilation. *Eur J Anaesthesiol* 2004;**21**:558–65.

Shah NB, Der E, Ruggerio C, *et al.* Prevention of hospitalizations for heart failure with an interactive home monitoring program. *Am Heart J* 1998;**135**: 373–8.

Shapiro PA, Levin HR, Oz MC. Left ventricular assist devices. Psychosocial burden and implications for heart transplant programs. *Gen Hosp Psychiatry* 1996;**18**(6 Suppl):30S–5S.

Sharma UC, Pokharel S, Evelo CT, Maessen JG. A systematic review of large scale and heterogeneous gene array data in heart failure. *J Mol Cell Cardiol* 2005;**38**:425–32.

Siegenthaler MP, Westaby S, Frazier OH, *et al.* Advanced heart failure: feasibility study of long-term continuous axial flow pump support. *Eur Heart J* 2005;**26**:1031–8.

Simon D, Fischer S, Grossman A, *et al.* Left ventricular assist device-related infection: treatment and outcome. *Clin Infect Dis* 2005a;**40**:1108–15.

Simon MA, Kormos RL, Murali S, *et al.* Myocardial recovery using ventricular assist devices: prevalence, clinical characteristics, and outcomes. *Circulation* 2005b;**112**(9 Suppl):I32–6.

Singh SN, Fletcher RD, Fisher SG, for the Survival Trial of Antiarrhythmic Therapy in Congestive Heart Failure. Amiodarone in patients with congestive heart failure and asymptomatic ventricular arrhythmia. *N Engl J Med* 1995;**333**: 77–88.

Sinha P, Chen JM, Flannery M, *et al.* Infections during left ventricular assist device support do not affect posttransplant outcomes. *Circulation* 2000;**102** (19 Suppl 3):III194–9.

Sladen RN. Oliguria in the ICU. Systematic approach to diagnosis and treatment. *Anesthesiol Clin North America* 2000;**18**:739–52.

Slaughter MS, Silver MA, Farrar DJ, *et al.* A new method of monitoring recovery and weaning the Thoratec left ventricular assist device. *Ann Thorac Surg* 2001;**71**:215–8.

Slaughter MS, Sobieski MA, Koenig SC, *et al.* Left ventricular assist device weaning: hemodynamic response and relationship to stroke volume and rate reduction protocols. *ASAIO J* 2006;**52**:228–33.

Smart K, Jett GK. Late tamponade with mechanical circulatory support. *Ann Thorac Surg* 1998;**66**:2027–8.

Smits JMA, De Meester J, Deng MC, on behalf of the COCPIT Study Group and the Eurotransplant Heart Transplant Programs. Mortality rates after heart transplantation: how to compare center-specific outcome data? *Transplantation* 2003a;**75**:90–6.

Smits JMA, Deng MC, Hummel M, on behalf of the COCPIT Study Group. A prognostic model for predicting waiting list mortality for a total national cohort of adult heart transplant candidates. *Transplantation* 2003b;**76**:1185–9.

Song X, Throckmorton AL, Untaroiu A, *et al.* Axial flow blood pumps. *ASAIO J* 2003;**49**:355–364.

Spanier T, Oz M, Levin H, *et al.* Activation of coagulation and fibrinolytic pathways in patients with left ventricular assist devices. *J Thorac Cardiovasc Surg* 1996;**112**:1090–7.

Spanier TB, Chen JM, Oz MC, *et al.* Time-dependent cellular population of textured-surface left ventricular assist devices contributes to the development of a biphasic systemic procoagulant response. *J Thorac Cardiovasc Surg* 1999;**118**:404–13.

St. John Kolar D. Cardiovascular news: heart transplantation survival rate best in high-risk group. *Circulation* 2000;**102**:e9024.

Stevenson LW. The evolving role of mechanical circulatory support in advanced heart failure. In: Frazier OH, Kirklin JK (eds.). *Mechanical Circulatory Support* (ISHLT Monograph Series, Vol. 1). Elsevier, Philadelphia, 2006.

Stevenson LW, Hamilton MA, Tillisch IH, *et al.*; Decreasing survival benefit from cardiac transplantation for outpatients as the waiting list lengthens. *J Am Coll Cardiol* 1991;**18**:919–25.

Stevenson LW, Kormos RL, Bourge RC, *et al.*; Mechanical cardiac support 2000: current applications and future trial design. *J Am Coll Cardiol* 2001;**37**:340–70.

Stevenson LW, Miller LW, Desvigne-Nickens P, *et al.*; REMATCH Investigators. Left ventricular assist device as destination for patients undergoing intravenous inotropic therapy: a subset analysis from REMATCH (Randomized Evaluation of Mechanical Assistance in Treatment of Chronic Heart Failure). *Circulation* 2004;**110**:975–81.

Stevenson LW, Shekar P. Ventricular assist devices for durable support. *Circulation* 2005;**112**:e111–5.

Stevenson LW, Steimle AE, Fonarow G, *et al.* Improvement in exercise capacity of candidates awaiting heart transplantation. *J Am Coll Cardiol* 1995;**25**:163–70.

Suman A, Barnes DS, Zein NN, *et al.* Predicting outcome after cardiac surgery in patients with cirrhosis: a comparison of Child–Pugh and MELD scores. *Clin Gastroenterol Hepatol* 2004;**2**:719–23.

Swartz MT, Lowdermilk GA, McBride LR. Refractory ventricular tachycardia as an indication for ventricular assist device support. *J Thorac Cardiovasc Surg* 1999;**118**:1119–20.

Swedberg K, for the CONSENSUS Trial Study Group. Effects of enalapril on mortality in severe congestive heart failure. *N Engl J Med* 1987;**316**:1429–35.

Swedberg K, Kjekshus J, Snapinn S. Long-term survival in severe heart failure in patients treated with enalapril. Ten year follow-up of CONSENSUS I. *Eur Heart J* 1999;**20**:136–9.

Sweeney MO, Ruskin JN, Garan H, *et al*. Influence of the implantable cardioverter/defibrillator on sudden death and total mortality in patients evaluated for cardiac transplantation. *Circulation* 1995;**92**:3273–81.

Teerlink JR, Massie BM. The role of beta-blockers in preventing sudden death in heart failure. *J Card Fail* 2000;**6**(Suppl 1):25–33.

Texereau J, Pene F, Chiche JD, *et al*. Importance of hemostatic gene polymorphisms for susceptibility to and outcome of severe sepsis. *Crit Care Med* 2004;**32**(5 Suppl):S1313–19.

Thakar CV, Arrigain S, *et al*. A clinical score to predict acute renal failure after cardiac surgery. *J Am Soc Nephrol* 2005;**16**:162–8.

Thalmann M, Schima H, Wieselthaler G, Wolner E. Physiology of continuous blood flow in recipients of rotary cardiac assist devices. *J Heart Lung Transplant* 2005;**24**:237–45.

Thoratec Corporation. Nutrition Management in Advanced Practice Guidelines for HeartMate® Destination Therapy. Report No. 1, 2004.

Tisol WB, Mueller DK, Hoy FB, *et al*. Ventricular assist device use with mechanical heart valves: an outcome series and literature review. *Ann Thorac Surg* 2001;**72**:2051–4.

Tjan TDT, Kondruweit M, Scheld HH, *et al*. The bad ventricle — revascularization versus transplantation. *Thorac Cardiovasc Surg* 2000;**48**:1–6.

Topkara VK, Dang NC, Barili F, *et al*. Predictors and outcomes of continuous veno-venous hemodialysis use after implantation of a left ventricular assist device. *J Heart Lung Transplant* 2006;**25**:404–8.

Topkara VK, Dang NC, Martens TP, *et al*. Bridging to transplantation with left ventricular assist devices: outcomes in patients aged 60 years and older. *J Thorac Cardiovasc Surg* 2005;**130**:881–2.

Toumpoulis IK, Anagnostopoulos CE, Swistel DG, DeRose JJ Jr. Does EuroSCORE predict length of stay and specific postoperative complications after cardiac surgery? *Eur J Cardiothorac Surg* 2005;**27**:128–33.

Van den Berghe G, Wouters P, Weekers F, *et al*. Intensive insulin therapy in the critically ill patients. *N Engl J Med* 2001;**345**:1359–67.

Veenhuyzen GD, Singh SN, McAreavey D, *et al*. Prior coronary artery bypass surgery and risk of death among patients with ischemic left ventricular dysfunction. *Circulation* 2001;**104**:1489–93.

Vincent JL, Angus DC, Artigas A, *et al*.; Recombinant Human Activated Protein C Worldwide Evaluation in Severe Sepsis (PROWESS) Study Group. Effects of drotrecogin alfa (activated) on organ dysfunction in the PROWESS trial. *Crit Care Med* 2003;**31**:834–40.

Vinsonneau C, Camus C, Combes A, *et al.*; Hemodiafe Study Group. Continuous venovenous haemodiafiltration versus intermittent haemodialysis for acute renal failure in patients with multiple-organ dysfunction syndrome: a multicentre randomised trial. *Lancet* 2006;**368**:379–85.

Wang JE. Can single nucleotide polymorphisms in innate immune receptors predict development of septic complications in intensive care unit patients? *Crit Care Med* 2005;**33**:695–6.

Wegner JA, DiNardo JA, Arabia FA, Copeland JG. Blood loss and transfusion requirements in patients implanted with a mechanical circulatory support device undergoing cardiac transplantation. *J Heart Lung Transplant* 2000;**19**:504–6.

Weissman C. Pulmonary complications after cardiac surgery. *Semin Cardiothorac Vasc Anesth* 2004;**8**:185–211.

Weitkemper HH, El-Banayosy A, Arusoglu L, *et al.* Mechanical circulatory support: reality and dreams — experience of a single center. *J Extra Corpor Technol* 2004;**36**:169–73.

Wieselthaler GM, Schima H, Hiesmayr M, *et al.* First clinical experience with the DeBakey VAD continuous-axial-flow pump for bridge to transplantation. *Circulation* 2000;**101**:256–9.

Wilhelm CR, Ristich J, Kormos RL, Wagner WR. Monocyte tissue factor expression and ongoing complement generation in ventricular assist device patients. *Ann Thorac Surg* 1998;**65**:1071–6.

Williams MR, Oz MC. Indications and patient selection for mechanical ventricular assistance. *Ann Thorac Surg* 2001;**71**(Suppl 3):S86–91.

Winkel E, Piccione W. Coronary artery bypass surgery in patients with left ventricular dysfunction: candidate selection and perioperative care. *J Heart Lung Transplant* 1997;**16**:S19–24.

Wright JC, Weinstein MC. Gains in life expectancy from medical interventions — standardizing data on outcomes. *N Engl J Med* 1998;**339**:380–6.

Wudel JH, Hlozek CC, Smedira NG, McCarthy PM. Extracorporeal life support as a post left ventricular assist device implant supplement. *ASAIO J* 1997;**43**:M441–3.

Yokomuro H, Li RK, Mickle DA, *et al.* Transplantation of cryopreserved cardiomyocytes. *J Thorac Cardiovasc Surg* 2001;**121**:98–107.

Yoo KJ, Li RK, Weisel RD, *et al.* Autologous smooth muscle cell transplantation improved heart function in dilated cardiomyopathy. *Ann Thorac Surg* 2000;**70**:859–65.

Young JB, Dunlap ME, Pfeffer MA, *et al.*; Candesartan in Heart Failure Assessment of Reduction in Mortality and Morbidity (CHARM) Investigators and Committees. Mortality and morbidity reduction with candesartan in patients with chronic heart failure and left ventricular systolic dysfunction:

results of the CHARM low-left ventricular ejection fraction trials. *Circulation* 2004;**110**:2618–26.

Young JB, Rogers JG, Portner PE *et al.* Bridge to eligibility: LVAS support in patients with relative contraindications to transplantation. *J Heart Lung Transplant* 2005;**24**:S75.

Zimpfer D, Wieselthaler G, Czerny M, *et al.* Neurocognitive function in patients with ventricular assist devices: a comparison of pulsatile and continuous blood flow devices. *ASAIO J* 2006;**52**:24–7.

Ziv O, Dizon J, Thosani A, *et al.* Effects of left ventricular assist device therapy on ventricular arrhythmias. *J Am Coll Cardiol* 2005;**45**:1428–34.

# APPENDICES

## APPENDIX 1: EVIDENCE-BASED MEDICINE CRITERIA

| Level | Therapy/Prevention, Etiology/Harm | Prognosis | Diagnosis | Differential diagnosis/Symptom prevalence study | Economic and decision analyses |
|---|---|---|---|---|---|
| 1a | SR (with homogeneity) of RCTs | SR (with homogeneity) of inception cohort studies; CDR validated in different populations | SR (with homogeneity) of Level 1 diagnostic studies; CDR with Level 1b studies from different clinical centers | SR (with homogeneity) of prospective cohort studies | SR (with homogeneity) of Level 1 economic studies |
| 1b | Individual RCT (with narrow confidence interval) | Individual inception cohort study with >80% follow-up; CDR validated in a single population | Validating cohort study with good reference standards; or CDR tested within one clinical center | Prospective cohort study with good follow-up | Analysis based on clinically sensible costs or alternatives; systematic review(s) of the evidence; and including multiway sensitivity analyses |

*(Continued)*

297

**Appendix 1.**  (*Continued*)

| Level | Therapy/Prevention, Etiology/Harm | Prognosis | Diagnosis | Differential diagnosis/Symptom prevalence study | Economic and decision analyses |
|---|---|---|---|---|---|
| 1c | All or none | All-or-none case series | Absolute SpPins and SnNouts | All-or-none case series | Absolute better-value or worse-value analyses |
| 2a | SR (with homogeneity) of cohort studies | SR (with homogeneity) of either retrospective cohort studies or untreated control groups in RCTs | SR (with homogeneity) of Level >2 diagnostic studies | SR (with homogeneity) of Level 2b and better studies | SR (with homogeneity) of Level >2 economic studies |
| 2b | Individual cohort study (including low-quality RCT; e.g. <80% follow-up) | Retrospective cohort study or follow-up of untreated control patients in an RCT; derivation of CDR or validated on split sample only | Exploratory cohort study with good reference standards; CDR after derivation, or validated only on split sample or databases | Retrospective cohort study, or poor follow-up | Analysis based on clinically sensible costs or alternatives; limited review(s) of the evidence, or single studies; and including multiway sensitivity analyses |

(*Continued*)

**Appendix 1.** (*Continued*)

| Level | Therapy/Prevention, Etiology/Harm | Prognosis | Diagnosis | Differential diagnosis/Symptom prevalence study | Economic and decision analyses |
|---|---|---|---|---|---|
| 2c | Outcomes research; ecological studies | Outcomes research | | Ecological studies | Audit or outcomes research |
| 3a | SR (with homogeneity) of case-control studies | | SR (with homogeneity) of Level 3b and better studies | SR (with homogeneity) of Level 3b and better studies | SR (with homogeneity) of Level 3b and better studies |
| 3b | Individual case-control study | | Nonconsecutive study; or without consistently applied reference standards | Nonconsecutive cohort study, or very limited population | Analysis based on limited alternatives or costs and poor quality estimates of data, but including sensitivity analyses incorporating clinically sensible variations |

(*Continued*)

**Appendix 1.** (*Continued*)

| Level | Therapy/Prevention, Etiology/Harm | Prognosis | Diagnosis | Differential diagnosis/Symptom prevalence study | Economic and decision analyses |
|---|---|---|---|---|---|
| 4 | Case series (and poor-quality cohort and case-control studies) | Case series (and poor-quality prognostic cohort studies) | Case control study; poor or nonindependent reference standard | Case series or superseded reference standards | Analysis with no sensitivity analysis |
| 5 | Expert opinion without explicit critical appraisal; or based on physiology, bench research, or first principles | Expert opinion without explicit critical appraisal; or based on physiology, bench research, or first principles | Expert opinion without explicit critical appraisal; or based on physiology, bench research, or first principles | Expert opinion without explicit critical appraisal; or based on physiology, bench research, or first principles | Expert opinion without explicit critical appraisal; or based on economic theory or first principles |

From: http://www.cebm.net/levels_of_evidence.asp

**ACC/AHA levels of evidence/strength of recommendation (Hunt *et al.*, 2001; Hunt *et al.*, 2005)**

- **High-level evidence:** Data from multiple randomized clinical trials (Level A ACC/AHA), systematic reviews of RCT with narrow confidence intervals, single randomized study with narrow confidence intervals, or all-or-none studies (Levels 1a, 1b, 1c EBM Oxford).
- **Medium-level evidence:** Data from other individual randomized clinical trials or nonrandomized studies (Level B ACC/AHA) or cohort studies, outcomes research, case series (Levels 2a, 2b, 2c, 3, 4 EBM Oxford).
- **Low-level evidence:** Consensus opinion of experts (Level C ACC/AHA) or first principle (Level 5 EBM Oxford).
- **Uniformly recommended:** Intervention for which there is evidence and/or general agreement that it is safe, effective, and useful.
- **Nonuniformly recommended:** Intervention for which there is conflicting evidence and/or divergence of opinion that it is safe, effective, and useful.
- **Not recommended:** Intervention for which there is evidence and/or general agreement that it is not safe, effective, or useful.

# APPENDIX 2: CONTACTS (INDUSTRY, EXPERT SOCIETIES, AGENCIES)

| Company website | | Comments |
|---|---|---|
| http://www.thoratec.com/ | | Thoratec Company info |
| | http://www.thoratec.com/about-thoratec/profile.htm | Products |
| | http://www.thoratec.com/ventricular-assist-device/index.htm | Professional info |
| | http://www.thoratec.com/medical-professionals/index.htm | |
| | http://www.thoratec.com/ventricular-assist-device/heartmate_lvas.htm | HeartMate I |
| | http://www.thoratec.com/ventricular-assist-device/heartmate_lvas.htm | Paracorporeal Thoratec |

*(Continued)*

**Appendix 2.** (*Continued*)

| Company website | | Comments |
|---|---|---|
| | http://www.thoratec.com/ventricular-assist-device/thoratec_imp.htm | Implantable Thoratec |
| | http://www.thoratec.com/thoratec-patients/index.htm | Patient info |
| | http://www.thoratec.com/news/index.htm | News |
| | http://phx.corporate-ir.net/phoenix.zhtml?c=95989&p=irol-irhome | Investors |
| | http://www.thoratec.com/heartmate-destination-therapy/index.htm | Destination MCSD |
| http://www.berlinheart.de/englisch/ | | Berlin Heart |
| | http://www.berlinheart.de/englisch/patienten/index.php | Patient info |
| | http://www.berlinheart.de/englisch/medpro/index.php | Professional info |

(*Continued*)

**Appendix 2.** (*Continued*)

| Company website | | Comments |
|---|---|---|
| | http://www.berlinheart.de/englisch/allgemein/index.php | Company info |
| | http://www.berlinheart.de/englisch/allgemein/news/Newsletter/ | Newsletter |
| | http://www.berlinheart.de/englisch/patienten/ INCOR/ | INCOR |
| | http://www.berlinheart.de/englisch/patienten/ EXCOR/ | EXCOR |
| http://www.abiomed.com/ | | Abiomed |
| | http://www.abiomed.com/patients_families/patient_stories.cfm | Patient stories |
| | http://www.abiomed.com/about_abiomed/index.cfm | Clinical info |
| | http://www.abiomed.com/about_abiomed/index.cfm | Company info |

(*Continued*)

**Appendix 2.** (*Continued*)

| Company website | | Comments |
|---|---|---|
| | http://www.abiomed.com/products/index.cfm | Product overview |
| | http://www.abiomed.com/news/press_releases.cfm | Newsletter |
| | http://www.abiomed.com/products/ab5000.cfm | Abiomed AB 5000 |
| | http://www.abiomed.com/products/bvs5000.cfm | Abiomed BVS 5000 |
| | http://www.abiomed.com/products/heart_replacement.cfm | AbioCor II |
| http://www.syncardia.com/ | | CardioWest |
| | http://www.syncardia.com/patients.php | Patient |
| | http://www.syncardia.com/physicians.php | Physician info |
| | http://www.syncardia.com/about.php | Company info |

(*Continued*)

**Appendix 2.**  (*Continued*)

| Company website | | Comments |
|---|---|---|
| http://www.jarvikheart.com/<br>home.asp | http://www.syncardia.com/<br>newsletters.php | Newsletter |
| | | Jarvik Heart |
| | http://www.jarvikheart.com/<br>basic.asp?id=27 | Patient info |
| | http://www.jarvikheart.com/<br>basic.asp?section=<br>Treatment+Options | Professional info |
| | http://www.jarvikheart.com/<br>basic.asp?section=About+Us | Company info |
| | http://www.jarvikheart.com/<br>basic.asp?id=21 | Product info |
| | http://www.jarvikheart.com/<br>news.asp | Newsletter |
| | http://www.jarvikheart.<br>com/basic.asp?section=<br>Jarvik+2000 | Jarvik 2000 |

(*Continued*)

**Appendix 2.** (*Continued*)

| Company website | | Comments |
|---|---|---|
| http://www.medos-ag.com/ | | MEDOS |
| | http://www.medos-ag.com/VAD-Training_en.html | Professional info |
| | http://www.medos-ag.com/enterprise.html | Company info |
| | http://www.medos-ag.com/medos_vad_system.html | Product info |
| | http://www.medos-ag.com/news_en.html | Newsletter |
| | http://www.medos-ag.com/medos_vad_pump-chambers_ventricles_.html | MEDOS |
| http://www.micromedtech.com/ | | DeBakey |
| | http://www.micromedtech.com/videos.htm | Professional info |
| | http://www.micromedtech.com/companyhistory.htm | Company info |

(*Continued*)

**Appendix 2.** (*Continued*)

| Company website | | Comments |
|---|---|---|
| | http://www.micromedtech.com/<br>productprofile.htm | Product info |
| | http://www.micromedtech.com/<br>micromednews.htm | Newsletter |
| http://www.worldheart.com/ | | Novacor |
| | http://www.worldheart.com/<br>patients/index.cfm | Patient info |
| | http://www.worldheart.com/<br>clinical_information/<br>index.cfm | Professional info |
| | http://www.worldheart.com/<br>about/index.cfm | Company info |
| | http://www.worldheart.com/<br>products/index.cfm | Product info |
| | http://phx.corporate-ir.net/<br>phoenix.zhtml?c=117539&<br>p=irol-news&nyo=0 | Newsletter |

(*Continued*)

**Appendix 2.** (*Continued*)

| Company website | | Comments |
|---|---|---|
| | http://www.worldheart.com/products/novacor_lvas.cfm | Novacor |
| | http://www.worldheart.com/products/heartquest_vad.cfm | Novacor Rotary |
| | http://www.worldheart.com/products/novacor_2_lvas.cfm | Novacor II |
| http://www.heartware.com.au/ | | HeartWare |
| | http://www.heartware.com.au/IRM/content/clinical_glpanimal.html | Patient info Professional info |
| | http://www.heartware.com.au/IRM/content/about_heartware.html | Company info |
| | http://www.heartware.com.au/IRM/content/products_tech.html | Product info |

(*Continued*)

**Appendix 2.** (*Continued*)

| Company website | | Comments |
|---|---|---|
| | http://www.heartware.com.au/IRM/content/index.htm | Newsletter |
| | http://www.heartware.com.au/IRM/content/products_hvad.html | HVAD |
| http://www.evaheart-usa.com/ | | EVAHEART |
| | http://www.evaheart-usa.com/publications.cfm | Professional info |
| | http://www.evaheart-usa.com/company_emusa.cfm | Company info |
| | http://www.evaheart-usa.com/deviceInfo.cfm | Product info |
| | http://www.evaheart-usa.com/newEvents-2_events.cfm | Newsletter |
| http://hdz-nrw.de/en/center/press/details.php?id=1062&anzeige=2005 | | CorAide Terumo |

(*Continued*)

**Appendix 2.** (*Continued*)

| Company website | Comments |
|---|---|
| http://www.terumoheart.com/ | DuraHeart Terumo |
| http://www.terumoheart.com/failure_lvas.asp | Patient info |
| | Professional info |
| http://www.terumoheart.com/aboutus.asp | Company info |
| http://www.terumoheart.com/tech_duraheart.asp | Product info |
| http://www.terumoheart.com/news.asp | Newsletter |
| http://www.terumoheart.com/tech_how.asp | DuraHeart Pump |
| http://cardiactransplantresearch.cumc.columbia.edu/ | Website of Dr Mario Deng |
| http://www.a-s-t.org/ | American Society of Transplantation |
| http://www.global-good.org/ | Global Organization for Organ Donation |
| http://www.unos.org/ | United Network for Organ Sharing |

(*Continued*)

**Appendix 2.** (*Continued*)

| Company website | Comments |
| --- | --- |
| http://www.hearthope.com/ | Heart Hope |
| http://www.intermacs.org/ | Interagency Registry for Mechanically Assisted Circulatory Support |
| http://www.nhlbi.nih.gov/ | National Heart, Lung, and Blood Institute |
| http://www.sts.org/ | Society of Thoracic Surgeons |
| http://www.aats.org/ | American Association of Thoracic Surgeons |
| http://www.acc.org/ | American College of Cardiology |
| http://www.fda.gov/ | Food and Drug Administration |
| http://www.nih.gov/ | National Institutes of Health |
| http://www.ctsnet.org/ | Cardiothoracic Surgeon Network |
| http://www.abouthf.org/ | Heart Failure Society of America |
| http://www.americanheart.org/ | American Heart Association |
| http://www.asaio.com/ | American Society of Artificial Implantable Organs |

(*Continued*)

**Appendix 2.** (*Continued*)

| Company website | Comments |
| --- | --- |
| http://www.eacts.org/ | European Association of Cardio-Thoracic Surgeons |
| http://www.esao.org/ | European Society of Artificial Organs |
| http://www.escardio.org/ | European Society of Cardiology |
| http://www.eurotransplant.nl/ | EuroTransplant |
| http://www.d-t-g-online.de/ | German Organ Transplantation Society |
| http://www.gstcvs.org/ | German Society for Thoracic and Cardiovascular Surgery |
| http://www.ncbi.nlm.nih.gov/entrez/query.fcgi?CMD=search& DB=PubMed/ | National Library of Medicine |
| http://www.ishlt.org/ | International Society of Heart and Lung Transplantation |
| http://www.isrbp.org/ | International Society of Rotary Blood Pumps |

# APPENDIX 3: INFECTION PROTOCOLS

## Columbia Infection Monitoring Protocol (Status July 2006)

### (A) Patient selection issues:

    a. All conditions that might enhance the risk of fungal infection should be considered and properly managed. Acute systemic infection should be considered a contraindication (III/A) (Mehra *et al.*, 2006).

### (B) Preoperative infection management:

    a. Management of preoperative infection sources

        i. Odontological care

           1. Considerations

        ii. Preimplant invasive procedures: prophylaxis

           1. Guidelines

        iii. Immunizations

           1. Compliance with standards of practice

    b. Management of infections not contraindicating MCSD implantation

        i. Prior isolated bacteriemia

        ii. Asymptomatic bacteriuria

        iii. Skin ulcers

        iv. Dental septic foci

    c. Definition of "able to be implanted": time of treatment before MCSD implantation

### (C) Intravenous catheters:

    a. All unnecessary intravenous catheters should be removed and all others replaced 12–24 h preoperatively.

    b. Follow the recommendations for IV catheter insertion as per guidelines.

### (D) Urinary catheters
### (E) Antimicrobial prophylaxis:

    a. Vancomycin 15 mg/kg IV 1 h preop, then q 12 h × 48 h

    b. Levofloxacin 500 mg IV 1 h preop, then q 24 h × 48 h

c. Rifampin 600 mg PO 1–2 h preop and QD × 48 h

d. Fluconazole 200 mg IV preop, then q 24 h × 48 h

e. Nasal mupirocin (Bactroban™) application the evening prior to surgery

**(F) Preoperative scrubs:** Night and morning before when possible

**(G) Clip body hair:** Clarify not to razor it for risk of skin microlacerations as port of entry for staph.

**(H) Operating room (OR) precautions:**

a. Personnel

   i. Fresh scrubs

   ii. Booties

   iii. Headwear that covers all hair

   iv. Mask

b. Restricted traffic near pump assembly table

c. Sterile field out-of-reach rule with barriers to protect field

d. Air ultrafiltration system (HEPA)

**(I) Intraoperative management:**

1. Prior to the procedure, review the plans for driveline and exit-site positions to minimize manipulation of the aseptic site during surgery.

2. Prepare with antiseptic scrub, alcohol, and Betadine gel (or equivalent), and drape with steridrapes (e.g. Ioban).

3. Minimize exposure of the LVAD by the following:

   i. Not opening device too early and eliminating unnecessary traffic

   ii. Using fit model for device positioning, not the actual device

   iii. Wrapping implantable materials in antibiotic-soaked lap sponges

4. Percutaneous lead management:

   i. Tunnel percutaneous lead to the upper right quadrant, subcostal region exiting in the midclavicular line 4–6 cm below costal margin (with the percutaneous lead passing through a long intramuscular tunnel); orient the 5–7 cm of exteriorized percutaneous lead towards the anterior axillary fold.

5. Immobilize the LVAD with fixation at two or more points.

6. Secure meticulous hemostasis.
7. Irrigate all surfaces with antibiotic solution prior to closing (vancomycin 2 g/L and gentamycin 160 mg/L in NS).
8. Place thoracic tubes and consider LVAD pocket drains.
9. Immobilize percutaneous lead (consider retaining suture) with exit-site dressing.

## (J) Postoperative management:

1. Systemic antimicrobials: continue antimicrobial prophylaxis for 48 h or modify regimen as clinically indicated.
2. All indwelling catheters require aseptic precautions and early removal or frequent rotations.
3. Drains/Securing suture:

    i. Remove thoracic tubes as per institutional protocol, followed by LVAD pocket drains when drainage is <30–50 cc/day (usually 3–7 days).
    ii. Remove percutaneous-lead–securing suture when good tissue ingrowth is seen.

4. Exit site dressing changes and exit site monitoring:

    i. Always employ aseptic techniques.
    ii. Follow the dressing change protocol as per institutional guidelines.
    iii. Dressing change frequency depends on the length of time postop; degree of tissue ingrowth; and freedom from exit-site problems like drainage, infection, or recent trauma (QD, BID, or >BID as clinically indicated).
    iv. Routine monitoring is essential to evaluate exit-site healing, rule out infection, and assure proper positioning and immobilization to avoid tissue-driveline separation.

5. Percutaneous lead immobilization:

    i. Use occlusive dressing initially postop, then immobilize with driveline dressing sponges held in place by a Montgomery strap.
    ii. As drainage tapers and patient activity increases, transit to custom percutaneous-lead–immobilizing binder.

6. Bathing:

   i. For the first 30 days postop, until the exit site has healed well with good tissue–percutaneous lead ingrowth, take sponge baths while protecting the wound from contamination and moisture.

   ii. After 30 days postop and when the exit site has healed, shower per MicroMed instructions while covering the exit site with a gauze pad and plastic wrap.

7. General medical issues:

   i. Maintain nutritional needs, especially during the immediate postoperative period; ensure good control of diabetes mellitus and avoid immunosuppression whenever possible.

## APPENDIX 4: ANTICOAGULATION PROTOCOLS

| Type | Platelet | Plasma proteins | Fibrinolysis monitoring |
|---|---|---|---|
| AbioCor | Aspirin | Coumadin | INR |
| Abiomed | Aspirin | Coumadin | INR |
| CardioWest | Aspirin | Coumadin | INR |
| Jarvik 2000 | Aspirin | Coumadin | INR |
| LionHeart | Aspirin | Coumadin | INR |
| Medos | Aspirin | Coumadin | INR |
| MicroMed DeBakey | Aspirin | Coumadin | INR |
| Thoratec HeartMate I | Aspirin Dipyridamole | | INR |
| Thoratec HeartMate II | Aspirin Dipyridamole | 10% dextran Heparin Coumadin | PTT 60–80 s INR 2.5–3.5 |
| Thoratec WorldHeart Novacor | Aspirin Dipyridamole | Coumadin | |

**Novacor (Status April 2004)**

**Operative management**

| | |
|---|---|
| **Antifibrinolytic agent:** | Aprotinin, tranexamic acid, or $\varepsilon$-aminocaproic acid |
| **Heparin:** | Standard CPB dose |
| **Protamine:** | Full reversal (TEG or check heparin levels) |
| **Blood products:** | TEG guidance (leucodepleted products only) |
|    **RBC:** | Standard HCT measurements (do not infuse pericardiotomy suction blood) |
|    **Platelets:** | Standard lab measurements for numbers |
|    **Platelet function:** | TEG, aggregometry, or PFA-100 |
|    **Clotting factors:** | TEG guidance for specific factors and fibrinolysis |

**Early postoperative management**

| | |
|---|---|
| **Blood products:** | |
|    **RBC:** | Standard HCT measurements (do not infuse mediastinal shed blood) |
|    **Platelets:** | Standard lab measurements for numbers |
|    **Platelet function:** | TEG, aggregometry, or PFA-100 |
|    **Coagulation clotting factors:** | TEG guidance for specific factors and fibrinolysis |

**When chest tube drainage is <60 mL/h for 3 consecutive hours:**

| | |
|---|---|
| **Heparin:** | Start with unfractionated heparin at 10 U/kg/h, and target a PTT of 50–64 s (APTT ratio of 1.5–2.0) for first 48 h and then 65–85 s (ratio 2.0–2.5). *(Use heparin infusion nomogram.)* |
| **Aspirin:** | Start with 81 mg daily. Monitor the effect by using TEG. Target inhibition is >50%. Maximum dose is 324 mg. |

*(Use TEG antiaggregant monitoring chart.)*

Alternatively, perform aggregometry using arachadonic acid as an activator and aim for complete inhibition. Nonresponders should be switched to clopidogrel or dipyridamole. Partial responders should have clopidogrel or dipyridamole added to aspirin.

**Clopidogrel:** Start with 75 mg. Monitor the effect by using TEG. Target inhibition is >30%. Maximum dose is 300 mg.

*(Use TEG antiaggregant monitoring chart.)*

Alternatively, perform aggregometry and aim for >30% inhibition of ADP-activated platelet aggregation. Full effect takes approximately 4–5 days. Monitor until 4–5 days after starting or after dose change. Use dipyridamole in case of resistance to both aspirin and clopidogrel, or when target percentage inhibition is not achieved. Maximum dose is 300 mg.

## Chronic management

Change from heparin to coumadin when platelet function is stabilized, chest tubes are removed, patient is stable, and hepatic function has returned to near-normal (usually after 2–4 weeks).

**Heparin:** Continue until INR >2.0.

**Coumadin:** Start with standard loading dose. Target INR is 2.0–3.0.

**Aspirin and/or clopidogrel** Use TEG or aggregometry to achieve above levels of inhibition. Use dipyridamole in case of aspirin and/or clopidogrel resistance. Combined therapy is preferable to monotherapy.

## Notes

- Increased vigilance and monitoring are required during any inflammatory or low-output condition. Diabetics require greater levels of platelet inhibition.
- Continue TEG surveillance monitoring indefinitely at intervals according to patient status, but at least quarterly.

## APPENDIX 5: COLUMBIA UNIVERSITY WEANING PROTOCOL

| Author | Method | Variables | Outcome |
| --- | --- | --- | --- |
| **Mancini** *et al.* **(1998b)** | Exercise testing using pneumatic LVAD (auto mode) interface<br>Heart rate decrease to 20 cycles/min<br>Serial hemodynamics<br>Repetition of exercise test if patient remains stable | Maximal exercise test<br>Hemodynamic monitoring<br>Respiratory gas analysis ($VO_2$)<br>LVAD flow<br>Cardiac output<br>PCPW | 39 consecutive patients<br>18 patients studied<br>15 patients exercised on maximal device support<br>7 patients remained normotensive and exercised at 20 cycles/min, but peak $VO_2$ declined<br>1 patient explanted |

# APPENDIX 6: COLUMBIA UNIVERSITY EVALUATION FORM

## COLUMBIA UNIVERSITY
## CARDIAC TRANSPLANT EVALUATION CHECKLIST

| Date | Patient name | MR# | Date of birth | Age | MD |
|---|---|---|---|---|---|
| | | | | | |

| Blood type | Weight | Height | Race | Gender | BSA |
|---|---|---|---|---|---|
| | | | | | |

| Telephone # | Address | | Referring MD | MD telephone # |
|---|---|---|---|---|
| | | | | |

| Re-op | Etiology | Social security # |
|---|---|---|
| | | |

### *PAST MEDICAL HISTORY*

|  |
|---|
| |

### *MEDICATIONS*

| Dig | Lasix | ACE | $\beta$-blocker | Amio | NTG | Coumadin | Other |
|---|---|---|---|---|---|---|---|
| | | | | | | | |

| Dobutamine | Dopamine | Milrinone | Levophed | Pitressin | IABP | | VENT |
|---|---|---|---|---|---|---|---|
| | | | | | | | |

### *PSYCHOSOCIAL DATA*

| Tobacco | ETOH | Illicit drugs | Occupation | Marital status | Pregnancies |
|---|---|---|---|---|---|
| | | | | | |

### *PHYSICAL EXAM*

| HR | BP | Rales | S3 | S4 | MR | TR | Edema |
|---|---|---|---|---|---|---|---|
| | | | | | | | |

### *HEMODYNAMICS*

| | RA | PA | mPA | PCW | CO | PVR | PA sat |
|---|---|---|---|---|---|---|---|
| Baseline | | | | | | | |
| Post-nipride | | | | | | | |

## *CORONARY CATH*

| Native: |
|---|
| |

| EKG: | Thallium: |
|---|---|
| | |
| CXR: | MUGA: |
| | |

| LVEF | Method |
|---|---|
| | |

| VO$_2$ | ECHO |
|---|---|
| | |

## *PULMONARY FUNCTION TESTS*

| VC | % | FEV1 | % | Ratio | DLCO | % |
|---|---|---|---|---|---|---|
| | | | | | | |

## *VIABILITY STUDY*

| |
|---|
| |

## *NIFS*

| |
|---|
| |

## *LOWER EXTREMITY VEIN DOPPLER – BILATERAL*

| |
|---|
| |

## *CAROTIDS*

| |
|---|
| |

## *ABDOMINAL ULTRASOUND*

| |
|---|
| |

## *LABORATORY DATA*

| Date | NA | K | Cl | CO$_2$ | Glu | BUN | Creat |
|---|---|---|---|---|---|---|---|
|  |  |  |  |  |  |  |  |

| Creat Cl | Urine Prot | Ca | Phos | Mg | UA | Alb | T Prot |
|---|---|---|---|---|---|---|---|
|  |  |  |  |  |  |  |  |

| Alk Phos | T Bili/DBili | GGT | ALT | AST | LDH | Chol | Trig |
|---|---|---|---|---|---|---|---|
|  |  |  |  |  |  |  |  |

| WBC | Hgb | Hct | Plt | PT | PTT | ESR | PSA |
|---|---|---|---|---|---|---|---|
|  |  |  |  |  |  |  |  |

| Fe | Ferritin | TIBC | T4 | T3 uptake | TSH | FTI | T3 |
|---|---|---|---|---|---|---|---|
|  |  |  |  |  |  |  |  |

| HBsAg | HBcoreAb | HBsAb | HCV | Toxo | CMV | EBV | HSV |
|---|---|---|---|---|---|---|---|
|  |  |  |  |  |  |  |  |
|  |  |  |  |  |  |  |  |

| VZV | HIV | PPD | ANA | RF | RPR | CPK | HbA1c |
|---|---|---|---|---|---|---|---|
|  |  |  |  |  |  |  |  |
|  |  |  |  |  |  |  |  |

*HEART FAILURE SURVIVAL SCORE:* ☐ *(low risk >8.1)*

$$[(0.69 \times \text{CAD: } \textbf{YES} = \textbf{1}; \textbf{NO} = \textbf{0}) + (0.022 \times \text{HR}) + (-0.046 \times \text{LVEF})$$
$$+ (-0.026 \times \text{mBP}) + (0.61 \times \text{IVCD: } \textbf{YES} = \textbf{1}; \textbf{NO} = \textbf{0}) + (-0.055 \times$$
$$\text{VO}_2) + (-0.047 \times \text{Na})]$$

## *IMMUNOLOGY DATA*

| PRA(%) | HLA-A | HLA-B | HLA-Dr | HLA-Dq | Transfusions |
|---|---|---|---|---|---|
|  |  |  |  |  |  |

*Psychiatry:*

|  |
|---|

*Social Work:*

| |
|---|

*Other:*

| |
|---|

*Insurance:*

| |
|---|

## <u>OUTCOME:</u>

Listed:

       Date:

       Status:

Rejected:

       Date:

       Reason:

Deferred:

       Reason:

# PATIENT/FAMILY EXPERIENCE VIGNETTES

| | |
|---|---|
| **Case summary: Robert R (born 1947)** | Robert R, born in 1947 and working as an engineer developing the HeartMate I MCSD, suffered a massive heart attack following occlusion of his left main coronary artery while fishing in Ohio in spring 2004. He was admitted to Ohio State University, underwent emergency left heart catheterization and reopening of his left main coronary artery, and received a HeartMate I MCSD. Subsequently, he was transferred to Columbia University Medical Center and underwent orthotopic heart transplantation in October 2004. Since then, he has returned to a quasi-normal life. He lives with his partner Jill. |
| **Jill (partner of Robert R, born 1947)** **Introduction** | Dr Deng, in October, you asked Robert and I for our "war stories" as it were. Like your other patients, I'm sure we have quite a few, and I am just as sure that we learned lessons from a lot of them (sometimes not so pleasantly). |
| **Jill (partner of Robert R, born 1947)** **MCSD surgery** | I cannot begin to tell you how difficult it was waiting all that time for Robert to be conscious enough for me to tell him that he had 8 lbs of titanium in his chest, and the best way I could describe it was that it looked like a water pump from an old car! Those were anxious days in more ways than one. Would he be angry? Would he be outraged? What would he be? As it turned out, he took the news quite well. I was much impressed and greatly relieved. |

| | |
|---|---|
| **Jill**<br>**(partner of**<br>**Robert R,**<br>**born 1947)**<br><br>**Postoperative**<br>**recovery** | As his recovery progressed, we learned how to manage the LVAD, me more so as Robert's short-term memory had been much incapacitated. At 56 years of age, being on the cutting edge of technology was daunting to say the least. I'd only just learned how to use a computer, and I had to be hauled out of the primeval swamps and into the 21st century by my children to do that!<br><br>I read that book from cover to cover. I practiced hand pumping, changing the batteries, identifying alarms, even changing the controller if need be — surely the most awkward set of instructions ever. I began to feel confident; I could manage this. Then came the day that they told me to make arrangements for him to go home; he was going to be discharged. I would have done anything to stay in that hospital. |
| **Jill**<br>**(partner of**<br>**Robert R,**<br>**born 1947)**<br><br>**Discharge**<br>**planning** | The sheer contemplation of going home was a nightmare. I have never felt so alone as I did the day he was discharged. That was when learning to live with the LVAD really began. Just getting used to the noise (surely it was never that loud in the hospital) and sleeping with it. The first night, I was so relieved when I woke up the next morning and he was still alive. |
| **Jill**<br>**(partner of**<br>**Robert R,**<br>**born 1947)**<br><br>**Learning the**<br>**battery supply**<br>**logistics** | But I/we learned, sometimes very fast. I had developed a system to make sure that each day when we left for the office 80 miles away, I had adequate batteries and supplies and Robert's batteries had enough juice in them to get him to the office. I was his driver, and at that time he was still having problems remembering the sequence of events when changing his batteries. Heaven knows I didn't want to fight four lanes of I-80 E traffic to the shoulder to change them. It only happened once. |

**Jill**
**(partner of**
**Robert R,**
**born 1947)**

**Emergency at**
**home: power**
**outage**

We learned to keep a flashlight by the bed the hard way too. One Saturday night, we were awakened from a sound sleep by the loudest alarm I have ever heard. I fell out of bed and groped for the light switch. Nothing. Total darkness. We realized that a power cut had occurred. Trying to remember which end of the power unit the charged batteries were, I managed to change Robert from the power unit to his batteries. We both fled the room before we went insane.

I returned to shut off the alarm, but nothing I did worked. I called the hospital, who alerted the person on duty, Margaret Flannery. She suggested other things, but nothing would shut the alarm off. So on her advice, I covered it with pillows and blankets and shut the door. I called the electric company, who I may add had already been advised of Robert's situation. They had assured me that they had heard and inwardly digested what I had said. However, when I reminded them, they had no record of it and the lady on the phone didn't understand what I was saying.

A car wreck just up the road from us had taken out a power line. So we waited. Robert and the dog went to sleep, I chewed on my fingernails, and Margaret kept checking on the situation. Eventually, after several hours and still no word from the electric company, I called them back. No, they had no idea when the power would be back on. I reiterated that I needed to know. "Why?" she said somewhat exasperatedly, "What will happen if it doesn't?" "He could die," I said. There was a long silence before she said, "I think I better call the foreman." "I think you'd better," I said. The power came back on an hour or so later.

**Jill**
**(partner of**
**Robert R,**
**born 1947)**

**Kids' interest**

On a lighter note, it amused us that children were so fascinated by the noise. They'd be near him, trying not to stare at this man who made funny noises. Sometimes we explained and, believe me, Robert would be right up there with the Power Rangers.

| | |
|---|---|
| **Jill**<br>**(partner of**<br>**Robert R,**<br>**born 1947)**<br><br>**Daily life**<br>**restrictions** | We livened up a couple of restaurants whenever the alarm to change the batteries went off. It was difficult to tell sometimes just how much they were charging, and it seemed as though we were always changing them for new ones. Robert, ever the engineer, questioned from the start the type of batteries used. "Why so big? Why so heavy?"<br><br>Water loomed large in our lives. Robert never did feel secure about the shower kit. He opted for very thorough washing. The day the garden hose covered him with water gave us a few anxious moments until we were quite sure that the controller hadn't been soaked. He missed fishing from his boat and swimming. The summer of 2002 was very hot. We had a pool, but Robert couldn't go in it. I dressed the driveline exit wound in absolutely sterile conditions and it paid off: we have had no infection problems that I am aware of. |
| **Jill**<br>**(partner of**<br>**Robert R,**<br>**born 1947)**<br><br>**Love life** | Sometimes, Dr Deng, I thought you had an overly healthy interest in our love life. I cannot think why. The LVAD is not conducive to the most romantic of sex lives. As the pace mounts, so does the noise. The first time, I was convinced that he would expire before he ever reached a climax. After a while, we became less anxious. What with drivelines, power lines, and batteries, the whole act could resemble a comedy routine. |
| **Jill**<br>**(partner of**<br>**Robert R,**<br>**born 1947)**<br><br>**Daily life** | Then there was the clothing situation. We never really have solved the problem of not bending the lines back. As for carrying those batteries, I bet we bought every type of fishing vest under the sun, but the holsters made Robert's back ache. |
| **Jill**<br>**(partner of**<br>**Robert R,**<br>**born 1947)**<br><br>**Philosophical**<br>**reflection** | The LVAD had a most profound effect on our lives. But we were most grateful to get it, for without it Robert would not be alive today. Despite its problems, awkwardness, and inconvenience, we managed to cope. After a while, our lives took on some semblance of normality. Upon reflection and looking on the positive side, for me it was a very |

affirming time. I felt that in bringing him through it all, I/we had really achieved something. A small victory over middle age. But to be honest, the one thing that helped to make it bearable was the knowledge that a heart transplant would happen in the future.

**Jill (partner of Robert R, born 1947)**

**Heart transplant is coming up**

After some "dry runs", he got his new heart. In true Rob's fashion, he drove himself to his own transplant. We had just 2 hours to get from our home in Pennsylvania to the hospital, and the low-battery alarm went off as we crossed the George Washington Bridge. He wouldn't stop for me to reach over and change them. "Great", I thought, "he is going to die before we get there." But we made it, and to this day I am in awe of his courage that night. I asked him how he could be so calm, and his answer was, "I am an engineer, Jill. It is very logical. I see the problem, I know what has to be done, and I'm going to do it."

**Jill (partner of Robert R, born 1947)**

**Conclusion**

We are so grateful to all of you for everything you have done and continue to do. Dr. Deng, I wish you a very happy new year and may all your dreams come true.

**Case summary: Helen M (born 1969)**

Helen M, born in 1969 and a married lawyer with one daughter, was diagnosed with dilated cardiomyopathy (likely caused by viral myocarditis) in 1997. She had an embolic stroke in 2000, and was listed for heart transplantation in 2002. Since her heart failure severity progressed, she required biventricular MCSD implantation in June 2002 (Thoratec PVAD BiVAD) with a post-MCSD course complicated by bleeding, kidney failure, and infections. In August 2002, she underwent heart transplantation and went home 3 weeks later. Since then, she has founded a patient support group focusing on young female heart transplant recipients and their specific situations, and has traveled to Italy with her husband and daughter.

**Helen M
(born 1969)**

**Experience
on BiVAD**

Dr. Deng, I apologize for taking so long to write this vignette about my experiences on the BiVAD. Obviously, there was a huge psychological barrier that I needed to overcome before I could write this (being on the BiVAD was, bar none, the worst experience of my life). My father said it best: "Why can't we just forget it ever happened?" Not an option for me, of course, but an interesting idea. So, here are some words about my experiences on the BiVAD.

**Helen M
(born 1969)**

**Filtered
information
during BiVAD
support**

My husband has told me that I was only the 13th person in the northeast to be on a biventricular assist device (BiVAD). I possess a sarcastic sense of humor, so my first inclination was to wryly say, "Lucky number thirteen." Truth be told, I am lucky. I know from other sources that Number 12 did not make it.

This is what characterizes my time spent on the BiVAD: information received secondhand, from other sources, filtered, sterilized, in the same way people bathed themselves in disinfectant when they came to visit me. I could not gather my own information, much to my chagrin, due to weakness and immobility. So, I waited for the information to make its way to me, slowly, piece by piece, especially the one piece of information I so fervently craved: that I would be free of the BiVAD because a heart had been found for me.

**Helen M
(born 1969)**

**Concepts of
disease**

The first information I received on the BiVAD came just after I opened my eyes. My husband leaned over me, as if he had been waiting for me to awaken, I think because he wanted me to know immediately before I realized on my own what had happened. He said, "Helen, they had to put two pumps on you and they couldn't put them on the inside." I was confused, thinking that this would be the way I would have to spend the rest of my life, with these pumps outside my body. How would I dress? I'd have to buy all new clothes. Where do you buy clothes with stretchy waistbands? How would I go to the beach? Would I wear a muumuu to hide my pumps?

I spent a lot of time being confused, wracked with pedestrian thoughts. For example, my kidneys failed while I was on the BiVAD. The doctors came and told me, almost offhandedly, not to worry, for they would give me a heart-kidney transplant. And I wondered, how would you lie in bed with a heart-kidney transplant? You can't lie on your back because of the kidney, and you can't lie on your stomach because of the heart. I resolved not to get a heart-kidney for this reason: I did not want to recuperate standing up.

| | |
|---|---|
| **Case summary: Joseph Y (born 1930)** | Joseph Y, born in 1930 and a married IBM engineer in retirement with three adult children, underwent coronary artery bypass grafting and mitral valve surgery in 2002. He underwent destination MCSD implantation with the Heart-Mate I in May 2004, after researching the internet for possible options and referring himself (upon consultation with his local cardiologist) to Columbia for this reason. After the HeartMate I device failed in November 2005, he required an exchange to the HeartMate II MCSD. He now leads a happy and productive life, appearing on TV shows to promote destination therapy and helping his wife do the dishes. |
| **Joseph Y (born 1930)** **Big batteries and quality of life** | My life during the day evolves in segments of 5–6 hours, i.e. the time before I have to change the batteries. There is great discomfort in carrying two 2-lb batteries and in fitting into normal clothing. The batteries bulge, and make you look obese and uncomfortable. |
| **Joseph Y (born 1930)** **General hospital and LVAD** | I had a mishap not related to the heart, and had to be taken by ambulance to my local hospital. The emergency room physician wanted to check me in, but insisted that either my wife or son, both of whom have been trained to handle the LVAD equipment, stay with me round the clock because no one in the hospital knew about the LVAD. |

| | |
|---|---|
| **Joseph Y (born 1930)**<br><br>**Noise and LVAD** | People I meet, friends, and physical therapists ask me, "What is the noise you're making?" I have to explain to them that it is the pump that makes the noise. That leaves them bewildered. They ask if this is a permanent noise or a temporary noise. |
| **Joseph Y (born 1930)**<br><br>**Philosophy** | All of this is worthwhile, because my quality of life has improved dramatically and I am able to write about it!! |
| **Joseph Y (born 1930)**<br><br>**The role of the caregiver** | One of the essentials I have learned is that the caregiver (my wife) must not only have knowledge of the LVAD equipment, know how to change the dressing, and handle matters such as vital signs and other related procedures; but must also be patient, efficient, and dedicated. In addition, my wife has to be understanding regarding the limitations of our lifestyle. |
| **Wife of Joseph Y (born 1930)**<br><br>**Husband living with destination LVAD** | Observation from caregiver: There is a tendency (on the part of the patient) to want prompt and immediate attention given to any matter that comes up, making things (sometimes of little significance) urgent that must be handled on his terms. This seems to be in the context of making life significant every moment; hence, an awareness of the ultimate reality for a patient in this predicament (i.e. with an LVAD).<br><br>My husband (the patient) cannot or will not go to the following: the theater, movies, libraries, professional meetings, supermarket checkout lines — all because of the noise of the pump. He feels that it keeps him from going to places that are quiet. In his words, "If I'm in the proximity of people in a quiet place or even in the waiting room of doctors' offices, people stare at me because they wonder where the sound (the pump) comes from." |

He is frustrated about going on cable at night and not being able to walk into another room of the house. For example, "If I want a drink from the kitchen or if I want to join the family in another room, I can't because I am tied to the PBU." The caregiver has to become accustomed to what I term sedentary behavior. Activity is limited or carefully selected by my husband.

**Case summary: Peter P (born 1947)**

Peter P, born in 1947, suffered a myocardial infarction in 1999, for which he underwent emergency bypass surgery at an outside hospital. Unfortunately, he required transfer to Columbia University Medical Center for HeartMate I MCSD implantation in August 1999, followed by heart transplantation in November 1999. After discharge, he now leads a happy and productive life.

**Peter P (born 1947)**

**LVAD and noise**

While in a crowded elevator, there were a few moments of silence. My LVAD became the only sound heard by the passengers. A young lady at the back became very alarmed and asked, "Oh my, what is that sound? Is there something wrong with the elevator?" I quickly replied in my best southern drawl, "No, honey, it's my heart going pitter-patter over you." My traveling companion, aware of my condition, started laughing out loud.

**Peter P (born 1947)**

**Return to normal life: car racing**

As I have always been an avid car enthusiast and racer, I participated in an autocross (a high-speed course navigated through pylons in a large parking lot). Some of the participants who were aware of my condition moved jokingly to create a special handicapped class for me. I subsequently led the field with first place in my usual class and forgot about any handicaps.

| Peter P (born 1947) LVAD and love life | A few weeks after returning home from all the operations and wearing an LVAD, my wife and I attempted to have sex. I wore the battery packs to give me more flexibility, but that proved to be dangerous as I bruised my wife with them. So, I quickly unplugged them and connected myself to the charger. Now, I was limited to a 5-foot radius from the equipment. |
| --- | --- |
| Peter P (born 1947) Movie theatre | One day, my wife and I decided to go to a movie theatre. As the audience settled down and became silent to await the beginning of the movie, the sounds from my LVAD became very noticable. People directly in front of us started to look around in search of the sound. I quickly grabbed my winter leather jacket and suffocated the noise as best as I could. Luckily, the movie started and nobody took further notice. |
| Peter P (born 1947) After heart transplantation | Five months after my heart transplant, my family decided to go on vacation to Club Med at Columbus Isle. Both my wife and I are avid scuba divers. So I checked with Columbia, and they reluctantly agreed to let me go. We went out with a group to a famous reef location where we could see sharks, barracudas, and other sea creatures. The dive was wonderful. |
| | When I returned to the boat and removed my wetsuit jacket, the dive master noticed the very long scar on my chest. He asked what had happened to me. I promptly answered, "I had a heart transplant a few months ago." His jaw dropped to the floor and he asked with trepidation, "Does your doctor know what you just did?" I asked him if he could keep a secret (in jest). |
| Peter P (born 1947) Battery charge emergency | About 2 months after my quadruple bypass and LVAD surgery, I was sent home. I went to work and commuted about half an hour to my office. One day, as I joined the rush hour crowd and entered the ramp to the New Jersey Turnpike, I noticed that it was not moving. The average |

timeline for my batteries was about 4 hours. I had replaced them with my last set of charged batteries, as usual, about 3 hours before the end of the workday. I sat in the car counting the minutes as they went by and worrying about my batteries.

An hour later, I had progressed about halfway home. I got the pump out of the pouch within inches of where it was supposed to be hooked up, and got everything loose and ready for a quick transfer. Luckily, I made it home with a few minutes left on my batteries. After that, I got an extra pair of batteries from the hospital and they have remained in the car.

**Case summary: Eric G (born 1950)**

Eric G, born in 1950 and married with two grown-up daughters, suffered a heart attack in 1990 and a repeat heart attack in October 2005 that nearly killed him. He underwent emergency transfer to Columbia University Medical Center, followed by short-term MCSD implantation with the Impella in October 2005, and converted to the HeartMate I for long-term MCSD implantation in November 2005 after being listed for heart transplantation. After the heart transplantation in February 2006, he was discharged home and has since returned to a normal life.

**Eric G (born 1950)**

**Decision by family for LVAD**

It wasn't exactly like I had a choice in the matter, the matter being the actual use of the equipment. I had a heart attack one Saturday afternoon in the fall of 2004. Although I appeared to those around me as if I had my wits about me, the fact is that I have no recollection of anything that happened over a 2-week period. The memory lapse spans from the moment I passed out at home, while waiting for the paramedics to take me to the hospital, until 2 weeks later, when I woke up in a coronary care unit in one of New York's most prestigious hospitals. My wife and children made the decision for me and I'm going to have to live with it for the rest of my life.

| Eric G (born 1950) Accepting the LVAD decision | Somewhere in the fog of semiconsciousness, my family and the medical staff repetitiously explained to me what had happened and the medical treatment that had been given to me. But I don't recall any of it. I do recall being aware of wires and "stuff", perhaps even that something had been implanted in my system to supplant my failed heart. The fact that my heart was so damaged that I now needed a transplant was somehow just part of the scheme. No terror, no panic, no shock, just acceptance: it is what it is. An term unknown to me before this point in time — LVAD — is now my primary focus in life. |
|---|---|
| Eric G (born 1950) Description of HeartMate I device | It sounds simple and I suppose it is. Then, there's the reality: the realization that for my immediate (and possibly longer-term) future, I have a leash. In my chest is a titanium drum about 4 inches in diameter and about 2 inches thick. It's attached via tubing to my heart and my aorta. Then, there's that tube sticking up out of my belly that connects to an air vent and the controller unit, which in turn connects to the power for this device. During the day, I have batteries that have to be charged and ready 24/7. Even to walk down the block to see my neighbors, I need a hand pump just in case the batteries die, a cable breaks, or a controller fails; if I don't manually pump the device in these scary scenarios, I will die. The controller is the brain behind the pump's ability to keep me alive. It is directly and securely attached to the tube that is sticking out of my belly. It is always with me. On the positive side, it isn't terribly large (perhaps $4.5'' \times 5'' \times 1''$) and it weighs practically nothing. The controller requires two power connections. |

In order to maximize living with an LVAD, the developers gave the unit two ways to be powered. During the day, the unit uses two rechargable batteries. Remove one or the other without replacing it quickly, and an alarm will sound: the system will admonish you. There are two power sources, even though one might be strong enough; there's no "safety" with just one power source. The first time you hear the alarm, you will panic, although you know what it means (change the battery a little faster). Really, is it just the battery or have I accidentally ended my life? Just the battery, whew.

At night, my leash is electric. A power base unit (PBU) is plugged into the wall. It has two cords that plug into the two cords on my controller. By changing one battery to AC and then the second battery to the AC, a continuity of power is maintained and no alarms sound. I have a range of about 20 feet at my disposal. Luckily, we worked out how to include both the bed and the bath inside that length.

But wait, there is no battery! What if the power fails tonight? Storms can happen at any time, a tree could fall and snap the power lines; through no fault of my own, I would be dead. However, the base unit has a safety battery built in. If the unit stops improperly, alarms sound and an internal battery that isn't obvious from the outside takes over, thus giving me precious minutes to reattach batteries. The rechargable batteries last only 4–6 hours; even with several sets, the batteries last for just 20—24 hours. Therefore, as another safety measure, there's a massive battery pack (almost the weight of a car battery) that is good for 24 hours.

**Eric G
(born 1950)**

**Daily life with
HeartMate I**

Sleeping with an LVAD isn't as challenging as one might suppose. It takes time to position the wires and to comfortably move them, so that you can turn a bit without pulling on anything critical and waking yourself up. As the chest heals, more and more movement becomes possible. Within days, comfortable sleep is possible. After 2 months, I was almost on my stomach, but not quite! That titanium drum is formidable.

After a short time, it's easy to become comfortable with the unit, much like the comfort one experiences in the presence of a recently tamed wild animal: unfailing trust, but with one eye always open. You can't forget that you have an LVAD, not even for a minute. Are the batteries charged? Am I connected to the base unit? Where is the manual pump and what if I have to use the damn thing?

A normal daily life is attainable, but there is the constant reminder of the reality. A fair analogy would be Poe's "The Telltale Heart": 80 times a minute, 60 minutes an hour, 24 hours a day, you can hear the pump moving your blood. But unlike the silent pounding in your chest that you're accustomed to, this sound is broadcast to everyone around you. At home, it's a constant reminder to you and to your family of what has transpired and what is to be.

Each day becomes a little better than the last. In the beginning, the idea of leaving the house is absurd. The fear of the device, the awareness of the noise, and not wanting to be noticed are all very much in the forefront of your mind. Then one day, it happens. You go out. Someone looks at you in a strange way and you realize that they are hearing the LVAD, but you aren't. Unabashedly, you say something out loud to answer their silent question: "It's a pump helping my heart." This may end the conversation or it may not. In either case, you are living with this beast in your chest and you're okay with that.

If you're very lucky, you get to the point of full acceptance by both you and your family. That point came for me one night when we were watching TV. My daughter turned to me and said, "I can't hear my show, and you're going to have to either turn that thing off or go in the other room." It's a good thing she loves me; she made sure I could watch what I wanted to in the other room.

It's a challenge, but it's not insurmountable. Once things fall into place, it is workable. Sometimes frustrating, sometimes infuriating; but always workable. Bathing in a tub and swimming are forbidden and for good reason. Movies and quiet restaurants might be difficult. However, with a little planning, most of everything else is possible.

I was able to exercise and regain my strength. I was able to work, play, and drive. I went shopping, and I went to Christmas dinner with my family. Assume that there's a way to do what you want, and then find the way. Ask for help; this is no time to go it alone.

I didn't make the original decision, but in hindsight it was the right decision. There's a balance between staying alive and quality of life. My heart attack was as serious as it gets, but the LVAD gave me the opportunity to recover. I wanted to recover. In the end, my quality of life was not seriously impacted and I am staying strongly alive.

I said that my family made the decision for me. The doctors were concerned about how I would react. My older daughter caught the essence of it. She told them, "He loves all those technical things and he'll think it's totally neat." To think it's "totally neat" might be extreme, but clearly she knows me well. Rarely does a day pass that I don't think, "Unbelievable, it's working."

If you want to keep the LVAD in perfect perspective, consider this very simple question: what's the alternative? To accept the LVAD and all that it entails requires a very simple philosophy: "It is what it is." The device is installed, it's working, and it's helping to make me stronger for the long term. With little exception, the LVAD does not stop me from doing anything that I could do before the implant. It may take creativity, but that's okay. Without it, however, life as I know it would be over and I'm just not ready to go.

**Janice (wife of Eric G, born 1950)**

**Referral for MCSD**

I first heard the word LVAD when we were at Mountainside Hospital, where my husband was taken by EMTs after he passed out at our home. The on-call cardiologist came out and told us that this hospital had done all they could for him, but they were just not equipped to provide any more assistance. His heart attack was much more serious than we thought. My husband was sitting up, talking to our children and seemingly stable. He was fooling us. The staff ensured us that he was absolutely **not** stable. He was about as critical as one could get.

The doctor called Columbia Presbyterian Hospital and had him transported there because it is one of the premier transplant hospitals. They also had this device that might be able to help my husband, something called an LVAD. Two things in that statement terrified me: "transplant", a term I was familiar with; and "LVAD", a term unknown to me, which was even scarier. My husband would end up needing both of these things. The LVAD would come first and would be a bridge to an eventual heart transplant.

**Janice (wife of Eric G, born 1950)**

**MCSD training**

First came the training for the LVAD. In the beginning, it was scary, especially when things had to be done speedily. There was also the worry that the controller would malfunction. Hopefully, I would not have to be the one to change it if it did fail. That was the most difficult and potentially dangerous part of the training process.

Once my husband was home, I was more confident because he was quite capable of switching from battery to machine and back again. He is much more technologically savvy than me; his ability helped me get through it. The noise at times was loud and distracting; but for the most part, acceptable. At times, sleeping was quite a struggle because of the buzz of the machine and its projected light. But, as with anything else, we got used to it. He had to make more daily sacrifices than me, even down to the way he could shower. But this was a new life that we all had to accept, so that's what we did.

**Daughter of Eric G (born 1950)**

**Evaluation and preparation for MCSD**

My mother, my younger sister, and I waited with baited breath as the seconds ticked by to hear of any news or changes. Nothing was stable anymore. If my father, the most constant, indestructible force in my life, could be unconscious and in such critical condition, then everything was up for grabs. The world as I knew it was about to change, but his world ... his world was about to be flipped left, right, and upside down.

All I really heard when the doctors talked about the LVAD was that my dad would have to be attached to a machine. Oh my God. Oh my God. The tears poured out. Hooked up to a machine? My dad was 54, in great shape, and incredibly active. What kind of life could he possibly have now? Oh my God, please, no, no, no. My father had been unconscious for days now, after what should have been a fatal heart attack. It was overwhelming to me that he had no idea what was going on. I hoped that he was having wonderful dreams because when or if he woke up, it would be into the middle of a nightmare. I just wanted him to sit up and ask, "What's for dinner?" (This, by the way, was what my father said to the doctors while he was on the stretcher having his first heart attack, a mild one though it was, 15 years ago. Yup, always the funny guy.)

**Daughter of Eric G (born 1950)**

**Preoperative consent for MCSD**

The doctors asked for our consent to put my father on the LVAD "just in case". They were going to try and do a bypass, but they wouldn't be able to discern what needed to be done until they opened him up. They sort of explained what the LVAD was, but we all had such faith in my dad's strength that we believed it wouldn't be necessary. However, when the doctors saw his heart, they had no choice. I felt so bad for him. I pitied him. I was so upset for him, or rather for his upcoming struggle.

It took some time (and sleep) to give me a bit of clarity on the matter. I realized that if he did have to live with the LVAD, well, at least he'd be living — the most important thing, after all. My dad is so inventive and a relentless fighter; I knew he'd figure out a way to deal with the LVAD, both physically and emotionally. In fact, being a computer whiz, he'd probably think it was kind of cool. For the battery packs that he would have to wear if he wanted to be mobile, I imagined him concocting some sort of harness/sling to better carry the weight. And you know what? When my father woke up after the LVAD had given him another chance at life, that's <u>exactly</u> what he did.

**Daughter of Eric G (born 1950)**

**MCSD–transplant transition**

My dad just had a heart transplant 3 weeks ago. Three months on the LVAD made that possible. It is still a struggle. He'll have to constantly be on medication to prevent his body from attacking his new heart, but at least he won't be attached to something every waking (and sleeping, for that matter) moment of his life ... right? Well, maybe.

The thing is, the LVAD was seemingly and comfortingly fail-safe. There were always options: the batteries, the base unit, the independent power generator in case there was a blackout, even the hand pump. It is a machine, and I think my dad trusts technology more than he trusts his own body's capabilities. He knows electronics and programs; he has mastery over them. The body's mechanics, though, will do what they will. With the removal of the LVAD, my dad's life is back in the hands of the doctors; he has been stripped of his control.

So even though the LVAD is not the most convenient lifestyle accessory, it has its benefits, living being the primary one of course. Having a new, healthy heart was always the goal of placing my father on the LVAD; but now that he has one, he almost misses that titanium metronome and the semi–sense of control it brought with it. Well, almost!

**Case summary: Abraham M (born 1940)**

Abraham M, born in 1940, underwent bypass surgery and, after a repeat heart attack, required HeartMate I MCSD implantation in August 2004. Subsequently, he underwent heart transplantation in October 2004, and has since returned home to lead a normal life.

**Betty (wife of Abraham M, born 1940)**

**Referral for MCSD**

Our story begins on the morning of July 22, 2004. When my husband awoke very early, we had breakfast and he went back to bed. When he reawoke, he complained of feeling chilly; he said that he was cold. My daughter called and I told her, "I don't know what's happening with daddy, he says that he has the chills." She advised me to call an ambulance. My husband did not want us to fuss.

My daughter and son-in-law ran over to appraise the situation. A short while later, Abe was taken to South Nassau Hospital with my son-in-law. While we waited for him to be transported to Columbia Presbyterian Hospital, we went through a large pallet of feelings.

Finally, under the directions of Dr Simon Maybaum, Abe was transferred to Columbia. We all knew that Columbia was our only hope. As excited, happy, tense, and nervous as we were, the sight of two ambulances surprised us. You may wonder and ask why two as we did, and the answer that we were given was just in case something broke down. We can't even begin to tell you how nervous we were at a time like this. However, the kindness and the gentle way of the cardiac staff at South Nassau Hospital and the ambulance drivers gave us strength. The sight of the two ambulances was an assurance that my husband was in good hands.

**Betty (wife of Abraham M, born 1940)**

**Evaluation for MCSD**

When we arrived at Columbia Presbyterian Hospital, Dr Farr was covering for Dr Simon Maybaum. She made sure she spoke to the whole family. Dr Farr advised us that the committee would decide if Abe would be a candidate for the LVAD. The next day, we were called and told that he was going to be operated on, and that I needed to get there as soon as possible to sign the release form for him to be operated on. We were very happy that they had approved him for the LVAD. We did not know that this was a last resort.

Dr Naka did not want to operate because he thought that there was another factor to Abe's condition, and he was correct. Abe had an infection, so they put the LVAD operation on hold and the group began taking care of Abe to get rid of the infection. Within a few days, he was taken off the respirator and started to come back to himself. He was stable and moved to a regular room. On August 5, we found out that he would have the LVAD operation the next day.

| | |
|---|---|
| **Betty (wife of Abraham M, born 1940)** **Meeting the LVAD** | The next day, Dr Oz came and sat with my husband and the family, and explained everything to us. He brought an LVAD with him to show my husband what would be going into his body. He went over how the LVAD works, and he made sure to allow my husband to discuss anything that was on his mind. He made him feel how heavy the LVAD was, and he explained that he would have this 3-pound machine in his body. I remember one specific question that Dr Oz asked my husband: "Are you afraid?" Abe answered, "No, you have to trust the doctors and the technology that the LVAD will work." Dr Oz went on to explain to my husband that the LVAD makes a sound and that he wouldn't be able to play poker, because when the machine works harder and faster, you can hear it. |
| **Betty (wife of Abraham M, born 1940)** **MCSD surgery** | The next morning, Friday, August 6, Abe was taken in and was given an LVAD. Dr Naka and Dr Oz performed the operation. In the middle of the night, they retook Abe into the OR because he was getting blood clots near his lungs. Dr Naka performed the operation, after which Abe started doing better. A few days later, Abe had arrhythmias and needed to be given the paddles. Had he not had the LVAD ... well, let's just say thank God he had the LVAD prior to the arrhythmias. |
| **Betty (wife of Abraham M, born 1940)** **Post-MCSD recovery** | After that, he began to improve. One day, we asked Dr Maybaum how he was doing and he said, "Because of the LVAD, we have rolled back 4 years of his heart's deterioration." After a while, he was able to go to rehabilitation. Abe was a new person. Physically, he was able to get his body back in shape. Although he was tethered to the machine and batteries, he was able to move around. I can't tell you that it wasn't scary and that we didn't have any questions. |

**Betty
(wife of
Abraham M,
born 1940)**

**View of the
MCSD concept**

The bottom line is that had the LVAD not existed, my husband would not have been around when a heart became available. The LVAD enabled him to get his body physically ready for when the heart became available. He was physically ready for it.

We owe a lot to the LVAD. It is a remarkable device. My family and I owe our future to the LVAD for three reasons. The first reason is the simple fact that the LVAD exists; the LVAD gave my family and me hope to endure while we waited for the heart. Secondly, the LVAD acted as a bridge until the doctors were able to find him a heart to replace his heart. Lastly and most important of all, the LVAD made his body strong enough to undergo the transplant operation.

Thank you to Dr Maybaum, Dr Naka, Dr Oz, the committee, the transplant group, and the staff who were there for us during the last few months every step of the way. You cannot imagine how nice and respectful everyone treated my family at Columbia Presbyterian Hospital. Columbia Presbyterian Hospital is a very special place.

**Case
summary:
Peter E
(born 1964)**

Peter E, born in 1964, suffered from dilated cardiomyopathy and required HeartMate I MCSD implantation in February 1997, followed by heart transplantation in October 1997. He subsequently returned home to lead a normal life.

**Peter E
(born 1964)**

**Living with
an LVAD**

My LVAD experiences, lets see … I was on the golf course that I manage with my then wife Christy chasing the geese (a big problem for sports turfs, parks, and golf courses). I was using a starter-like pistol that shoots whistlers to scare the geese. After we finished, we left the golf course, and we were driving along the road when an off-duty sheriff's officer who had been jogging at the nearby college campus cut me off and pulled me over. He had his gun drawn, thinking that my battery holsters were gun holsters!

The scariest and yet funniest incident, I guess, was at the September 1997 Rolling Stones concert at the Giants Stadium. I had tickets for two nights. The first night's seats were in the third row center. The opening band was fine; but when the Rolling Stones took to the stage, they were just into the beginning of the first song when my LVAD went into the fixed rate of 40 bpm with the alarm going off! Panic city!

I then proceeded to run under the stage with Christy to the first aid tent. I still felt very good. I found a doctor who knew what an LVAD was. He checked me and got me on an ambulance to Columbia Presbyterian. The pump was still alarming on the fixed rate. By the time I reached the George Washington Bridge, the pump had reset itself! I arrived at the emergency room (you know how nice that is!) with Margaret Flannery screaming at me, "Why the hell are you in the emergency room? Go to Milstein!!" I went home after being checked.

Needless to say, I had tickets to the next night's concert that were not quite as close to the stage, so I went. No sooner had the opening band (Foo Fighters) gone on when my pump began alarming and went to the fixed rate again. This time, we called the service and spoke to Dr Oz, asking him what we should do. We decided that although I felt fine, it would be better to go back to the hospital. Dr Oz's comment was, "I will meet you outside for the ticket stubs, okay?" He had me laughing! Another ambulance ride to NY. This time, the pump did not reset itself, and a tech was flown down from Boston to analyze the machine to find the problem. The pump reset itself the next morning. Two weeks later, I received the call from the hospital for the transplant.

Needless to say, I had spent a lot of money on those tickets, so I wrote a letter to the Stones' management to see if I could get my money back. Didn't happen.

**Case summary: Ed S (born 1956)**

Ed S, born in 1956, was diagnosed with heart muscle disease in 2000 after a viral flu-like disease. His heart failure condition worsened from July 2004 onwards, requiring listing for heart transplantation. He underwent MCSD implantation in September 2004, and heart transplantation in July 2005. After heart transplantation, he was discharged home and now leads a happy family and professional life.

**Ed S (born 1956)**

**Referral for MCSD**

I am a recipient of the HeartMate LVAD. I was diagnosed with cardiomyopathy in March 2000, and was told that I had an ejection fraction of 18%. I had caught a flu virus along with the rest of my family on New Year's Eve 1999. The rest of the family recovered, but I started to have the symptoms of congestive heart failure shortly after the new year. I was treated using drug therapy and functioned quite well for 5 years, save for a few hospitalizations with bronchitis, etc.

In June 2004, I was in the best physical shape I had been in for quite a while. I was swimming laps, working out on exercise machines, and doing quite a bit of walking and biking. In July, I went on vacation with my wife and 6-year-old son. I had a slight congestion sensation in my lungs. Within 2 weeks, I was laying on a couch for 2 weeks, not able to eat and only able to take sips of water without feeling bloated. To compound the problem, I knew of at least six people who were going through an intestinal virus of sorts, so I just assumed that I was going through the same things that they were experiencing. But, my liver and kidneys weren't functioning properly due to a lack of proper blood flow.

I have been a patient at Columbia Presbyterian Hospital since being recommended by my local cardiologist in 2001. I was admitted to the hospital on August 8, 2004, in serious condition. I responded to the intravenous medication, and after a month went home on the automatic pump system. I got sicker day by day, and after 10 days was readmitted back to the hospital, coughing constantly, damn near 24 hours a day, and unable to sleep for 3 days at a clip.

I walked into the CCU and was admitted. They told me they don't get many patients who walk into the CCU. Ha! Shortly after I arrived, the doctors who examined me said that I was in dire need of an LVAD and that I was on the heart transplant list.

**Ed S
(born 1956)**

**MCSD decision**

It was a pretty tough decision. The doctors and my family told me that it was the next logical step, a necessity. But I was the one who had to have the operation. And the thought of having my rib cage cracked open, having the doctors tap into my heart and aorta to install a 4-lb titanium pump in my chest cavity, was not appealing. I felt like I was a science experiment, and it sparked a bit of fear in me to say the least!

My doctor, Dr Rachel Bijou, was on her weekend off. I waited until she got back, because I wanted to hear her opinion as to whether I should have the pump installed and where I stood as far as options went. I took a leap of faith and agreed to the operation. The doctors here at Columbia Presbyterian have not steered me wrong, and I have a lot of faith in them.

**Ed S
(born 1956)**

**Postoperative
recovery**

I had the HeartMate installed on September 20, 2004. It was definitely not a walk in the park. I had never been sicker in my entire life before I had the operation; I was death warmed over! I was knocked down even lower after I had the procedure. My recovery was slow and painful. I needed 4 mg of morphine as needed to overcome the pain for about 2 months after the operation. I had trouble sleeping for a while after getting the pump. I've seen other patients who had the operation recover faster than myself, patients slightly older than myself. I turned 48 years old here in the hospital. I was given a box of Cheerios as a birthday present from the nursing staff! It took quite a while, but after 3 months or so the pain completely subsided.

| | |
|---|---|
| **Ed S (born 1956)**<br><br>**Living with MCSD** | I also wasn't too happy about not being able to swim anymore. But I have a 6-year-old son who is more important to me than being able to swim; and if I hadn't had the pump installed, I'm convinced that I would be doing the dead man's float anyway. Showering was a little difficult at first, but I've learned how to use the shower kit quite well with practice. I needed a lot of help at first, but I can do it by myself now and it doesn't take me as long. My lovely wife helps me with the dressing change. I've been fortunate in the fact that I haven't had an infection near the line that comes out of me for the pump. I'm careful to keep the site as clean as possible.<br><br>Slowly but surely, I have regained a lot of my muscle tone and my stamina has increased. My sleeping has returned to normal; after a month or two, I was able to sleep on my side without discomfort. Looking back over the last 7 months since I've had the pump, I can clearly see that it has saved my life. I was coughing so badly before I received the pump that I prayed to Almighty God that I would do anything if He would stop me from constantly choking and hacking. Well, He answered my prayers and sent me to Columbia Presbyterian Hospital! |
| **Ed S (born 1956)**<br><br>**Long-term social impact of MCSD** | I've had to go on total disability since I had the pump. The line of work I was doing required some physical prowess. I wasn't fortunate enough to have a profession that I could go back to with the LVAD, so I haven't figured out what to do yet. I'm in the hospital right now waiting for a heart transplant, but I'm one of the healthier patients here on the seventh floor. I'm alive, and that's a miracle of modern science. |
| **Ed S (born 1956)**<br><br>**Evaluation and patient decision** | While I was waiting to have the pump installed, I wasn't lucky enough to have someone who had had an LVAD installed and had recovered come in to see me so as to show me that it worked and that it wasn't as bad as I perceived it to be. I have gone to see a lot of patients |

awaiting the operation while I've been waiting here in the hospital for my transplant, and they usually light up with a little hope when they see someone walking around and functioning quite well with the pump.

If you saw me, you'd say that I don't even appear to be sick, which wasn't the case 7 months ago. The way I feel now, I don't think the recovery from the transplant will be as bad as the LVAD because the pump has allowed me to become a lot healthier than I was before. I'm glad I decided to go through with the process because there wasn't much hope any other way.

**Case summary: Joel L (born 1969)**

Joel L, born in 1969, suffered a rare form of acute inflammatory heart muscle disease called giant cell myocarditis in early 2002, requiring transfer to Columbia University Medical Center for emergency HeartMate I MCSD implantation in February 2002. Unfortunately, he suffered a stroke while on the MCSD, but underwent heart transplantation in April 2002 and returned to a normal life with chronic rehabilitation thereafter. In October 2005, he required retransplantation of the heart because of chronic rejection. He now wants to get married and win the Tour de France.

**Joel L (born 1969)**

**Living with the MCSD**

Dr Deng, I am here writing you with my thoughts on my LVAD experience from February 12, 2002, to April 6, 2002. I liked it since the device did the job of keeping me alive until a donor heart could be found. But during the time the unit was in me, it was very painful, causing me to need large doses of morphine and sleeping pills to get some rest at night. The size of it also kept me from eating a normal amount of food during mealtimes. I lost 50–60 pounds while I was a patient at Columbia. I would take just a few bites, and not be able to stomach any more. Being a small-framed man with a small body, the size of the unit was big in comparison to the size of the area in my abdomen. Patients with larger body types may not experience this, since they have more room to place the device. The noise of the LVAD was a bit distracting and loud, but I don't think much could be done about that. You can't really expect a chainsaw to be quiet, I suppose. All in all, I'm happy that it was used and that I'm alive to tell you my thoughts on its time in me.

**Deborah (mother of Joel L, born 1969)**

**Referral for MCSD**

You had asked quite some time ago for both Joel and I, and also his father and sister, to send you our thoughts about the LVAD. I had avoided this, as the emotions generated by putting onto paper those terrible months in 2002 were more than I could bear. But after reading Candy's book (Moose, 2005), I realized that we too had a story that should be shared.

From the moment I received the phone call from Dr Shuster on Monday, February 11, 2002, all color went out of my life and I saw the world in shades of gray. Joel had myocarditis, he said, and I was savvy enough to know that this meant Joel would need a heart transplant if he had any chance to survive at all. How did I know this so immediately, Joel's father had often asked. Probably from an article in *Women's Day* or *Ladies' Home Journal* about the courage of a family whose son got viral myocarditis. I can't be sure of the publication.

I was sitting at work at Beth Israel Deaconess Medical Center in Boston when the call came in. I immediately called my boss in the OR to tell him that I was leaving for an indefinite time, called Joel's father to tell him the news, and then walked out of my office, never to return again as an employee. I can't remember if I drove to my apartment in my own car or if I took a cab home. I remember throwing clothes in a bag, feeding my cat and leaving a key and a note for my neighbor to look after my cat, and then off I went to Stamford.

It was snowing heavily that day, the first snowstorm of 2002, and the road conditions were poor. At various points during the trip, I thought about pulling into a train station to take the train, but I knew I could not tolerate waiting for connections, and so I ignored the nearly white-out conditions and speeded along Route 95. I think I made it in record time even with the storm, arriving in Stamford just about 3 hours later.

Joel was in intensive care at Stamford Hospital when I arrived. He was upbeat, joking as he always was, and was busy watching the Winter Olympics. His major topic of discussion was whether the poster boy of those games, a speed skater, was going to win all that was predicted by the media.

Signs of Joel being ill? Some shortness of breath and the inability to urinate. Wow, maybe the doctor had over-called this one and all would be right in a few days. Joel was scheduled for an angiogram the next morning, and the results of this would tell us what the next step would be. Maybe this was only endocarditis with damage to one of the valves. Maybe he only needed a valve replacement, and he would be up on his bike again and back to normal. I prayed for this diagnosis, but foolishly worried about the sound that a mechanical valve makes and how that would impact on Joel's psyche. How naive I was!

The angiogram the next morning showed the worst-case scenario: Joel had myocarditis and needed to be transported to Columbia Presbyterian Hospital ASAP. Ironically, I had worked at CPMC in clinical pathology from 1965–1968, and his father had graduated from P&S in 1968. We met there while he was a medical student and I was working in the third-year medical students' clinical pathology laboratory on the medical floor. Now, all these years later, this was a sort of unwelcome homecoming for us.

Joel was transported by ambulance and his father, sister Alicia, and I drove to NYC after picking up a change of clothing. We had not been to the Medical Center in well over 20 years and had no idea of how it had changed. We instinctively went to Admitting Emergency on Broadway and 168th St., only to be told that he was in Cardiac Intensive Care of Milstein, a building that certainly did not exist during our tenure at CPMC. We ran down 168th St. to Fort Washington, and somehow made our way to the fifth floor of Milstein and Joel's cubicle. Gathered around him were interns, residents, medical students, and nurses.

Just a few days before, I had been given an article from the NY Times on "The Practice of Medicine" written by a young resident from Harvard. She had gone into great detail about how medical students learn to put in a central line and how painful this was to the patients. There, in the middle of this gaggle of medical personnel, was my son, crying out while a student/intern/resident was trying to put in a central line. "Stop!" I screamed. "You will not practice on my son!" I was quickly grabbed and pulled from the room, and was told that Joel was in grave condition and that this procedure was necessary to save his life. Soon after this, my niece who is a physician in NYC arrived at the hospital. She had been called from Stamford, told of Joel's condition, and she had alerted doctors she knew at CPMC that he was going there.

**Deborah (mother of Joel L, born 1969)**

**MCSD decision**

Dr Oz was the cardiothoracic surgeon on call that day, and he arrived, examined Joel, and explained Joel's condition of heart failure to us and to Joel. He explained that if Joel continued to fail and a heart was not available, then an LVAD could be implanted in him to augment his failing heart and hopefully keep him alive until a donor could be found. He asked for my permission to use the device and I could not give it. Joel was an adult. He needed to decide for himself if he wanted such a device put in him. He was the one to determine what his quality of life would be like, and whether this was what he could live with. To me, this was all too surreal and I could not deal with such a choice.

Dr Oz spoke with Joel, showed him pictures of the device, and told him that in all probability he would be up and walking with the device; if a heart was not immediately available, Joel could still go home with the device and maybe even go to work. Talk about naiveté. Joel called my niece Gail in and they discussed this. Gail felt strongly that this was Joel's only chance and she told him this, but emphasized that it was ultimately his choice. Within a very short time, his breathing became so labored that he asked for the device to be implanted. Much later, I discussed this time with Joel only to find out that he has no memory of any of this.

**Deborah (mother of Joel L, born 1969)**

**Preoperative situation**

I was called into his room to say goodbye to him and he was quickly sedated, intubated, and rushed off to the OR. Then the waiting began. We as a family waited on the fifth floor. After many hours, we got pillows and blankets and laid on the floor, trying to sleep. Some time in the early morning, Dr Argenziano (the surgeon who had implanted the LVAD) came to tell us that he was out of surgery, all had gone well, and we could see him briefly in the CTICU. I don't think any of the three of us was prepared for what we were about to see.

**Deborah (mother of Joel L, born 1969)**

**Postoperative situation**

Joel was hooked up to so many monitors and machines. He was intubated, and IVs were running into veins and arteries in his extremities and neck. Various machines were bleeping and blinking. And then there was the LVAD. This bigger-than-a-bread-box black box that had wires going into a wound in Joel's abdomen, whooshing and clicking; each whoosh and click keeping my beautiful son alive. I found myself staring at the machine, watching the digital read-out count beats and whatever else it counted. For the next 2 months, I guarded that machine, making sure no one touched it or tripped over its cord, looking at it as the essence of Joel's life.

Joel was a competitive cyclist before the myocarditis and he was extremely strong. He was able to ride 100 miles on his bike in the daytime and still go to work in the afternoon for a full 8 hours without missing a beat. He could carry in one hand things that took two men to carry. His postop nurse was a tiny Filipina and, although he was unconscious, he grabbed her and threw her across the room. Those first 24 hours, I delighted in his grabbing my hand and squeezing it until it blanched and I struggled to free myself. I would walk from one side of the bed to the other to have him grab at me. Joel was still unconscious and intubated, but I was assured that this was within normal range.

On the second day, I noticed that he was no longer grabbing with his left hand. I checked his reflexes on his left foot and found no reaction. I quickly called the staff, and after a gross examination he was taken for a CT scan, where it was horribly discovered that he had suffered an ischemic stroke. Oh God! My son! Paralyzed, unconscious, unresponsive, being kept alive by an ominous black box. Who was inside that body? Would Joel want to continue being that person? By now, his medical team had expanded to include neurologists and nephrologists. He was still not voiding. His creatinine was dangerously high and he was put on continuous dialysis. He was still unresponsive and unconscious. The neurologists called for another CT scan because they felt that he may have suffered another stroke.

The only sign of responsiveness Joel showed was to grimace in pain. I cried and prayed for him. I asked God to give him the strength to come back from all this, to wake up, to speak, to live, to just be Joel. Alicia and I sat for hours in the waiting room talking to other families and asking everyone to pray for Joel, as we would pray for their family members. I asked strangers on the street to please pray for him.

The CT scan showed that there was no further progression of the stroke, and all that was needed was time for him to regain consciousness. One morning, I walked into the room and saw a crash cart in his room. I turned to his medical student and asked why this was being stored in Joel's room, and he told me that Joel had to be cardioverted during the night. I remember falling into the wall and crying out with the realization that Joel was going to die. No one could assure me that this would not happen. No one knew and Joel was unconscious. In my mind, Joel was unconscious for weeks, but in reviewing his chart at a later date it seems that it was less than 2 weeks. Not for his family it wasn't; for us, it was an eternity.

I remember coming in one morning and finding him awake. He was still intubated and was not focused, but he was awake. We still did not know who was in Joel's body, and he was giving us no indication that he could think or recognize. Multiple times over the course of the next few days, the staff tried to extubate him, but he would bite down on the tube and they could not get his jaw to open. I am not sure when he was finally extubated, but it was a huge milestone. But even then, he would not speak, nor did he appear to know who we were or what was happening.

Finally, on a Sunday, with our dear Reb Terry present, he spoke his first words. I asked him as I did daily, "Do you know who I am?" "You are effing mom," he said. Yes, effing; not fucking because Joel did not swear: effing. That's Joel. He was there inside that poor, weak body, hooked up to all those machines, paralyzed, confused and scared, in pain; but Joel nonetheless.

I was overjoyed. If he never walked again, I would take care of him forever. I had my son back. But I had him tethered to that box, the LVAD. Although Joel was such a strong man, he is not a large man and the LVAD was really too big for his body. It constantly caused him pain. It took up too much space inside him and he was unable to eat more than one bite at a time. Not being able to move his left side made it impossible for him to get out of bed, but I am not sure that he could have anyhow. The device was causing him too much discomfort.

He was losing weight daily. His weight when he arrived at the hospital was somewhere around 155–160 pounds; by the end of March, it was around 103. He would feel hungry and ask that we bring him sandwiches and treats, and Alicia and I would gladly bring them in only to have him take one bite and stop eating. His body was breaking down and his heart was quickly failing.

**Deborah (mother of Joel L, born 1969)**

**Discharge**

Joel was transferred briefly to the seventh floor. During this time, I was asked to learn to care for the LVAD at home. I went through the motions of being shown how to clean the wires and check the machine, but I was saying to myself, "I don't think so." There was no way I was going home with Joel attached to that thing. I slept very little during this time, and I imagined sleeping even less were he able to come home. I imagined sitting there watching the digital read-outs, listening to the sounds and praying that there never be a blackout. To all the patients on an LVAD who went home and to all their families who cared for them during this time, I salute you. You have my utmost admiration. I have no idea how these people could withstand that kind of pressure.

Joel was not to go home. After just a short time on the seventh floor, he was transferred back to the CTICU for heart failure, to either await a heart transplant or die.

**Deborah (mother of Joel L, born 1969)**

**Pre-heart transplant**

On April 5, 2002, one of the cardiologists told me that if there was no heart over the weekend, there would probably be no Monday for Joel. They were willing to take an old heart, even a not completely healthy heart, just to allow Joel to live. That evening, Alicia and I were sitting in the third-floor waiting room, away from the tumult of the fourth-floor waiting room, when I picked up a newspaper lying on the table. The paper was open to the horoscopes page and I looked at Joel's. "You will have a change of heart," it read. How ironic!

Blessedly, on April 6, 2002, a heart became available. Not just a heart, but a healthy heart, a perfect match. Sadly of course, a family had lost someone, but they had made the decision to donate this person's organs so that others might live and so that the death of a 35-year-old man in NYC would not be in vain.

At Joel's bedside, waiting for the move to the OR with me was Alicia, my nephew and his significant other, my niece, and Alicia's girlfriend from Massachusetts who wanted to be there to give Joel strength. We chatted and joked and cheered Joel on throughout the day, and then some time before 7 PM they came to take Joel to the OR. The medical staff looked at me and asked me to pull the LVAD plug from the wall for the last time. I remember shaking as I went to the wall socket. I pulled the plug, and immediately we were all overwhelmed with the sound of silence. No whooshing, no clicking. The battery pack that controls the device does not make the same sound. Joel was free, and in a few hours his new life would begin.

You know the rest of the story. Joel has had his ups and downs since the transplant. He has regained so much of his strength, but not his balance from the stroke. He walks with a slight limp, and cannot move his hand and fingers as swiftly or deftly as before. His cognitive function is good, but not 100%. However, he works, he lives alone, he drives, he hikes, he plays the piano and guitar, and he knows more about sports then the whole of ESPN. He is being treated for a recurrence of the giant cell, and he will beat this as he has beaten everything else. He feels down, especially when the weather is good and the cyclists are out, but his will to live is so strong.

What you don't know and should know is that he answers questions on Jeopardy that we have no idea from where he would have learned the answers. For this reason, he has invented a biography of his transplanted heart: the brilliant 35-year-old man who worked on Wall Street, enjoyed decorating and cooking, and was educated in the humanities (probably with a Phi Beta Kappa). Joel, being the person that he is, does not want to know any reality of the soul who gave him his second chance at life. This would be too disturbing for him, and I and everyone else respect his wishes.

When you asked us to send you our thoughts on the LVAD, he asked me what you were looking for. I told him to send you his feelings about having had the device in him. I asked him if he was happy to be alive, and he unequivocally said yes. "Then the ends justified the means," I said. And that is the bottom line. Joel is alive.

We have him with us to share his life, to hear his laughter, to share his knowledge, to just be with him. For this, we are all grateful.

**Case summary: Travis B (born 1979)**

Travis B, born in 1979, fell ill with acute leukemia and underwent chemotherapy that included the drug adriamycin, which caused progressive heart failure. For this reason, Travis B underwent long-term MCSD implantation as a destination MCSD therapy in October 2002 because his cancer history presented a (temporary) contraindication for heart transplantation. After the remission of his cancer, he was accepted on the waiting list for heart transplantation, which he underwent in April 2005.

**Travis B (born 1979)**

**Living with the MCSD**

I do not have many stories for someone who had the LVAD for over 2 years. All LVAD patients need to know how to change their LVAD controller, and the LVAD makers need to do a better job of checking the spare controllers before they give them to people. It was not a problem for me because I was in the hospital. The night I was put on the pneumatic pump, I thought my controller had gone bad. The controller that I was using was my backup because I had to change controllers once during my first year with the LVAD. When I went to change controllers that night in the hospital, the spare controller went right to the red heart when I hooked it up. I was lucky that I never had to change my controller a second time at home, because I would have had to hand pump my LVAD for over 3 hours while driving to the hospital.

During my first year with the LVAD, I felt good enough to play golf until my left hip started to become painful. I stopped playing that fall. The hip limited what I could do on the LVAD during the second year.

Before I was sent to Columbia to have the LVAD implanted, I was at Bassett Hospital. While I was there, one of the residents asked my father and me if we would like to have her Thursday tickets to the 2003 Masters golf tournament. We said that if I was feeling well enough, we would be interested. Shortly after that, I was transferred to Columbia, where I received my LVAD on December 10, 2002.

The following April, we went to the Masters. That Thursday was cold and rainy. The play was canceled that day. On the way out of the golf course, we were interviewed by a reporter from an Atlanta newspaper. It was the first time ever that a day at the Masters had been totally canceled due to rain. During the trip, we also went to Nashville to visit my dad's family. On the way to Nashville, we called the family of the resident to thank them for letting us use her tickets and to tell them that we had made it into the newspaper. They felt so bad because we did not get to see any golf that they said that we could have their tickets for Sunday of the 2004 Masters. We went the next year and the weather was perfect.

We drove to Augusta and Nashville because flying presented too many problems. I did not think flying would be very safe because the PBU could get lost or damaged during the flight. The PBU would probably have been too big to take as a carry-on. I did not want to take the risk of getting to our destination and having the PBU broken in another city. You know how airlines tend to treat your luggage.

**Case summary: Herbert E (born 1930)**

Herbert E, born in 1930, underwent bypass surgery twice in 1973 and 2003, followed by worsening heart failure. Since he was not a heart transplantation candidate because of advanced age, destination MCSD implantation was recommended and performed with the HeartMate I in April 2005. Postoperatively, the patient suffered several complications, including refractory (untreatable) infection associated with the MCSD. His quality of life continuously deteriorated, and he requested the termination of MCSD support to be allowed to die peacefully. After consultation with the Columbia University Ethics Committee, his wish was granted. The MCSD support was turned off, and he died in January 2006 in the presence of his family.

| | |
|---|---|
| **Eileen (daughter of Herbert E, born 1930)** **Post-MCSD** | My father has mentioned to me that you would like to receive a copy of my son's essay about his grandfather. It is attached. My son's name is Jacob and he is 9 years old. We're flattered by your interest.

As you may know, Dr Naka is in the process of attempting to obtain a HeartMate II device for my father. Due to excessive scar tissue from many previous surgeries, the opening necessary to accommodate the HeartMate I cannot close and infection has resulted. Dr Naka feels that the HeartMate II is small enough to allow the skin to close, thereby avoiding constant infection.

Without the HeartMate II, it's pretty clear that my father has little or no chance of survival, as the infection will remain and only get worse. We understand that Dr Naka is going to present his case to the IRB in the next day or so. I should note that Dr Naka's efforts on behalf of my father have been extraordinary.

In addition to the medical considerations involved, you are well aware of the emotional and psychological aspects, as evidenced by your interest in my son's essay. Please consider whether you can be of any assistance to Dr Naka in fighting for a HeartMate II for my father.

Thank you very much for your interest, concern, and help. |
| **Jacob, age 9 years (grandson of Herbert E, born 1930)** **Post-MCSD** | **Trying to Fly**

Grandpa was sitting on a wooden patio chair, loafers on his feet. It was a sunny, breezy, hot day, the sun beating down from the baby blue sky. Beads of sweat danced down my face as I ran barefoot all the way across the lawn, all the way to Grandpa. I rested myself on Grandpa's lap, his face so close his breath tickled my ears. "Want to learn a lesson, Jakey?" Grandpa asked. All enthusiastically, I nodded my head, bouncing up and down, the only way a 4-year-old knows how to. So Grandpa said, "Everyone can fly in their own way ... everyone." Grandpa told me, for the very first time that day. I got all excited and flapped my arms, trying to fly. |

Grandpa and I were sitting on a satiny blue couch, flipping through picture albums, the black-and-white torn pictures haphazardly collaged on each page. My 5-year-old hands delicately turned the yellowing pages of the album, knowing how much it meant to Grandpa. A brisk winter storm was whipping outside, but Grandpa and I were safe and warm by the fire. I sat close, resting my head on his clean white polo shirt, it smooth against my cheek. And then, while we were staring at those old pictures, the faces staring back, faces I vaguely knew, in that silence so precious, Grandpa said, "Everyone can fly in their own way ... everyone." Grandpa told me, his voice soothing and calm. At that moment, I started to wonder what Grandpa meant.

As I tiptoed up the polished wooden stairs, my socks slipping and sliding, I saw Grandpa sleeping peacefully, curled up like a ball, wearing red plaid boxers and a thin white undershirt. I crawled into the blue-and-white patterned covers, thumping down, waking him from his doze. When he first woke up, he looked startled. He smiled widely at me, his silver hair messy and knotted, and gave me a tight good morning hug. Grandpa took one look at my 6-year-old head and exclaimed, "The wolf has arrived!" gleaming at his own joke. Though I didn't say it, his hair was worse than mine. Gingerly, Grandpa patted down my hair, I ruffled his, and thus the hair war began. At the end, we always had a contest on whose hair was messier. Grandpa usually won, but I'm not too unhappy about that, for it is a contest for the worst looks. When we were lying in bed, hushed for a moment, Grandpa said, "Everyone can fly in their own way ... everyone." Grandpa told me. "What do you mean, Grandpa?" I asked. Grandpa told me that the meaning would come when the time was right.

Grandpa sat on the cushioned strawberry silk chair, a newspaper covering his face, the headlines screaming. The autumn leaves were thick and many on the backyard lawn, brilliant yellows, rich crimsons, and dazzling oranges. I was playing with an antique perfume bottle, and even though it was empty, the smell of lavender perfume wafted off my hands. Grandpa said, "Hey! Watcha doing with my perfume?!" We both laughed, his laugh louder and richer than anybody else's; mine just a 7-year-old laugh, nothing special. I secretly admired Grandpa's laugh. I went to sit by him, me on the arm of the chair, Grandpa in the middle. He looked down and smiled a sweet Grandpa smile. "Everyone can fly in their own way ... everyone." Grandpa told me, his voice blanketed with love and emotion. The time was not yet right. Little did I know the time would come soon.

Grandpa sat on the green booth, a blue shirt on, bright against the dreary day outside. My mouth tingled from the warmth of the hot chocolate. We chatted about what we wanted, the news, ourselves, our feelings ... anything. The only Saturday morning I had ever imagined, chatting, sipping, nibbling, and being with Grandpa. Perfect. Grandpa called me over, ran his soft hands through my hair, and said, "Everyone can fly in their own way ... everyone." Grandpa told me. At the tip of my tongue, the answer was there, but I couldn't grab hold of it. The questions kept coming, but were left unanswered.

Grandpa was lying on the hospital bed, starched white sheets gauntly laid over him. Tubes and wires snaked out of him and down to the floor. A worn look washed across his face, a sorrow-sweet smile. I stood up, went over to Grandpa, and sat by his side. Tightly, Grandpa gave me a hug, his arms cradled around me. At that moment, I never wanted to let go, feeling safe in Grandpa's arms. But I did let go, and when I did Grandpa said, "Everyone can fly in their own way ... everyone." Grandpa told me, his voice a whisper. And at that very moment, it all made sense. Everything. All those years of wondering, and now it had finally come to me. "The right time is here, Jacob," Grandpa said to me. And on that day, I flew. I flew to the top of the world with Grandpa.

**Case
summary:
Ted L
(born 1943)**

Ted L, born in 1943 with a congenital heart disease called hypertrophic cardiomyopathy, spent his early years fully functional and became symptomatic as an adult. After having received consultations from leading experts in the country, he was placed on the waiting list of Columbia University Medical Center, and underwent HeartMate I MCSD bridge-to-transplantation implantation in April 2004 and subsequent heart transplantation in June 2005. He returned home as an activist for the cause of organ donation and patient communication.

**Ted L
(born 1943)**

**Perspective of
gratefulness**

My name is Ted and on June 24, 2005, I received a heart transplant. It was a miracle from God and a gift of life from a very generous 51-year-old woman and her immediate family, who at a time of profound grief found it in their hearts to donate their loved one's organs. I was told by the hospital that seven lives were saved because of their generous offer.

I want to thank the Columbia Presbyterian Hospital's heart transplant team — the cardiologists, surgeons, nurses, and staff. They are terrific specialists and wonderful, caring people. Over the last 18 months, they have become my family and friends.

**Ted L
(born 1943)**

**Living with
heart failure:
preoperative
perspective**

### My Early Years

I was born with a congenital heart disease that kept me from keeping up with my little playmates. But as I reached my high school years, I began to outgrow the problem and went on to enjoy college intramural sports and upon graduation skiing, squash, sky diving, and golf.

After graduating from Rollins College, I went to Wall Street to make my fame and fortune. I spent 20 hectic years in a bond-trading room, jumping up and down, yelling "buy!" "sell!" "you're done!" Then, I spent 16 years working as a financial planner with individuals and their corporations to develop a plan to cover all of life's contingencies.

During this time, in 1973, I met Trina Richner and within 5 weeks we were engaged. Since I had not seen a heart specialist in 20 years, I thought it best to get an updated diagnosis for my future bride and myself.

Dr Steve Scheidt at New York Presbyterian Hospital–Cornell Medical Center was recommended to me, and I spent several days undergoing diagnostic tests. His conclusion: I had a form of cardiomyopathy called idiopathic hypertrophic subaortic stenosis — an enlarged heart muscle. But since I was asymptomatic, there was little I needed to do. I had annual checkups with him for the next 20 odd years.

## My Medical Journey

In the early 1990s, I experienced my first heart problem: dizzy spells and skipped heart beats. Over the next decade, my cardiologist mixed and matched various medications as the problems grew progressively worse. By early 2003, I knew I was really in trouble as I was having difficulty walking a New York City block, having to stop four or five times to catch my breath. I developed the typical symptoms of a person with chronic heart failure. I had shortness of breath and edema that was particularly obvious when one looked at my ankles. Dr Steve Scheidt came to the conclusion that I should have a consultation with a leading heart specialist in cardiomyopathy, Dr Barry Maron at the Minneapolis Heart Institute. In May 2003, I spent a day undergoing tests with his team of six, and late in the afternoon we convened in his office to hear the results.

Let me read a few sentences from a recent correspondence of his.

> Dear Ted ... I often think about the day of our consultation and how awkward I felt about hitting you with such bad news that I know you didn't expect ... and using such severe medical terms as "end-stage hypertrophic cardiomyopathy" to emphasize the point that you needed to move fast ... which you did ... fortunately. Best Regards, Barry Maron.

I only had one question for Dr Maron: "The words 'end-stage' don't sound good to me. Just what are you telling me?" "Ted, you have 6 months to a year to live with that heart of yours."

Within a week upon return, I was interviewed by members of the Columbia Presbyterian Hospital's heart transplant team. I was told that I would make a good transplant candidate, but at that moment I was too healthy to be put on the heart transplant list. They would be most happy to follow my case. In 5 days, I went from "go home, move fast, you are dying and need a heart transplant" to "you're too healthy to be put on the list." Go figure!

At first I got mad, then I got angry and went into denial. But reality finally came upon me, and I began to ask God "why me?" Hadn't I spent the last 20 years as an active member of my church being as good a Christian as I could? I was even helping my community by serving on my cooperative building's Board of Trustees.

I also began to question my own body. Why had my body suddenly deserted me? For my entire life, my heart, mind, and body had all gone along together. If something bad happened to me, my body took care of it. Now, it was going off in a different direction and I had no control over it.

I began an emotional journey that has continued to this day. Once I began to learn about organ transplantation, I found that one out of three persons die while waiting for a new heart. Would I live long enough to get a new heart? I felt sorry for myself. Would the new heart take if I got one? How would it work? How long would it last? I thought a lot about my wife. If I died, was I leaving her in good financial shape? Who would she turn to for help? We had to make plans together.

One day, I came to the sudden realization that for me to live someone else had to die. I had been praying for God to get me a new heart from the beginning, but I couldn't imagine asking God to have someone else die so that I could live. I came around to the realization that if God wanted me to live, then he had a plan for me. What was it? If I was to get a new heart, what did he want me to do with it? That began a dialog between us that has continued right up to the present.

Dr Maron was right. My heart deteriorated rapidly to the point where I was having trouble walking from my bedroom to my kitchen by March 2004. Due to chronic heart failure, my body filled with 30 pounds of fluid surrounding my heart, lungs, and other bodily functions. It was most pronounced to the casual observer in my very swollen ankles.

**Ted L (born 1943)**

**The heart pump**

### The Heart Pump

On April 1, 2004, I was rushed to Columbia Presbyterian Hospital and almost checked out before I checked in. I was one very sick fellow. Dr Donna Mancini, the head of the heart transplant unit, and Dr Yoshifumi Naka, one of the specialists in heart surgery, told my wife that I was too sick for a transplant and that the only course of action was to implant a heart assist device in my chest: an LVAD (left ventricular assist device). It would take over for my heart's main pumping chamber, the left ventricle. Dr Naka did this on April 13, 2004.

The LVAD was implanted in my chest and was very obvious to anyone within 15 feet of me. First, it was physically intimidating. It was just under the skin of my chest and weighed 5 pounds. It was 5 inches in diameter, 2 inches thick, and had an external tube coming out of my chest for the electrical wires to the motor and as an exhaust for the pump. Most notable was the sound and feel of the pump. With each heartbeat, it went "wish, wish, wish". Besides hearing the exhaust, I could hear and feel the pump with each beat of my heart. What fantastic state-of-the-art equipment! Each day, the nurses meticulously cleansed the opening and put new bandages over the wound to make sure that I did not get infected. I became amazed at just how hard the heart works every moment of every day.

Once I recovered and had completed my physical therapy, the doctors discharged me on May 26, 2004 — 56 days after arriving. Over the next 14 months, with the help of the heart pump, I recovered all my bodily functions and went on to get myself in the best physical shape I had been in for a decade or so. I worked out 3 days a week at the Cornell Cardiac Fitness Center on stationary bicycles, treadmills, and rowing machines. I kept this up until the day I got my call for a new heart. I basically got myself into better shape than I had been in the previous 10–15 years through exercise, carefully sticking to the prescribed diet, and keeping myself mentally and physically active.

Before leaving the hospital, both my wife and I were trained in the use of the LVAD. Trina became an expert in cleansing and changing my bandages, and she followed my exercises and dietary activities each day. I began calling my wife Dr L. When I first came home and was just recuperating around the apartment, the set of batteries would run the pump for about 7 $^1/_2$ hours, but as I became more active this dropped to about 5 hours. When I was going to bed at night, I used a 25-foot extension cord from my power unit that limited my movements to the bed, the chair, and the bathroom. The power unit charged my four sets of batteries each night while I slept.

It is quite an experience to carry an implanted 5-pound pump, two external batteries weighing 10 pounds, and a computer regulating the pump and sending messages about the state of its operation. I also had to carry with me a beeper for instant communications with the hospital and a cell phone to call anyone.

Since the pump continually needed new batteries and could possibly malfunction, I carried an extra set of batteries, an extra computer, and a hand pump. The LVAD, if necessary, could be operated with a hand pump should something happen to the electrical system; however, that would be the ultimate emergency.

The biggest concern was that the batteries would run out of juice before I could get home and get to my backup batteries. Most people leave home each morning with the idea that if plans change, they will adapt. But if I was stuck somewhere and was unable to get home to replace and recharge my batteries, I would be in severe trouble, having to rely on the hand pump.

Learning how to take a shower properly became a challenge. No water could ever get into the exhaust tube, or the electrical motor could short-circuit and stop. Not good, as they say. After cutting up plastic shower curtains and using tape, my wife and I realized that it wouldn't work. The tape always came loose. After much trial and error, I settled on large sheets of tegaderm bandages — totally adhesive-backed and water-repellent. Before you knew it, I was enjoying 20-minute showers without any concern.

I will never forget the first time my wife and I went to the opera. We found our places, the lights went dim, and all noises stopped, with one exception: my heart pump kept going "wish, wish, wish". People to the left, right, behind, and in front of us began to wonder what that irritating noise was. One fellow turned around and said, "Would you turn off whatever it is that's making the noise?"

In the summer of 2004, there were bomb scares by terrorists at several buildings in New York City. One was my favorite haunt, the Citicorp Center building, because the Barnes & Noble bookstore was located there — my home away from home while I was on the LVAD. Two policemen were stationed at every door, and you should have seen their reaction to my equipment. Carrying two black boxes in a shoulder holster and a black box on my belt got their attention. Eventually, they came to know me and asked how I was coming along. They became quite interested in the heart pump, as they had never heard of such a thing.

The highlight of my life on the LVAD came at a charitable dance at Mt. Sinai Hospital. My wife's firm had taken a table and we were invited to attend. I told Trina that I would try to get out on the dance floor, but was not sure how long I would last. We started with a waltz, but before you knew it the band was doing more upbeat rhythms. We began jitterbugging and I was able to keep up. Meanwhile, back at the table, my wife's associates began asking themselves, "Tell me again, who is it that is waiting for a heart transplant?"

Many people have asked me how I withstood the waiting, never knowing when the call would come. My answer to that was this: I set a schedule each day and stuck to it, just as if I were in college and had classes to attend. I filled each day reading books, studying about medications and transplantation, took courses on geopolitics, went to New York University School of Continuing and Professional Studies for a certificate in foundation management, volunteered at the New York Organ Donor Network, and made sure to meet and talk to friends about my heart pump.

**Ted L**
**(born 1943)**

**The heart**
**transplant call**

### The Call

The miracle from God and the gift of life came on June 23, 2005. The transplant team called and said, "We have a donor heart for you, come right away." While I had thought about this moment for over a year, the next few hours were a blur. I was wheeled into the operating room at about midnight, and $5\frac{1}{2}$ hours later Dr Naka told Trina that all had gone well and that I had gotten a good heart. It was as close a match as could have been possible. Within a day, the nurses had me up and walking. By the fifth day, I was doing physical therapy on a stationary bicycle for 20 minutes at a time.

While it took me a number of hours to come around after the operation, my body immediately recognized that it now had a foreign object in it. The brain sent out an all-points message: "Every antibody get to the heart area; we have a foreign object that must be eliminated." My body wanted to reject my new heart and will keep this up as long as I live.

Therefore, the doctors and nurses began an educational program to make me understand the very big responsibility that I had going forward. I would have to take many very powerful medications to suppress my immune system in order to reduce the body's efforts to eliminate my new heart. Since my immune system would be compromised, I would be subject to the slightest cold, flu, or virus. I would have to make sure to avoid sick people and large crowds.

I now take various antibiotics and antiviral medications to fight infections, and will do so for the rest of my life. I also need medications to offset the effects of these strong drugs. There are always trade-offs in life, and a heart transplant patient may possibly get diabetes, coronary artery blockage, or osteoporosis. As time passes from the day of transplantation, many patients can have these medications reduced, but never eliminated.

Twelve days after being admitted to the hospital for the transplant, I was discharged on my wife's birthday. She says it was the best present she has ever received.

## Your Help

Have any of you ever had someone say to you, "If you could come back to earth a second time and do it all over again, what would you do?" God and I have been having many long chats about what I will do with my new life. I quickly decided that I would not go back to Wall Street. Instead, I would dedicate myself to helping other people by dedicating my life to raising the awareness of the need for and benefits of organ donation. Today, I am continuing my volunteer work at the New York Organ Donor Network and have joined the Board of Trustees of the Transplant Speakers International, an organization that educates the public on the need for organ donation.

According to the latest statistics from the UNOS (the federal agency responsible for organ transplants), there are just over 90000 people waiting for an organ transplant and not nearly enough donors. One hopeful organ recipient dies every 17 minutes. If we could just get everyone to sign up to donate their organs and to let their wishes be known and accepted by their families, then there would be no waiting lists and everyone would get a transplant.

There is a saying that goes like this:

> Don't take your organs to heaven
> Heaven knows, we need them here on earth!

Would each of you be willing to become an organ donor? Would you be willing to encourage your family, neighbors, and friends? Would you be willing to be ambassadors at your place of work to encourage this?

May God bless each and every one of you, and may you appreciate your good health and that of your family and friends. Not everyone is as lucky as you.

**Case summary: Carl K (born 1939)**

Carl K, born in 1939, developed idiopathic dilated cardiomyopathy with dangerous ventricular arrthymias refractory to defibrillator therapy, requiring HeartMate I bridge-to-transplantation MCSD implantation in September 2004. This was followed by heart transplantation in July 2005. Subsequently, he was discharged and has since returned to a productive and happy life.

**Carl K (born 1939)**

**LVAD experience**

My experience with the LVAD, which was implanted in September 2004, was rather unique. My wife and I did not have an opportunity to familiarize ourselves with the device I was to receive or the surgical procedure involved. I was in the hospital as a result of a PICC-line infection that developed 2 days after its insertion, which was to have a dobutamine drip administered to help my heart failure. While in the hospital on intravenous antibiotics, I began experiencing what I perceived to be fainting spells, but fortunately an episode of rapid and repeated attacks of tachycardia occurred while a doctor on rounds and my wife were in my room.

I remember waking up with approximately 15 people around me and a nurse with paddles both under and above my heart while I was being transported to the intensive care unit. Apparently, I was saved by my defibrillator/pacemaker. My condition was so critical that Dr Naka recommended I have immediate surgery to implant an LVAD as soon as I was stabilized. While its function was explained to me, I really did not take it all in, nor did my wife, and we only discovered the true nature and size of the device after it was implanted.

Our first real exposure to it was when an LVAD nurse came to my room with a tote bag and placed what appeared to be a beating canteen with a snorkel hose on top of my blanket. My first reaction was, "That's inside of me? Take it away!" My wife and I were in a state of shock. Whether or not we would have consented to its installation had we known how it operated and the care required to keep it running is an unanswered question.

The device improved my condition tremendously. For the first time in months, I could walk for extended periods without being out of breath. I could eventually taste my food and generally felt better than I had in at least 3 years. However, the recovery period from the surgery was quite painful. The LVAD was to remain implanted until such time as I could receive a heart transplant, for which I had previously qualified and was at Level 1B.

I subsequently found, while waiting for a new heart, that my wife was very troubled by the device and the possibility that we would lose the electrical power necessary to run the pump. In fact, a problem occurred after about 3 months of usage. I discovered that the manufacturer or distributor of the LVAD had shipped us the wrong strength of solution used for cleaning the vent site in my side. The antiseptic given to me was 3% strength, but it should have been 40%. I attribute this error to the development of a Serratia infection at the site, which could not be cured until I got a new heart.

The LVAD ran effectively for approximately 9 months, when it started to develop warning signals and began to fail. I was changing batteries every $2\frac{1}{2}$ hours and the alarm (gold wrench) was always on. After many trips back and forth to Columbia Presbyterian, it was determined that I could not be sustained on the LVAD as an outpatient, and I was connected to a pneumatic device to keep the pump operating. Since I was then hospitalized, my transplant status was elevated to 1A, and amazingly after 2 weeks a new heart became available for me.

All in all, I would say that the experience with the LVAD was not the best nor was it the worst that I have ever had.

**Elaine (wife of Carl K, born 1939)**

**Wife's perspective on husband's LVAD experience**

Carl and I both have living wills and healthcare proxies. I am his proxy. When he was coded and the crash cart came, everyone in the hospital who knew us met me in the waiting area. Our transplant coordinator at the time, Kim Hammond, sat with me along with a chaplain (after sending a priest and a rabbi away). At the time, it wasn't clear if Carl would pull through.

The next day, I was in touch with the transplant coordinator at Robert Wood Johnson in NJ who was advising me <u>not</u> to let an LVAD be implanted and to transport Carl by ambulance to Robert Wood Johnson. In fact, Carl may not remember this, but they brought him a phone outside the operating room and he said it was too late; I know that he wouldn't have wanted to be anywhere but Columbia because he always says "it's the best in the world." So, I went to sit in the cardiac/thoracic ICU and was given a pamphlet with a "happy-face little clock", which is supposed to represent an LVAD — you don't get the big binder of material until the surgery is over. I watched the nurse assigned to him after surgery operate this console and about 27 different bags and bottles going into his neck, groin, chest — every orifice. And I thought, "What have I done? He's on a respirator, so I can't ask him!"

You can ask Rosie about my "training". She'll remember because I was the worst person she ever had to teach. In fact, I refused to learn and said that Carl had to go to a nursing home. I asked what would even happen if there was no one to train, and was told that that had been factored in without even asking me. After a tremendous scene with a nurse named Eileen and Rosie, I stayed away for 3 days.

The day I came back to the hospital, Dr Drusin suggested to Carl to "go on battery and take your wife for a walk." So with the aid of a walker, we crawled around the hospital corridors and I thought, "Isn't this just great!" Carl said he would fake that I knew how to operate the hand pump when I told him he would have to die if the time came that he needed to be hand pumped, as long as I would just agree to change his dressing. So, so he took his "test" and we were cleared for discharge (but we really didn't know how to do anything complicated, like changing the controller).

I'll leave out my attempt to hire a public advocate and have the pump removed and my one session of psychotherapy, since I'm sure that you wouldn't want to include this in any paper you write. I was asked to talk to the wife of another patient getting an LVAD, Marjorie HG, and I thought, "What the hell am I supposed to say to her that's positive?" In hindsight, she did much better than I did living with the LVAD, and we intend to stay in touch.

Skipping to the day I brought Carl home and thereafter, I was constantly afraid of the device. Taking a shower was the worst, as was helping him put the batteries in that shower kit pouch. Once when he was in the shower, the nozzle came undone and I heard a tremendous sucking noise, and I was sure we were going to end up in the emergency room because water had gone in it, but it didn't. I bought him a police radio dispatcher belt so he could wear the batteries around his waist, but then his pants fell down, so he stuck with the shoulder holster.

The LVAD to lay people is kind of freakish. People who see Carl now comment on how disturbed they were by the noise the pump made (his hair stylist, tailor, dentist, dermatologist, etc.), and carrying a tote bag with the emergency equipment is a bit much. Once, Carl was at a restaurant and had to change batteries, but realized he had uncharged batteries in the bag, so not knowing how long he had before he was in real trouble, he had to race home. I don't know what would have happened if he was more than a half hour away and don't want to know.

I could go on and on, but I guess you get the drift. I am not an LVAD fan and I would never have one implanted in me. I know they say "never say never", but here it is: Never. Never. Never.

All's well that ends well!

# GLOSSARY

**Adrenergic receptors:** Also known as adrenoceptors. They are a class of G protein–coupled receptors that are targets of the catecholamines. Adrenergic receptors specifically are activated after binding with their endogenous ligands, the catecholamines adrenaline and noradrenaline (also called epinephrine and norepinephrine). Many cells possess these receptors, and the binding of an agonist will generally cause the cell to respond in a fight-or-flight manner (i.e. increase heart rate, pupil dilation, energy mobilization, and distribution of blood flow from other organs to skeletal muscle).

**Adrenergic system:** Sometimes referred to as sympathetic nervous system. It is a neurohormonal system that regulates multiple physiological responses mediated by catecholamines (see *catecholamines*), which are secreted by the central nervous system and the medullar aspect of the suprarenal glands, causing general physiological changes that prepare the body for physical activity/stress (fight-or-flight response). Some typical effects are increases in heart rate, blood pressure, and blood glucose levels.

**Adrenergic system blockade** (see *beta-blocker*)

**Advanced heart failure (AHF)** (see *heart failure*)

**Alanine aminotransferase:** Also known as alanine transaminase or ALT. It is an enzyme that catalyzes the reversible transfer of an amino group from alanine to a-ketoglutarate. It is found in serum and in various bodily tissues, but is most commonly associated with the liver. It is also called serum glutamate pyruvate transaminase (SGPT) or alanine aminotransferase (ALAT). Elevated levels of ALT often suggest the existence of other medical problems such as alcoholic or viral hepatitis, congestive heart failure, liver damage, biliary duct problems, infectious mononucleosis, or myopathy.

**All-or-none studies:** Observational nonrandomized studies in which the observed effect of comparing two interventions is huge (arm 1: everybody dies; arm 2: no one dies).

**Alternative to transplantation:** Also called destination therapy. It denotes the implantation of an MCSD as a permanent therapy, and is indicated when a patient is not a suitable candidate to receive a heart transplant.

**Angiotensin II receptor blockers:** Also known as angiotensin II receptor antagonists or angiotensin receptor blockers (ARBs). They are a group of pharmaceuticals/drugs that modulate the renin-angiotensin-aldosterone system. Their main use is in hypertension (high blood pressure), diabetic nephropathy (kidney damage due to diabetes), and congestive heart failure (sometimes as an alternative when patients are intolerant to ACE inhibitors, but also in addition to ACE inhibitors for patients with advanced heart failure; see *ACEI*).

**Angiotensin-converting enzyme inhibitor (ACEI):** The name of a group of pharmaceuticals that are used primarily in the treatment of hypertension, vascular disease, and congestive heart failure; in most cases, as the drug of first choice. ACE inhibitors inhibit the renin–angiotensin system and thereby lower arteriolar resistance and increase venous capacitance; increase cardiac output and cardiac index as well as stroke work and volume; and also lower renovascular resistance, leading to increased natriuresis (excretion of sodium in the urine). Epidemiological and clinical studies have shown that ACE inhibitors reduce the progress of diabetic nephropathy independently of their blood pressure–lowering effect. This action of ACE inhibitors is utilized in the prevention of diabetic renal failure. ACE inhibitors have been shown to be effective for indications other than hypertension even in patients with normal blood pressure, including the prevention of diabetic nephropathy and congestive heart failure as well as the prophylaxis of cardiovascular events. The use of ACEIs in these clinical conditions is justified because they improve clinical outcomes independent of their blood pressure–lowering effect.

**Antinuclear antibodies (ANAs):** Also referred to as autoantibodies. They are unusual antibodies, detectable in the blood, that have the capability of binding to certain structures within the nuclei of cells. They are found in patients whose immune system may be predisposed to cause inflammation against their own body tissues. ANAs indicate the possible presence of autoimmunity/autoimmune disease.

**Aspartate aminotransferase:** Also known as aspartate transaminase (AST) or aspartate aminotransferase (ASAT). It is an enzyme that catalyzes the reversible transfer of an amino group from aspartate to a-ketoglutarate. It is found in serum and in various bodily tissues, but is most commonly associated with the liver and is raised after liver damage. It is also present in red blood cells and cardiac muscle. AST was formerly called serum glutamic oxaloacetic transaminase (SGOT). When a body tissue or organ (e.g. heart, liver) is diseased or damaged, additional AST is released into the bloodstream. The amount of AST in the blood is directly related to the extent of tissue damage. After severe damage, AST levels rise in 6–10 hours and remain high for about 4 days. The AST test may be done at the same time as the ALT test. The ratio of AST to ALT (AST:ALT) can sometimes help determine whether the liver or another organ has been damaged. AST can also help determine the cause of the liver damage. Both ALT and AST levels are reliable indicators of liver damage.

**Asynchronous ventricular contraction:** Nonphysiological squeezing of the heart muscle because of heart muscle damage.

**Beta-blocker:** Sometimes also written as ß-blocker. It is a class of drugs used for various indications, including the management of cardiac arrhythmias and cardioprotection after myocardial infarction, but is the mainstay therapy for patients suffering from heart failure. Beta-blockers may also be referred to as beta-adrenergic blocking agents, beta-adrenergic antagonists, or beta-antagonists. The beta-adrenergic receptor mediates the stimulation of ß1 receptors by epinephrine, induces a positive chronotropic (increase in heart rate) and inotropic (increase in heart contractility) effect on the heart, and increases cardiac conduction velocity and automaticity. The stimulation of ß2 receptors induces smooth muscle relaxation, resulting in vasodilation and bronchodilation among other actions. The blockade of this mechanism has been shown to be favorable for the failing heart. Beta-blockers inhibit the normal epinephrine-mediated sympathetic actions, which are highly exacerbated in people with advanced heart failure. There are different classes of beta-blockers that vary according to the selectivity for each specific beta-adrenergic receptor (ß1 and/or ß2), but some of them also have activity against alpha-adrenergic receptors ($\alpha$1 and/or $\alpha$2).

**Biventricular support:** The implantation of a biventricular assist device in addition to the left ventricular support when patients have a failing right heart. The resulting system is complete mechanical assistance, in which both ventricles (right and left) are supported by independent devices.

**Body mass index (BMI):** Also known as Quetelet index. It is a statistical measure of the weight of a person scaled according to height, and is used as a simple means of classifying individuals with an average body composition. A BMI of 18.5–25 indicates optimal weight; a BMI lower than 18.5 suggests that the person is underweight, while a BMI above 25 indicates that the person is overweight; a BMI below 15 indicates that the person has an eating disorder; and a BMI above 30 suggests that the person is obese (over 40, morbidly obese). The BMI is meant to broadly categorize populations for purely statistical purposes. Its accuracy in relation to actual levels of body fat is easily distorted by such factors as fitness level, muscle mass, bone structure, gender, and ethnicity.

**Body surface area:** The measured or calculated surface of a human body. Several formulas can be used for this estimation, and might better reflect the metabolic mass than body weight because it is less affected by abnormal adipose mass.

**Bridge to recovery:** The implantation of an MCSD with the intention of replacing the function and alleviating the workload of the heart when the potential for functional recovery is foreseen.

**Bridge to transplantation:** The implantation of an MCSD with the intention of replacing the function of the heart until the patient becomes a candidate for heart transplantation.

**Calcium channel blocker:** A class of drugs with an effect on many excitable cells of the body, such as heart muscle cells, smooth muscle cells of vessels, and neuron cells. The main action of calcium channel blockers is to lower blood pressure; therefore, they are used in individuals with hypertension. Most calcium channel blockers decrease the force of contraction of the myocardium and are detrimental for heart failure.

**Cardiac transplantation:** The transplantation of a heart from one body to another for the purpose of replacing the recipient's damaged or failing heart with a working one from the donor.

**Cardiopulmonary bypass:** Also known as heart–lung machine. It is a device that temporarily takes over the function of the heart and lungs.

**Cardioversion:** The use of electricity or drug therapy to transiently change the electrical properties of the heart that resynchronize the cardiac beats being controlled by an abnormal impulse (i.e. low excitability thresholds in an ischemic/infarcted area) with the physiological pacemaker of the heart (i.e. sinus node). Cardioversion converts heart arrhythmias into normal rhythms.

**Case-control studies:** Studies that use patients who already have a disease or other condition, and that look back to see if the characteristics of these patients differ from those who do not have the disease. Case-control studies are a less expensive and often-used type of epidemiological study, which can be carried out by small teams or individual researchers in single facilities in a way that more structured trials often cannot.

**Case series:** The description of cases related to specific diseases, usually by single groups of researchers.

**Catecholamines:** Chemical compounds derived from the amino acid tyrosine, which circulates in the bloodstream. The most abundant catecholamines are adrenaline (epinephrine), noradrenaline (norepinephrine), and dopamine. They are produced mainly from the adrenal medulla and the postganglionic fibers of the sympathetic nervous system. Epinephrine acts as a neurotransmitter in the central nervous system and as a hormone in the blood circulation. High catecholamine levels in blood are associated with different forms of stress (see also *adrenergic system*).

**Cerebrovascular accident:** Also known as stroke. It is an acute neurological injury in which blood supply to a part of the brain is interrupted. A stroke involves a sudden loss of neuronal function due to a disturbance in cerebral perfusion.

**Chronic heart failure** (see *heart failure*)

**Clinical trial:** A research study.

**Cohort study:** A type of research study design. In medicine, it is usually undertaken to obtain additional evidence in order to refute or support the existence of an association between a suspected cause and a disease. The cohorts are identified prior to the appearance of the disease under investigation. The study groups, so defined, are observed over a period of time to determine the frequency of disease among them.

**Complete left ventricular support:** The dependence of blood flow on the contribution of the asset device alone when a patient is undergoing ventricular assistance of the left ventricle.

**Confidence interval (CI):** An interval between two numbers with an associated probability $p$ that is generated from a random sample of an underlying population, such that if the sampling was repeated numerous times and the CI was recalculated from each sample according to the same method, a proportion $p$ of the CIs would contain the population parameter in question.

**Congestive heart failure (CHF)** (see *heart failure*)

**Continuous venous-venous hemodialysis:** A method for removing waste products (e.g. potassium, urea) and free water (filtration) from blood when the kidneys are incapable of doing this, i.e. in renal failure. It is a renal replacement therapy. Hemodialysis is typically conducted in a dedicated facility or at the bedside in an intensive care unit setting. Although less typical, dialysis can also be done in a patient's home as home hemodialysis.

**Coronary artery bypass surgery:** A surgical procedure performed on patients with coronary artery disease (see *coronary artery disease*) for the relief of angina and possible improved heart muscle function. Veins or arteries from elsewhere in the patient's body — usually the veins of the leg, or the arteries of the internal thoracic cage (right or left internal mammary) or arm (radial) — are grafted from the aorta to the coronary arteries, bypassing coronary artery narrowing caused by atherosclerosis and improving blood supply to the myocardium.

**Coronary artery disease:** Also referred to as ischemic heart disease, coronary heart disease, or atherosclerotic heart disease. It is the end result of the accumulation of atheromatous plaques within the artery walls supplying the myocardium (heart muscle). While the symptoms and signs of coronary heart disease are noted in the advanced stage of the disease, most individuals with coronary heart disease show no evidence of disease for decades as the disease progresses until the first onset of symptoms (often a sudden heart attack) occurs. After decades of progression, some of these atheromatous plaques may rupture and (along with the activation of the blood-clotting system) start limiting blood flow to the heart muscle.

**Coronary heart disease** (see *coronary artery disease*)

**Cost-effectiveness:** A comparison of the relative expenditure (costs) and outcomes (effects) associated with two or more courses of action or interventions. Cost-effectiveness is typically expressed as an incremental cost-effectiveness ratio, i.e. the ratio of change in costs or change in effects.

**Creatinine:** The breakdown product of creatine phosphate in muscle. Serum creatinine measurement is the most commonly used indicator of renal function. A rise in serum creatinine levels is observed only with marked damage to functioning nephrons. The most accurate indicator is the estimation of the creatinine clearance, which considers some or all of the following variables: sex, age, weight, and race. In the US, creatinine is typically reported in mg/dL; while in Canada and Europe, $\mu$mol/L may be used. The equivalent of 1 mg/dL of creatinine is 88.4 $\mu$mol/L. The typical reference range for women is 0.5–1.0 mg/dL (about 45–90 $\mu$mol/L); for men, 0.7–1.2 mg/dL (60–110 $\mu$mol/L). While a baseline serum creatinine of 2.0 mg/dL (150 $\mu$mol/L) may indicate normal kidney function in a male bodybuilder, a serum creatinine of 0.7 mg/dL (60 $\mu$mol/L) can indicate significant renal disease in a frail old woman. More important than the absolute creatinine level is the trend in serum creatinine levels over time. A rising creatinine level indicates kidney damage, while a declining creatinine level indicates improving kidney function.

**Desmopressin (DDAVP):** Also known as arginine vasopressin (AVP). It is a synthetic drug that mimics the action of antidiuretic hormone.

**Ejection fraction (EF):** The amount of blood pumped divided by the amount of blood the ventricle contains. A normal EF is more than 55% of the blood volume. If the heart becomes enlarged, even if the amount of blood being pumped by the left ventricle remains the same, the relative fraction of blood being ejected decreases. The EF is a measurement of the heart's efficiency and can be used to estimate the function of the left ventricle, which pumps blood to the rest of the body. The left ventricle pumps only a fraction of the blood that it contains.

**Electrophysiological study:** Heart catheter study to understand and treat heart rhythm disorders.

**End-stage heart failure (ESHF)** (see *heart failure*)

**End-systolic volume index:** The volume of the heart at the end of systole relative to the body surface area.

**Epidemiological transition:** The patterns of diseases that occur across different geographical areas or across different times. Diseases tend to cluster together, and are associated with common etiologies such as poverty. For example, in the case of patterns that are consistent with the changing infectious disease rates, as infectious diseases go down, the population ages and noncommunicable diseases (e.g. cardiovascular disease, diabetes) emerge. In the early stage of the epidemiological transition, there is a marked variability of mortality rates due to disease epidemics. As the infectious disease burden is reduced, the epidemics occur less frequently and the variation in mortality rates goes down. The emergence of different causes of diseases is systematic and constant across the developing countries: first, trauma; followed by noninsulin-dependent diabetes mellitus, coronary heart disease, and finally cancer. In the specific case of cardiovascular disease, the augmented life expectancy related to improvements in medical treatments has led to the emergence of heart failure.

**Erythrocyte sedimentation rate (ESR):** The rate at which red blood cells sediment in a tube of anticoagulated blood. The test is used as an indication of underlying inflammatory processes. However, it is not specific for any particular disease or disease process.

**Erythropoietin:** Also called hematopoietin or hemopoietin. It is a hormone produced by the kidney that regulates red blood cell production. Erythropoietin is available as a therapeutic agent produced by recombinant DNA technology in mammalian cell culture. It is used to treat anemia resulting from chronic renal failure or cancer chemotherapy.

**Evidence-based medicine:** The application of scientific methods to medical practice. According to the Centre for Evidence-Based Medicine, "Evidence-based medicine is the conscientious, explicit and judicious use of current best evidence in making decisions about the care of individual patients."

**Extracorporeal life support:** Also known as extracorporeal membrane oxygenation (ECMO). It is a temporary extracorporeal technique that provides both cardiac and respiratory support oxygen to patients whose heart and lungs are severely diseased and can no longer serve their function.

**Hazard ratio:** The effect of an explanatory variable on the hazard or risk of an event (in survival analysis).

**Heart failure:** A condition resulting from any structural or functional cardiac disorder that impairs the ability of the heart to fill with or pump a sufficient amount of blood throughout the body. Because not all patients have volume overload at the time of initial or subsequent evaluation, the term "heart failure" is preferred over the older term "congestive heart failure". Heart failure is often undiagnosed due to the lack of a universally agreed definition and difficulties in diagnosis, particularly when the condition is considered mild (in contrast to advanced heart failure). However, the terminology of chronic heart failure in its advanced stages is not very precise. The terms "advanced", "severe", "congestive", "refractory", and "end-stage" heart failure are used in largely interchangable ways. The term end-stage heart failure reflects the impaired prognosis associated with it, and has been incorporated into the recent staging system for heart failure (Hunt *et al.*, 2001; Hunt *et al.*, 2005). The term congestive denotes the condition in which impairment of the heart muscle function leads to an abnormal accumulation of fluid within the body including the lungs and abdominal organs, compromising their functions. In this book, the term advanced heart failure is used to express the more recent insight into the partial reversibility of the heart failure remodeling process.

**Heparin-induced thrombocytopenia (HIT):** Thrombocytopenia (low platelet counts) due to the administration of heparin. While it is mainly associated with unfractionated heparin (UFH), it can also occur with the exposure to low-molecular-weight heparin (LMWH), albeit at significantly lower rates. Despite the low platelet count, it is a thrombotic disorder. HIT typically develops 4–14 days after the administration of heparin. Heparin (UFH) is used in cardiovascular surgery as a prevention or treatment for deep vein thrombosis and pulmonary embolism, and in various other clinical scenarios.

**Human leukocyte antigen (HLA):** Sometimes called human lympho-cyte antigen. It is the general name for a group of genes in the human major histocompatibility complex (MHC) region on human chromosome 6 (mouse chromosome 17) that encodes the cell-surface antigen-presenting proteins. The proteins encoded by HLAs are the proteins on the outer part of body cells that are (effectively) unique to that person.

**Idiopathic dilated cardiomyopathy:** A disease that causes dysfunction of the heart muscle (myocardium) and enlargement of the ventricular cham-bers. The term "idiopathic" is used to denote that there is no known cause for this condition.

**Implantable systems** (see *intracorporeal pumps*)

**International normalized ratio (INR):** A measure of the extrinsic path-way of coagulation. It is used to determine the clotting tendency of blood and to measure warfarin dosage, liver damage, and vitamin K status. The normal range for the INR is 0.8–1.2. It is used in conjunction with the activated partial thromboplastin time (aPTT), which measures the intrinsic pathway. Because of differences in the batches and manufacturers of tissue factor (a biologically obtained product), the INR was devised to standard-ize the results. Each manufacturer gives an international sensitivity index (ISI) for any tissue factor made. The ISI value indicates how a particular batch of tissue factor compares to an internationally standardized sample. The ISI is usually between 1.0 and 1.4. The INR is the ratio of a patient's prothrombin time to a normal (control) sample, raised to the power of the ISI value for the control sample used.

**Intracorporeal pump:** The chamber in assist devices that generates blood flow and is placed inside the patient's body, usually in the abdomen. Free movement/deambulation is generally possible with this kind of pump, and its implants can last for a long period.

**Intravenous immunoglobulin (IVIG):** A blood product mainly used as treatment for inflammatory and autoimmune diseases, immune deficien-cies such as X-linked agammaglobulinemia and hypogammaglobulinemia, and other diseases featuring low antibody levels. It contains the pooled IgG immunoglobulins (antibodies) extracted from the plasma of over 1000 blood donors. It is administered intravenously in autoimmune diseases, and its effects last between 2 weeks and 3 months. The precise mechanism by which IVIG suppresses harmful inflammation is unknown. The donor antibody may bind directly with the abnormal host antibody, stimulating its removal.

**Intraventricular conduction delay:** The delay in the time of conduction of the electrical impulse in the heart, frequently related to extensive myocardial disease involving disease of the heart's conduction (nervous) system. It can be appreciated as a prolonged duration of the QRS interval (a specific measurement of the electrocardiogram reading) that is beyond 12 ms.

**Kaplan–Meier analysis:** A nonparametric estimation from incomplete observations (see *Kaplan–Meier survival analysis*).

**Kaplan–Meier survival analysis:** Also known as Kaplan–Meier estimator or product limit estimator. It provides an estimate of the survival function from lifetime data. In medical research, it might be used to measure the fraction of patients living for a certain amount of time after a specific clinical intervention.

**Left ventricular diastolic dysfunction:** An impairment of the heart's ability to relax normally.

**Left ventricular ejection fraction (LVEF):** (see *ejection fraction*)

**Left ventricular end-diastolic diameter (LVEDD):** The diameter of the left ventricle at the end of the relaxation phase of the cardiac cycle (diastole) measured between both inner edges of opposite ventricular walls (interventricular septum and posterior wall). It is measured at the highest diameter, perpendicular to the major axis of the heart (transversal).

**Left ventricular end-systolic diameter (LVESD):** The diameter of the left ventricle at the end of the ejection phase of the cardiac cycle (systole) measured between both inner edges of the walls (interventricular septum and posterior wall). It is measured at the highest diameter, perpendicular to the major axis of the heart (transversal).

**Left ventricular internal diameter in diastole (LVIDd):** (see *LVEDD*)

**Left ventricular systolic dysfunction:** An impairment of the heart's ability to contract normally.

**Mechanical circulatory support device (MCSD):** Also known as ventricular assist device (VAD). It is a mechanical device that is used to partially or completely replace the function of a failing heart. The devices are designed to replace or assist cardiac function temporarily or permanently. VADs are designed to assist either the right or left ventricle, or both. Mechanical circulatory support is used to treat patients with advanced heart failure. A mechanical pump is surgically implanted to provide pulsatile or nonpulsatile blood flow to supplement or replace the blood flow generated by the native heart. Types of circulatory support pumps include pneumatic and electromagnetic pumps. Rotary pumps are also available.

**Mechanical circulatory support system** (see *MCSD*)

**Mitral regurgitation (MR):** The abnormal flow of blood from the left ventricle to the left atrium of the heart, caused by a leaky mitral valve. This abnormal flow can cause breathing problems, fatigue, irregular heartbeats, and potentially fatal congestive heart failure.

**Multisite biventricular pacing:** An electrical therapy technique to restore the synchronization of ventricular contraction. It emerged as a modality for the treatment of patients with dilated cardiomyopathy and congestive heart failure associated with major intraventricular and interventricular conduction disorders. Multisite ventricular pacing or resynchronization reduces the degree of electromechanical asynchrony by altering the pathways of spontaneous depolarization. Biventricular pacing improves hemodynamics in CHF patients with severe left ventricular systolic dysfunction and major left-sided intraventricular conduction disorders. A longer spontaneous QRS complex may be predictive of a greater positive response to pacing.

**Myocardial infarction:** Also called heart attack. It is caused by the sudden blockage of a heart artery with a blood clot, leading to progressive muscle injury over the next 6–12 hours. This is a medical emergency requiring early treatment to minimize heart damage.

**New York Heart Association** (see *NYHA functional class*)

**Nonsteroidal anti-inflammatory drugs:** A group of drugs with analgesic, antipyretic, and anti-inflammatory effects (e.g. aspirin).

**Nonsustained ventricular tachycardia:** An abnormally rapid beating of the heart, defined as a resting heart rate of 100 or more beats per minute in an average adult that is self-limited to 30 or less seconds.

**New York Heart Association (NYHA) functional class:** A simple way to classify the extent of heart failure. It places patients in one of four categories, based on how much they are limited during physical activity: I — no symptoms and no limitation in ordinary physical activity; II — mild symptoms and slight limitation during ordinary activity (comfortable at rest); III — marked limitation in activity due to symptoms, even during less-than-ordinary activity (comfortable only at rest); and IV — severe limitations (experience symptoms even while at rest).

**Outcomes research:** An evaluation of the trends and correlations between a specific condition and its association with specific events in a population which has been exposed to that condition in comparison to those that have not been exposed. The population that is not exposed to the condition is usually named the control population. Outcomes research is useful to guide the direction of intervention research (either clinical or basic). The process of generating hypotheses based on the results of current standards/practice or on specific trends in a population is known as translational research.

**Panel-reactive antibodies (PRAs):** The measure of a patient's level of sensitization to donor antigens. It is the percentage of cells from a panel of blood donors against which a potential recipient's serum reacts. The PRA reflects the percentage of the general population that a potential recipient makes antibodies (is sensitized) against. The higher the PRA, the more sensitized a patient is to the general donor pool, and thus the more difficult it is to find a suitable donor. A patient may become sensitized as a result of pregnancy, blood transfusion, or previous transplant.

**Paracorporeal pump:** The chamber in assist devices that generates blood flow and is located outside the body, in an adjacent position in relation to it. Free movement/deambulation is generally not possible with this kind of pump, and its implants can only last for a short period.

**Partial left ventricular support:** The dependence of blood flow on the ejection of the native heart and on the contribution of the assist device when a patient is undergoing ventricular assistance of the left ventricle.

**Peak oxygen uptake (VO$_2$):** Also called maximal oxygen consumption or maximal oxygen uptake. It is the highest rate at which oxygen can be taken up and utilized during exercise by a person. It is expressed either as an absolute rate (L/min) or as a relative rate (mL/kg/min).

**Peripheral vascular disease:** Also known as peripheral artery occlusive disease. It is a collator for all of the diseases caused by the obstruction of large peripheral arteries (e.g. legs, kidneys) as a result of atherosclerosis, inflammatory processes leading to stenosis (narrowing) of the arteries that in turn can lead to total occlusion by embolism or thrombus formation. It causes either an acute or chronic loss of blood supply (i.e. oxygen) to the tissues (ischemia).

**Power base unit (PBU):** The unit that provides the power (energy) for the functioning of the MCSD.

**Primary endpoint:** A disease, symptom, or sign that constitutes one of the target outcomes of a research trial. The results of a clinical trial generally indicate the number of people enrolled who reach the predetermined clinical endpoint during the study interval, compared with the overall number of people who are enrolled. Once a patient reaches the endpoint, he or she is generally excluded from further experimental intervention. Endpoints can be divided into primary, secondary, or exploratory endpoints if they are the main, secondary, or minor exploratory objectives for which the research is designed.

**Prothrombin time (PT):** A measure of the extrinsic pathway of coagulation. The reference range for PT is usually around 12–15 seconds (see also *INR*).

**QRS duration:** The duration of the QRS complex of the electrocardiogram. It refers to a group of deflections in the electrocardiogram (ECG) tracing caused by depolarization of the ventricles that leads to mechanical contraction of the myocardium.

**Randomization:** The assignation of cases to an intervention in a clinical study by chance to prevent selection bias (e.g. using random number tables).

**Randomized clinical trial:** A clinical trial study designed to elucidate whether a new intervention is effective and to measure the effect of that intervention in a controlled population. These are fundamental information in evidence-based medicine. To avoid selection bias (the tendency to include any patient in a predefined group), the investigator assigns the study subjects to an intervention in a randomized way (e.g. using random number tables).

**Refractory and end-stage heart failure** (see *heart failure*)

**Right ventricle systolic work index:** A useful marker of right ventricular function.

**Right ventricular support:** The implantation of a right ventricular assist device in addition to the left ventricular support when patients have a failing right heart.

**Signal-averaged electrocardiogram:** The acquisition of multiple ECG tracings (obtained over a period of approximately 20 minutes). All of the electrical signals from the heart are averaged, providing greater analytical information that can be correlated with the likelihood of developing sustained ventricular tachycardia or sudden (arrhythmic) death.

**Six-minute walk test:** A simple study that objectively quantifies the distance traveled by an individual during 6 minutes of constant walk. This measurement correlates with the functional capacity of the patient (i.e. peak oxygen uptake).

**Specialized Centers of Clinically Oriented Research (SCCOR):** An extensive research program funded by the NHLBI to foster translational research in order to improve the prevention, diagnosis, and treatment of particular diseases.

*Staphylococcus aureus*: A Gram-positive coccus (bacterium) that frequently lives on the skin or in the nose of a healthy person.

*Staphylococcus epidermidis:* A Gram-positive coccus (bacterium) that frequently lives on the skin or in the nose of a healthy person.

**Sudden cardiac death:** Also called cardiac arrest. It is a death resulting from an abrupt loss of heart function. The victim may or may not have been diagnosed with heart disease. The time and mode of death are unexpected. It occurs within minutes after the symptoms appear. The most common underlying reason for patients to suddenly die from cardiac arrest is coronary heart disease.

**Sustained ventricular tachycardia:** An abnormally rapid beating of the heart, defined as a resting heart rate of 100 or more beats per minute in an average adult that exceeds 30 seconds.

**Syncope:** The temporary loss of consciousness and posture, described as "fainting" or "passing out". It is usually related to temporary insufficient blood flow to the brain, often related to an abnormal supply of oxygen to the brain. Syncope may be caused by several benign causes, but serious causes may also result from several heart, neurological, psychiatric, metabolic, and lung disorders.

**Transcutaneous driveline:** The connection between the intracorporeal assist device and the extracorporeal computer/battery/power supply.

**Ventricular assist system (VAS)** (see *MCSD*)

**Ventricular tachycardia:** An abnormally rapid beating of the heart, defined as a resting heart rate of 100 or more beats per minute in an average adult.

# ABBREVIATIONS

ACEI: angiotensin-converting enzyme inhibitor
AHF: advanced heart failure
ALT: alanine aminotransferase
ANA: antinuclear antibody
ARB: angiotensin II receptor blocker
AST: aspartate aminotransferase
BB: beta-blocker
BMI: body mass index
BSA: body surface area
BTR: bridge to recovery
BTT: bridge to transplantation
BiVAD: biventricular assist device
CA: cancer
CABG: coronary artery bypass graft
CAD: coronary artery disease
CCB: calcium channel blocker
CD: cluster of differentiation
CFD: computational fluid dynamics
CHD: coronary heart disease
CHF: congestive heart failure
CI: confidence interval
CO: cardiac output
CPB: cardiopulmonary bypass
CPMC: Columbia Presbyterian Medical Center
Crea: creatinine
CT: cardiac transplantation
CTICU: cardiothoracic intensive care unit
CUMC: Columbia University Medical Center
CVA: cerebrovascular accident

CVP: central venous pressure
CVVH: continuous venous-venous hemodialysis
CXR: chest X-ray
DDAVP: desmopressin
DTT: destination therapy
EBM: evidence-based medicine
ECLS: extracorporeal life support; also known as extracorporeal membrane
    oxygenation (ECMO)
EF: ejection fraction
EPO: erythropoietin
ESHF: end-stage heart failure
ESR: erythrocyte sedimentation rate
ESVI: end-systolic volume index
HF: heart failure
HIT: heparin-induced thrombocytopenia
HLA: human leukocyte antigen
HR: hazard ratio
HT: heart transplantation
IABP: intra-aortic balloon pump
ICU: intensive care unit
IDC: idiopathic dilated cardiomyopathy
INR: international normalized ratio
ISHLT: International Society for Heart and Lung Transplantation
IV: intravenous
IVIG: intravenous immunoglobulin
KM: Kaplan–Meier
LVEDD: left ventricular end-diastolic diameter
LVEF: left ventricular ejection fraction
LVESD: left ventricular end-systolic diameter
LVIDd: left ventricular internal diameter in diastole
MCSD: mechanical circulatory support device
MCSS: mechanical circulatory support system
MI: myocardial infarction
MR: mitral regurgitation
NHLBI: National Heart, Lung, and Blood Institute
NIH: National Institutes of Health

NSAIDS: nonsteroidal anti-inflammatory drugs
NSVT: nonsustained ventricular tachycardia
NYHA: New York Heart Association
NYP: New York–Presbyterian
OMM: optimal medical management
OR: operating room
PAP: pulmonary artery pressure
PBU: power base unit
PCP: pulmonary capillary pressure
PPCM: peripartum cardiomyopathy
PRA: panel-reactive antibodies
PT: prothrombin time
PVD: peripheral vascular disease
PVR: pulmonary vascular resistance
QoL: quality of life
REMATCH: Randomized Evaluation of Mechanical Assistance for the
    Treatment of Congestive Heart Failure
RVAD: right ventricular assist device
RVD: right ventricular dysfunction
RVSWI: right ventricle systolic work index
SCCOR: Specialized Centers of Clinically Oriented Research
SD: sudden death
SVT: sustained ventricular tachycardia
TIA: transient ischemic attack
UNOS: United Network for Organ Sharing
VAS: ventricular assist system
$VO_2$: peak oxygen uptake
VT: ventricular tachycardia
WRF: worsening renal function
6WT: 6-minute walk test

# INDEX